THE ANATOMY OF GENERAL SURGICAL OPERATIONS

Commissioning Editor: Timothy Horne
Development Editor: Clive Hewat
Project Manager: Frances Affleck
Designer: Erik Bigland
Illustration Manager: Bruce Hogarth/Gillian Murray
Illustrator: Peter Cox

THE ANATOMY OF GENERAL SURGICAL OPERATIONS

Glyn G. Jamieson MD MS FRACS FACS

Dorothy Mortlock Professor of Surgery, Department of Surgery,
Royal Adelaide Hospital, Adelaide, South Australia

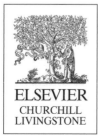

ELSEVIER
CHURCHILL
LIVINGSTONE

EDINBURGH LONDON NEW YORK OXFORD PHILADELPHIA ST LOUIS SYDNEY TORONTO
2006

ELSEVIER
CHURCHILL
LIVINGSTONE

First published 1992
Second edition 2006

ISBN(10):   0443100071
ISBN(13):   978-0-443-10007-9

British Library Cataloguing in Publication Data
A catalogue record for this book is available from the British Library

Library of Congress Cataloging in Publication Data
A catalog record for this book is available from the Library of Congress

Note
Neither the Publisher nor the Authors assume any responsibility for any
loss or injury and/or damage to persons or property arising out of or
related to any use of the material contained in this book. It is the
responsibility of the treating practitioner, relying on independent
expertise and knowledge of the patient, to determine the best treatment
and method of application for the patient.

 ELSEVIER   your source for books,
journals and multimedia
in the health sciences
www.elsevierhealth.com

Working together to grow
libraries in developing countries

www.elsevier.com | www.bookaid.org | www.sabre.org

ELSEVIER   **BOOK AID** International   Sabre Foundation

The
Publisher's
policy is to use
**paper manufactured
from sustainable forests**

Printed in China

Contents

Preface

When I wrote the first edition of *The Anatomy of General Surgical Operations*, I thought it unlikely that a second edition would be needed. A second printing I hoped for, but why would a second edition be needed, as gross anatomy doesn't change, and surgical procedures can evolve but change would be slow? Or so I thought. Well, anatomy has not changed, but the way we see it has. I am referring of course to minimal access surgery. Although I undertook my first laparoscopic cholecystectomy in France in 1990, during the study leave when I wrote the first edition of this book, I did not forsee the veritable explosion of minimal access techniques.

Therefore, for the new edition, I have incorporated what might be called `minimal access anatomy' whenever possible, and I specifically asked my collaborators (all of whom are experts in their field and some of international renown) to keep this in mind when reviewing and editing their chapters. Some of the chapters have been extensively rewritten, but many have changed less, with the addition of the minimal access material. The new edition has allowed many of the diagrams to be redrawn to produce a greater consistency of style, and some new ones have been added.

My thanks to my secretary Christine Bates-Brownsword for her typing (and retyping) and generally marshalling the contributions into order and to Clive Hewat of Elsevier for guiding the second edition to publication.

G.G.J   Adelaide, 2005

Contributors

Derek Alderson MBBS MD FRCS
Professor University of Bristol
Division of Surgery, Level 7
Bristol Royal Infirmary
Bristol, United Kingdom

Mehran Anvari MB BS PhD FRCSC FACS
Professor of Surgery
McMaster University
St Joseph's Hospital
Hamilton, Ontario
Canada

Robert Baigrie MD FRCS
Senior Surgeon
Groote Schuur Hospital
Capetown, RSA

Michael Berce MBBS FRACS
Senior Visiting Surgeon
Vascular Unit, Royal Adelaide Hospital
Adelaide, Australia

Leslie H Blumgart MD FACS FRCS
Professor, Chief, Hepatobiliary Service
Memorial Sloan-Kettering Cancer Center
New York, USA

Murray F Brennan MD FACS
Professor, Chairman, Department of Surgery
Memorial Sloan-Kettering Cancer Center
New York, USA

Jean-Marie Collard MD
Professor, Universite Catholique de Louvain
Cliniques Universitaires Saint-Luc
Service de Chirurgie de l'Appareil Digestif
Bruxelles, Belgium

Brendon J Coventry BMBS PhD FRACS
Associate Professor
Department of Surgery
Royal Adelaide Hospital
Adelaide, Australia

Andrew C de Beaux MD(Ed) FRCS(Ed) MB ChB (Aberd)
Department of General Surgery
Royal Infirmary of Edinburgh
Edinburgh, UK

Haile T Debas MD FACS
Professor of Surgery
Department of Surgery
University of California
San Francisco, USA

Leigh Delbridge MD FRACS
Professor, Head, Division of Surgery
The University Clinic
Wallace Freeborn Professorial Block
Royal North Shore Hospital
Sydney, Australia

Peter G Devitt MS FRCS FRACS
Associate Professor, Department of Surgery
Royal Adelaide Hospital
Adelaide, Australia

André CH Duranceau MD FRCS (Can)
Professor of Surgery
University of Montreal
Centre Hospitalier de l'Universite de Montreal
Montreal, Canada

Larry Ferguson MBBS
Director of Vascular Surgery
Vascular Unit, Royal Adelaide Hospital
Adelaide, Australia

Robert A Fitridge MBBS FRACS
Associate Professor
Vascular Surgery Unit
The Queen Elizabeth Hospital
Woodville, Australia

P Grantley Gill MD FRACS
Associate Professor, Head
Breast, Endocrine & Surgical Oncology Unit
Royal Adelaide Hospital
Adelaide, Australia

David Gotley MBBS FRACS MD
Professor, Department of Surgery
Princess Alexandra Hospital
Woolloongabba, Australia

S Michael Griffin MD FRCS
Professor of Gastrointestinal Surgery
Royal Victoria Infirmary
Queen Victoria Road
Newcastle upon Tyne, UK

Daniel Hains MBBS FRACS
Erstwhile Head of Ear, Nose and Throat Department
Royal Adelaide Hospital
Adelaide, Australia

Dudley C Hill MBBS DObstRCOG FRACGP FACD
Dermatologist, Wakefield Clinic
Adelaide, Australia

John Hunter MD
Professor and Chairman
Department of Surgery
Oregon Health Services University
Portland, Oregon, USA

Glyn G Jamieson MS FRACS FACS
Dorothy Mortlock Professor of Surgery
Department of Surgery
Royal Adelaide Hospital
Adelaide, Australia

Nigel R Jones MBBS FRACS DPhil (Oxf) FFPMANZCA
GH Michell Professor of Neurosurgery
Department of Neurosurgery
Royal Adelaide Hospital
Adelaide, Australia

James Katsaros MBBS FRACS
Director
Department of Plastic & Reconstructive Surgery
Royal Adelaide Hospital
Adelaide , Australia

Suren Krishnan MBBS FRACS
ENT Department
Royal Adelaide Hospital
Adelaide, Australia

Bernard Launois MD
Erstwhile Head
Centre de Chirugie Digestive et Unite de Transplantation
Hospital
Pontchaillou, Rennes, France

Guy J Maddern PhD MS MD FRACS
Jepson Professor of Surgery
Department of Surgery
The Queen Elizabeth Hospital
Woodville, Australia

Peter L Malycha MBBS FRCS FRACS
Consultant Surgeon
Breast Endocrine and Surgical Oncology Unit
Royal Adelaide Hospital
Adelaide, Australia

R Gwyn Morgan MBBS FRACS
Senior Lecturer
Department of Plastic Surgery
Flinders Medical Centre
Adelaide, Australia

Peter Morris FRS FRCS
Erstwhile Nuffield Professor of Surgery
Oxford, UK

Colm J O'Boyle MBBS MS
Department of General Surgery
Division of Upper Gastrointestinal &
Minimally Invasive Surgery
Hull & Castle Hill Hospital
Cottingham, UK

Frank G Quigley MBBS MS FRACS
Vascular Surgeon
Pimlico, Australia

Spero Raptis MBBS FRACS
Head of Unit
Vascular Surgery Unit
Royal Adelaide Hospital
Adelaide, Australia

Peter L Reilly MD BMedSc(Hons) FRACS FFPMANZCA
Professor, Director
Department of Neurosurgery
Royal Adelaide Hospital
Adelaide, Australia

Nicholas Rieger MBBS FRACS
Senior Lecturer in Surgery
Department of Colorectal Surgery
The Queen Elizabeth Hospital
Woodville, Australia

Michael G Sarr MD FACS
Professor, Gastroenterology Research Unit
Mayo Clinic
Rochester, USA

Nathaniel J Soper MD FACS
Professor and Vice-Chair for Clinical Affairs
Director of Minimally Invasive Surgery
Northwestern University Feinberg School of Medicine
Chicago, USA

Lee L Swanstrom MD MA FACS
Director
Division of Minimally Invasive Surgery
Legacy Health System
Portland, Oregon, USA

Jesper Swedenborg MD PhD
Professor of Surgery
Dept of Vascular Surgery
Karolinska Hospital
Stockholm, Sweden

David Watson MBBS MD FRACS
Professor, Head, University Department of Surgery
Flinders Medical Centre
Bedford Park, Australia

John Wayman MBBS MD FRCS
Consultant Surgeon
Cumberland Infirmary
Carlisle, UK

John Wong
Professor of Surgery
Department of Surgery
Queen Mary Hospital
Pokfulam Road
Hong Kong, China

ABDOMINAL OPERATIONS

Abdominal incisions: the anatomy of the abdominal wall. Laparoscopic access

Glyn Jamieson and John Wayman

The superficial and deep layers of the superficial fascia of the abdominal wall have little surgical relevance except where the deep layer fuses with the fascia of the thigh below the inguinal ligament. There is no such fusion with the fascia of the penis and scrotal contents or vulva and so blood from incisions in the abdominal wall sometimes tracks downwards and causes swelling and discoloration of the skin of the scrotum and penis or vulva postoperatively.

The deep layer of the superficial fascia is often quite well seen in young patients in the lower abdominal region and some surgeons like to close this layer when closing an incision made in the area, believing that wounds stretch less if this layer is closed.

THE EXTERNAL OBLIQUE MUSCLE (Fig. 1.1)

This muscle arises from the lower eight ribs or costal cartilages. Its upper four slips interdigitate with serratus anterior, its lower four slips with latissimus dorsi. The slips unite to form a wide flat muscle whose posterior fibres pass downwards to insert into the anterior half of the iliac crest and whose middle and anterior fibres insert into the aponeurosis, called the external oblique aponeurosis. This insertion takes place near the lateral edge of the rectus muscle and the aponeurosis passes in front of the rectus muscle to insert into the linea alba. The aponeurosis fuses with the anterior rectus sheath to a greater degree above than below where it is often quite separate from the rectus sheath.

The posterior border of the muscle between the 12th rib and the iliac crest is a free margin. The inferior border of the aponeurosis forms the inguinal ligament and this is considered elsewhere (see Ch. 16). Muscle fibres of the external oblique rarely descend below a line joining the anterior superior iliac spine and the umbilicus.

The muscle is supplied segmentally by the lower six intercostal (thoracic spinal) nerves with the nerves coming from the main nerves and entering the muscle wall laterally.

THE INTERNAL OBLIQUE MUSCLE (Fig. 1.2)

The external oblique muscle arises mainly above and sweeps downwards and forwards. The internal oblique on the other hand arises mainly behind and below and sweeps upwards and forwards. It arises from the thoraco-lumbar fascia, the anterior two-thirds of the iliac crest and the lateral two-thirds of the inguinal ligament. Its fibres posteriorly ascend to insert into the seventh to ninth costal cartilages, but the great majority of its fibres insert into the aponeurosis which forms the rectus sheath and the lowermost fibres are associated with the formation of the inguinal canal. This area is considered separately in Chapter 16. The muscle is supplied by the ventral rami of the lower six intercostal (thoracic spinal) nerves and the first lumbar nerve. Thus the nerve supply enters the muscle more anteriorly than the nerve supply to the external oblique which is supplied from the main trunks of the nerves.

THE TRANSVERSUS MUSCLE (Fig. 1.3)

This is the deepest of the three abdominal wall muscles and its origin, insertion and nerve supply are similar to the internal

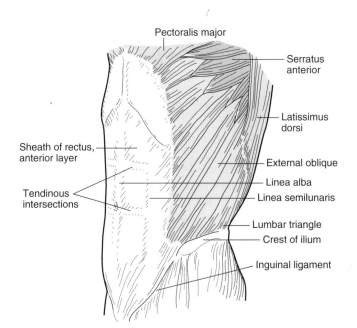

FIGURE 1.1 The external oblique muscle.

Labels: Pectoralis major; Serratus anterior; Latissimus dorsi; External oblique; Linea alba; Linea semilunaris; Lumbar triangle; Crest of ilium; Inguinal ligament; Sheath of rectus, anterior layer; Tendinous intersections

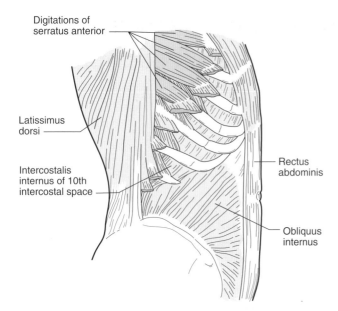

FIGURE 1.2 Muscles of the right side of the trunk. The external oblique has been removed to show the internal oblique (obliquus internus), but its digitations from the ribs have been preserved. The sheath of the rectus abdominis has been opened and its anterior lamina removed.

oblique. However, it arises above by fleshy slips which interdigitate with diaphragmatic muscle from the lower six ribs, then the thoracolumbar fascia, anterior two-thirds of the iliac crest and lateral third of the *ligament*. Its fibres run – as implied by its name – mainly in a transverse direction to end as the conjoint tendon below, but the majority of its fibres end as the posterior layer of the rectus sheath and linea alba. Above the level of the umbilicus, muscle often extends behind the rectus muscle before forming the sheath.

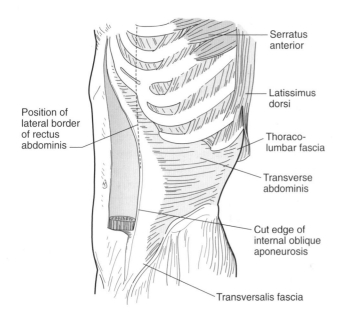

FIGURE 1.3 The transversus abdominis (transverse abdominis).

The muscle is supplied by the ventral rami of the lower five or six intercostal (thoracic spinal) nerves and the first lumbar nerve.

THE RECTUS MUSCLE (Fig. 1.1)

The rectus muscle arises from the pubic crest and pubic tubercle and anterior aspect of the pubic symphisis below and inserts into the fifth, sixth and seventh costal cartilages and the xiphoid process, above. It is partially interrupted by three or more tendinous intersections which are nearly always most marked in the upper half of the muscle (one at the xiphoid level, one at umbilical level and one about halfway between these two). These tendinous intersections rarely completely interrupt the muscle fibres posteriorly but do so anteriorly and furthermore are fused with the rectus sheath anteriorly. The nerve supply of the muscle is from the ventral rami of the lower six or seven intercostal (thoracic spinal) nerves and the nerves enter the lateral and posterior aspect of the muscle. The pyramidalis muscle is a small muscle arising from the front of the body of the pubis and symphysis and it ascends in front of the rectus to insert into the linea alba. It diminishes in size as it rises and inserts midway between umbilicus and pubis. It is often larger on one side than the other. It is supplied by the ventral ramus of the subcostal nerve (12th thoracic spinal nerve).

The actions of the anterolateral abdominal muscles

Acting together these muscles are the compressors of the abdomen and their tonic contraction helps to support the abdominal viscera. Acting individually they have other actions. For example, the rectus muscle flexes the spine and the oblique muscles assist lateral flexion and rotation of the spine.

THE RECTUS SHEATH AND THE LINEA ALBA

The rectus sheath is believed to be rather more complex in its formation than was previously held to be the case. However, its formation is of little consequence to the surgeon and the essential features remain time-honoured. Thus, above there is no sheath posteriorly, the muscle lying directly on the costal cartilages, and anteriorly it is formed by the external oblique aponeurosis only. Then from the point where the muscle passes below the costal margin to a variable point below the umbilicus the sheath has both anterior and posterior layers: the anterior layer is made up of the external oblique aponeurosis and the anterior lamina of the internal oblique aponeurosis, while the posterior layer is made up of the posterior layer of the internal oblique aponeurosis and the transversus aponeurosis (Fig. 1.4). At

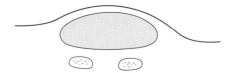

Rectus sheath - above costal cartilages

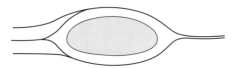

Rectus sheath - upper two-thirds

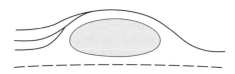

Rectus sheath - lower third
(note external oblique aproneurosis)

FIGURE 1.4 The mode of formation of the rectus sheath (right side).

some point below the umbilicus the posterior layer passes in front of the rectus muscle to fuse with the anterior layer. The free edge of the sheath behind the rectus muscle is called the arcuate line. The linea alba is a six-lamina structure with up to three decussations of the various layers, but from a surgical point of view, the important decussation is the midline one. Below the umbilicus the linea alba is narrow and the rectus muscles usually lie contiguous to each other. The fascia at the lateral edge of the rectus muscle in the area of the arcuate line is sometimes called Spigelius' fascia. As weaknesses occur at this point in some patients, hernias at the outer edge of the rectus muscle and below the level of the umbilicus are called Spigelian hernias. Sometimes small defects occur in the linea alba above the umbilicus, leading to small hernias known as epigastric hernias. It is unusual for them to contain other than extraperitoneal fat.

THE TRANSVERSALIS FASCIA

This is the layer of fibro fatty tissue which lies between the inner surface of the transversus muscle and the peritoneum. It is of importance in two regards. First, in making extraperitoneal approaches to various structures and second, in regard to the transversus aponeurosis and the conjoint tendon where a certain confusion exists. It is important to note that posteriorly the transversalis fascia fuses with the fascia

behind the psoas muscle (thoracolumbar fascia). The areas where the transversalis fascia assumes surgical importance are discussed in appropriate sections later.

NERVE COURSES IN THE ABDOMINAL WALL

The anterior abdominal wall and its skin are largely supplied by the lower six intercostal (thoracic) nerves and the subcostal (first lumbar) nerve. Below the costal region the nerves tend to run in the direction imparted to them by the intercostal space so that they run obliquely downwards and forwards. The periumbilical region is usually supplied by the 10th thoracic nerve. Clearly, in vertical incisions in the midline the nerves are uncut but if the incision is at the outer border of the rectus muscle then the rectus will be denervated over the length of the cut. If a vertical incision is made even further laterally then transversus and internal oblique may be denervated as well, hence the stricture on lateral vertical incisions in the abdominal wall. Transverse incisions rarely divide more than two or three nerves and such division does not lead to untoward clinical consequences.

VESSEL COURSES IN THE ABDOMINAL WALL

The arterial supply to the anterior abdominal wall is derived above from the superior epigastric artery, the continuation of the internal thoracic artery, and from anterior and collateral branches of the 10th and 11th intercostal and subcostal vessels. Inferiorly, the superficial circumflex iliac and superficial epigastric arteries arise from the femoral artery and course in the superficial fascia along the inguinal ligament and towards the umbilicus respectively. The inferior epigastric artery and deep circumflex iliac artery arise from the external iliac artery just above the mid point of the inguinal ligament. The deep circumflex iliac artery runs on the deep aspect of the anterior abdominal wall parallel with the inguinal ligament. The inferior epigastric artery runs superiorly and enters the rectus sheath below the arcuate line, travelling along a line which approximates from the mid inguinal point to a point 4–5 cm lateral to the umbilicus. Nevertheless, such things as body habitus, divarication of the rectus muscles and normal variation make the position of the artery difficult to pinpoint with certainty. Damage to these vessels in the abdominal wall by laparoscopic port insertion, particularly the inferior epigastric artery, can result in catastrophic haemorrhage but more usually abdominal wall haematoma. Sometimes the course of superficial vessels can be determined and avoided by transillumination and the inferior epigastric vessels can be identified laparoscopically by the lateral umbilical fold of peritoneum which covers them before they pass beneath the arcuate line.

CT scan mapping of the epigastric vessels has demonstrated that they are usually more than 4 cm from the midline and rarely more than 8 cm from the midline. As much as possible, the 4–8 cm zone should be avoided.

ABDOMINAL INCISIONS

Midline incisions

A midline incision is most easily performed above the umbilicus. If the patient is obese then the middle decussation of the linea alba is most easily found by forceful retraction of the skin edges. This causes splitting of the subcutaneous tissue and invariably leads to the decussation. Most surgeons skirt the umbilicus if extending the incision to the lower abdomen. The linea alba for all practical purposes disappears here and it is difficult to make a lower midline abdominal incision without seeing the rectus muscles. At the lowermost level the pyramidalis muscles are encountered.

Improvements in suture technology have led to this incision being the most popular incision for abdominal access, particularly for operations in the upper abdomen. Incision of the peritoneum is best commenced in the upper part of the incision as this is above the level of the small or large bowel and so the incision is safest at this level.

When an incision is made below the umbilicus it is as well to remember the bladder and its structures which lie between the rectus and the peritoneum. A patent urachus can be divided and closed with impunity. As the incision becomes more caudad, then the bladder itself can appear in the wound.

Paramedian incisions

These incisions are less used today. As the incision is made separately in the anterior and posterior rectus sheaths, the rectus muscle has to be dissected away from its tendinous intersections medially. These are fused with the anterior rectus sheath and have to be sharply dissected from it. The well formed upper intersections always convey blood vessels. The nerve supply to the rectus muscle enters laterally so that mobilization of the muscle from medial to lateral does not produce any denervation.

Subcostal incisions

A right subcostal incision is popular for gall bladder surgery and when combined with a left subcostal incision gives good exposure for liver surgery. The rectus muscle is divided and the superior epigastric artery is usually found embedded deeply in the rectus in its medial half. When the excision is extended beyond the lateral border of rectus – which is usual – one or two lower thoracic nerves and accompanying vessels are divided. If the incision is extended across the midline then the falciform ligament and ligamentum teres must be divided.

Transverse muscle-cutting incisions

When a transverse incision is made, because of the direction of the nerves and vessels in the abdominal wall it is unusual for more than two thoracic nerves to be divided, regardless of the site of a transverse incision. For incisions below the umbilicus which incorporate division of the rectus muscle, care must be taken to isolate and divide the inferior epigastric artery. It ascends outside the rectus muscle posteriorly to a varying level and even when it enters that muscle it tends to remain well posterior in position.

Muscle-splitting incisions

The most frequently used muscle-splitting incision is the so-called McBurney incision which is used in appendicectomy. In fact today the incision is usually made more transversely in the right iliac fossa, but still centred over McBurney's point. (This is the point centred over the junction of the middle and outer thirds of the line joining the anterior superior iliac spine to the umbilicus.) The first layer encountered is almost always the deep layer of the superficial fascia which in young people can be a respectable layer and can fool the inexperienced into thinking it is the first important layer, i.e. the aponeurosis of external oblique. (Remember that muscle fibres of this muscle are almost always above a line joining the anterior superior iliac spine and the umbilicus.) When the aponeurotic fibres are encountered they are easily split obliquely upwards and backwards and obliquely downwards and forwards.

The next layer encountered is the internal oblique muscle with muscle fibres crossing approximately at right angles to the line of direction of the split external oblique aponeurosis. Upon separating the internal oblique muscle fibres the transversely running fibres of the transversus muscle are seen. While the next important layer is the peritoneum it must be remembered that the transversalis fascia can be strong enough to be picked up and scratched at with a scalpel, with the inexperienced thinking it is peritoneum. This is of more than theoretical interest. If surgeons divide this layer thinking they have divided peritoneum, and then burrow in feeling for the appendix, they are likely to encounter an appendix 'feel-alike' and if they do not notice that the structure is pulsating then the scene is set for a disaster to occur. Although it may sound improbable to mistake the iliac artery for the appendix, such cases are reported around the world each year.

EXTRAPERITONEAL APPROACHES TO RETROPERITONEAL STRUCTURES

The extraperitoneal space can be opened using any one of the incisions described above. Most commonly used are an oblique iliac fossa muscle-cutting incision for an extra-peritoneal approach to the lower aorta and its iliac vessels and a muscle-splitting incision, like an appendiceal incision but at a higher level, for an extraperitoneal approach to the sympathetic chain for lumbar sympathectomy. Whatever its insignificance as an anatomical structure to anatomists, the surgeon has to pay special attention to the transversalis fascia in these incisions. The layer is not strong, it is true, but unless it is formally broken through, it puts the surgeon in the wrong plane for exposure of the iliac vessels. This is not usually much of a problem because the exposure is good and the vessels can be found by palpation. The wrong plane is more of a problem in approaching the lumbar sympathetic chain however, for it directs the surgeon to the plane *behind* the psoas muscle. It is only when the transversalis fascia is broken through that the correct plane, extraperitoneal and in front of the psoas, is found.

Although used infrequently, the midline or paramedian extraperitoneal approach to retroperitoneal structures can be a very useful approach. It is somewhat tedious to make, which probably accounts for its lack of popularity, but the peritoneum can be completely stripped away from the anterior and lateral abdominal wall muscles. Once again it is necessary to break the transversalis fascia posteriorly in order to gain the plane in front of the psoas muscle. This approach has the advantage of allowing the surgeon to approach directly a structure such as the abdominal aorta or renal artery without abdominal contents spilling into the field. Furthermore the fact that the abdominal cavity is not opened means that post-operative paralytic ileus is usually less of a problem.

LAPAROSCOPIC APPROACHES

There are several points worth making in regard to laparoscopic incisions. Perhaps first and most important is that instrumentation in the midline, or close to the midline and particularly from the umbilical level and above, has the potential to cause damage to the aorta or inferior vena cava. Even in relatively obese patients the distance between the abdominal wall and aorta or inferior vena cava is much shorter than most surgeons realize – because of the normal lordosis of the spine. For this reason a trochar and cannula should be angled away from the midline during insertion, even when the skin incision is in the midline.

Second is the fact that the linea alba and peritoneum are usually fused at the umbilical region so that an approach either immediately above or below the umbilicus is regarded as the simplest approach for insertion of a cannula, which is no doubt why this approach is much used. Conversely where an approach to the extraperitoneal space is required, as in the totally extraperitoneal laparoscopic hernia repair, a paramedian port-site is preferred, with intubation of the space between the rectus muscle and the posterior rectus sheath. By passing down in the space the surgeon passes out extraperitoneally, caudal to the arcuate ligament.

FURTHER READING

Saber A A, Meslemami A M, Davis R, Pimenter R 2004 Safety zones for anterior abdominal wall entry during laparoscopy. Ann Surg 239:182–185.

2

Liver resections and liver transplantation: the anatomy of the liver and associated structures

Glyn Jamieson and Bernard Launois

The usefulness of a precise knowledge of anatomy is well demonstrated with the anatomy of the liver. In the past 20 years or so, knowledge of the intrahepatic anatomy has been applied to surgery of the organ and this has led to the development of precise operations on the liver.

Surgical access to the liver can be through a generous midline abdominal incision or a bilateral subcostal incision, which is preferred by many surgeons. Division of the peritoneal attachments of the liver allows it to be displaced downwards for access to the hepatic veins and all surfaces of the liver.

THE PERITONEAL ATTACHMENTS

The falciform ligament and ligamentum teres

The falciform ligament attaches the front of the liver to the anterior abdominal wall and then descends attaching to the posterior aspect of the umbilicus. It is a vestige of the ventral mesogastrium of embryonic life and the ligamentum teres runs in its free edge. This is a supposedly fibrous *cord* which attaches from the umbilicus, runs in the free edge of the falciform ligament and joins the left branch of the portal vein. In fetal life it formed the left umbilical vein and it used to be thought that it became obliterated at birth. In reality its lumen is usually closed rather than obliterated and it can be dissected at the umbilicus, dilated and used for access to the left portal vein in more than 50% of patients. This channel occasionally opens up in portal hypertension, forming a collateral channel to bypass the liver and in these circumstances the umbilical vein can often reach quite large proportions. The ligamentum teres has surgical significance for several reasons. As it passes to the left from the midline, it tends to get in the way during upper abdominal surgery and so it is usually divided. Small paraumbilical veins extend from the portal system to the umbilicus and travel with the ligamentum teres; these should be ligated before being divided to prevent bleeding from these veins. The ligamentum teres can be divided near the liver and dissected towards the umbilicus or vice versa and its free end can then be used as an anchoring 'guyrope', if needed. It has been most used in this manner to anchor the oesophagus in the abdomen after antireflux surgery. The free umbilical end is passed around the mobilized oesophagus as a sling and then attached to its self, making the sling into a racket frame. Or it can be attached to the anterior wall of the stomach, making the sling a sort of shepherd's crook.

Perhaps more important, however, has been the use of ligamentum teres as a guide to the ductal system of segment III of the liver for biliary enteric drainage procedures (see Ch. 3). Once the ligamentum teres reaches the liver it passes in a fissure which separates segment III on the left (the anterior portion of the morphological left lobe of the liver) from segment IV (quadrate lobe) on the right. This fissure may be complete or it may contain some liver tissue which bridges over the ligamentum teres. A finger or large forceps can be insinuated through with the ligamentum teres deep to this bridge of tissue, which can then be divided with diathermy as it is relatively avascular. The ligamentum teres can be traced through to the point of entry into the left portal vein where it tends to fan out somewhat. The biliary duct from segment III usually joins the left hepatic bile duct behind and somewhat superior to this junction (Fig. 2.1).

The two layers of the falciform ligament fan out on the liver surface to blend with the peritoneum covering the liver. The ligament is a relatively avascular structure and can be divided back to its posterior most portion where its leaves separate and become the anterior leaves of the right and left coronary ligaments.

The triangle formed by the posterior part of the falciform ligament has the common trunk of the middle and left hepatic vein lying at the base on the left and a depression of liver tissue in front of the vena cava on the right. This depression lies between the right and left hepatic veins (Fig. 2.2).

The coronary and triangular ligaments

These are the ligaments which attach the posterior surface of the liver to the diaphragm. The coronary ligament lies mainly to the right and consists of a superior leaf which runs to the right and caudally; near the edge of the right side of the liver it is in close proximity to the inferior leaf. It turns to become the inferior leaf and at this point the two leaves together are called the right triangular ligament. The inferior leaf then passes back and runs behind the inferior vena cava

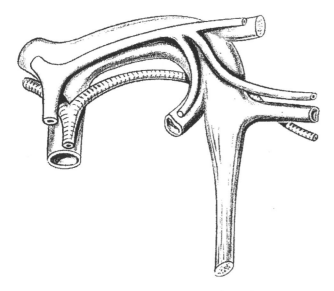

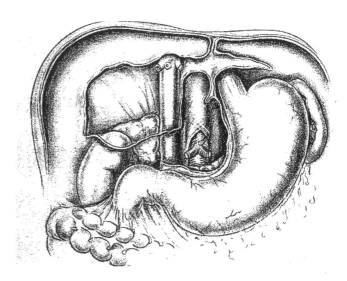

FIGURE 2.3 The ligaments of the liver.

FIGURE 2.1 The ligamentum teres joining the left portal venous system.

eventually to take part in the formation of the lesser omentum (Fig. 2.3).

The two leaves of the coronary ligament are widely separated and the posterior surface of the liver here lies against the diaphragm without any peritoneal covering, the so-called bare area of the liver (the liver here is attached to the diaphragm by fibroareolar tissue which varies in the density of the fibrous component. It is not avascular). The leaves of the coronary ligament passing to the left come into proximity almost immediately and form the left triangular ligament which suspends the posterosuperior surface of the left side of the liver to the diaphragm. The inferior vena cava and the entering hepatic veins lie within the bare area of the liver.

In order to gain mobility of the liver for resections it is necessary to divide these ligaments and it should be appreciated that, as the division reaches towards the midline, important venous structures are in close proximity and therefore are at risk. Therefore as one divides the left triangular ligament one approaches the left hepatic vein near the

midline. In dividing the superior leaf of the coronary ligament it is the right hepatic vein and inferior vena cava which are in proximity and for the inferior leaf of the coronary ligament it is the inferior vena cava which is in proximity.

THE LOBES AND SEGMENTS OF THE LIVER

Upon opening the abdominal cavity the falciform ligament appears to divide the liver into a large right and a small left hepatic lobe. In this and subsequent discussions the diagrams of the liver will be from the caudal aspect of the patient looking upwards, i.e. the CT scan view of the liver. When examined from below there are two other areas which are demarcated by anatomical structures (Fig. 2.4). First is the area bounded by the gall bladder and its bed on the right and the umbilical fissure with the ligamentum teres on the left. This is the quadrate lobe of the liver. It contains the portal fissure and the portal structures at its base. Second is the area which is posterior and superior to the portal fissure

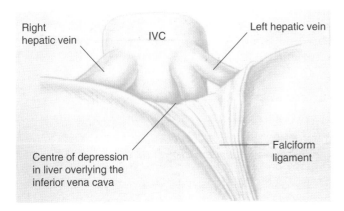

FIGURE 2.2 The triangular base of the falciform ligament. IVC = Inferior vena cava.

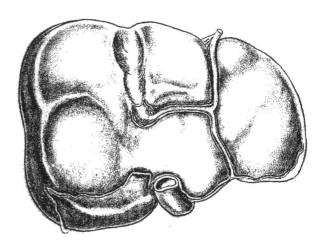

FIGURE 2.4 The boundaries of the caudate and quadrate lobe.

with the inferior vena cava to its right and the continuation of the umbilical fissure (called the fissure for the ligamentum venosum) on its left – the caudate lobe. The ligamentum venosum is the cord formed by the obliteration at birth of the ductus venosus which joined the left branch of the portal vein directly to the left hepatic vein, allowing fetal blood to bypass the liver.

The morphological lobes of the liver do not correspond to the right and left sides of the liver. In fact it has been known for many years that the portal trinity (portal vein, bile duct, hepatic artery) divides the liver into a right and left side. However, the dissemination of this knowledge in regard to its surgical importance was due to Ton That Tung (who first published in the field in 1936) and Claude Couinaud who in 1957 published a book entitled *The Liver: Anatomical and Surgical Studies*.

The division between the functional right and left sides is a line which runs inferoposteriorly through the middle of the gall bladder bed, passes slightly to the left at the porta hepatis to pass in the middle of the region where the portal structures bifurcate and then across the caudate process. On the anterosuperior surface this line runs from the middle of the gall bladder notch back to the middle hepatic vein or left side of the inferior vena cava. Thus, as viewed in the open abdomen, the line passes obliquely from the tip of the gall bladder to the point where the falciform ligament disappears posteriorly. This plane is known as the main fissure of the liver (Fig. 2.5).

The segmental anatomy of the liver which has led to such a rapid evolution of resectional surgery is based on the intrahepatic distribution of the portal trinity, the principal component of which is the portal vein and its divisions. The right branch of the portal vein supplies the right liver. This right branch divides into two, dividing the right liver into two parts, a medial part – the right medial sector, which is predominantly anterior – and a lateral part – the right lateral sector, which is predominantly posterior (Fig. 2.5). The plane between the two sectors is the right fissure of the liver and it is a vertical plane, the anterior border of which is parallel to the right edge of the liver. It lies somewhat variably between the tip of the gall

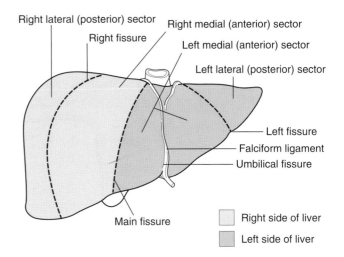

FIGURE 2.5 The fissures and sectors of the liver.

bladder and the right edge of the liver. The plane then passes back more or less in the coronal plane towards the right hepatic vein as it enters the inferior vena cava.

The left branch of the portal vein supplies the left liver and also divides it into two parts, an anterior and posterior sector, the plane between which is the left fissure and which approximately bisects the left morphological lobe at 45° to the coronal plane, posterior to the insertion of the ligamentum teres into the portal vein. Thus the liver consists of four sectors (Fig. 2.5). Each sector is divided into two segments, with one exception. Roman numerals are used to designate the segments, beginning at the inferior part of the liver and going around the portal vein in an anticlockwise direction (when viewed from below), or as Ronald Malt put it, in a spiral, like the *arrondissements* of Paris. There are eight segments (Fig. 2.6). When viewed from below, segment VIII is not seen as its posterior portion is narrow and lies in front of the inferior vena cava (Fig. 2.6b).

Because the plane between the right medial and right lateral sectors is coronal it means that the segments of the right

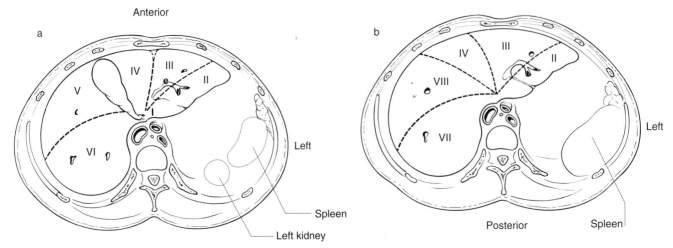

FIGURE 2.6 Diagrammatic representation of CT scan view of the liver. The level of (a) is more caudad than (b) (see text).

medial sector tend to lie in front of the segments of the right lateral sector. Thus when viewed from the front, segment VI tends to lie behind segment V (Fig. 2.6a).

It also means that the posterior surface of the right side is made up mainly of segments VII and VI. The confusion which has arisen in regard to segmental orientation is a result of the difference between the in situ liver and a liver lying on a flat surface outside the body (Fig. 2.7).

For the left liver the anterior sector is made up of segment IV (the quadrate lobe) medially and segment III laterally and these are separated by the umbilical fissure.

The posterior sector of the left side is the one exception to the rule and is made up of only one segment, segment II.

Segment I is the caudate lobe of the liver and it is an autonomous segment receiving branches of the portal trinity from both right and left sides. It also drains independently into the inferior vena cava. Its separateness from the right and left livers is demonstrated in hepatic venous occlusion where the liver is congested and functioning poorly. The caudate lobe hypertrophies perhaps also taking some of the hepatic venous drainage back to the inferior vena cava. The segments are shown schematically in Figure 2.8.

Therefore the terms right hepatectomy and left hepatectomy refer to removal of the right or left liver respectively. Right and left lobectomy refers to removal of the morphological lobes on either side of the umbilical fissure. On the right this involves removal of some of the left side of the liver and in the USA this is sometimes known as a trisegmentectomy.

It is possible to remove any single segment of the liver without jeopardizing the blood supply or biliary or venous drainage to the rest of the liver. However in practical terms it is sometimes easier to remove more than just the involved segment of liver. For instance, lesions in segment I are difficult of access and so are often approached via a right or left hepatectomy including segmentectomy IV. Also segment II or segment III lesions are more easily removed by left lobectomy although in the cirrhotic patient it may be important to conserve liver and any one of these three segments (I, II or III) can be removed alone. The anatomy of individual segments, as it relates to their removal, is considered in more detail later.

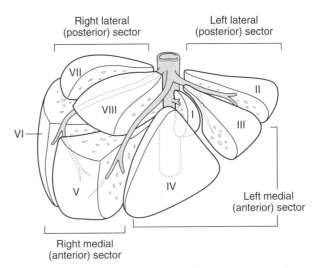

FIGURE 2.8 Diagrammatic representation of the eight segments of the liver.

GLISSON'S CAPSULE AND THE PORTAL TRINITY

Glisson's capsule condenses around the portal trinity structures and surrounds them as they enter the liver substance. Thus each bile duct, hepatic artery, portal vein unit is surrounded by a fibrous sheath which was called the valoean sheath by Couinaud, after Valoeus, an anatomist from the Middle Ages who first described the liver capsule. Within each sheath the portal vein is surrounded by loose areolar tissue making dissection of it relatively easy. The condensation of fibrous tissue around the bile duct and hepatic artery is tougher and dissection of these structures is therefore more difficult within the sheaths. When approached from within the liver substance the sheaths simplify a ligation of the portal trinity. In other words, the sheath is the structure which is mobilized with its contained three structures and this sheath can be ligated and divided as one structure (Fig. 2.9). This manoeuvre is made simpler with the larger sheaths by using a vascular automatic stapling device.

The diagram which shows the common pattern for the structures (Fig. 2.10) therefore gives some indications of the pattern for each of the branches of the portal vein, the bile duct and the hepatic artery. There are many variations however, which makes dissection of individual structures within the liver difficult and even hazardous. However if the sheath to a particular segment is taken it will only contain structures passing to or from that segment. Ligation of individual sheaths is therefore not only simpler, but safer (Fig. 2.11). Sometimes it is necessary to dissect structures individually within a sheath (this is particularly true for biliary-enteric anastomoses). The bile duct tends to be elliptical rather than round and the inferior aspect usually faces the corresponding artery (Fig. 2.12). The relationship between the three structures within the sheaths follows two general

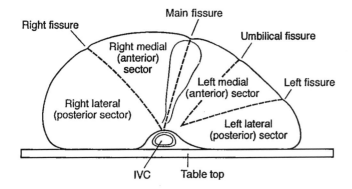

FIGURE 2.7 The ex vivo liver lying on a flat surface. IVC = Inferior vena cava.

a

b

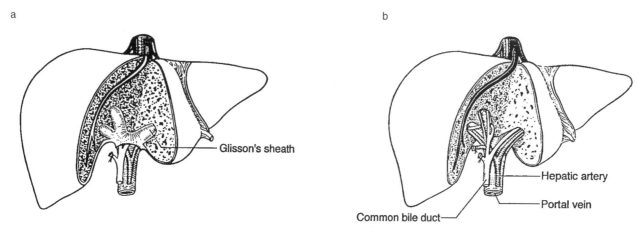

FIGURE 2.9   (a) Glisson's capsule and the manner in which it forms the portal sheaths. (b) The sheath has been cut away.

a

b

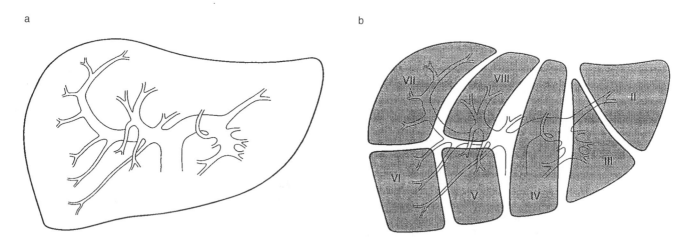

FIGURE 2.10   (a) Diagrammatic representation of the Glissonian sheaths. (b) The sheaths and segments they supply.

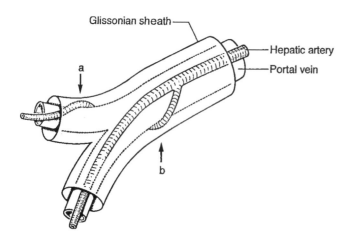

FIGURE 2.11   If the sheath is opened at (b) and the individual structures are dissected, then the abnormally branching artery may be ligated under the supposition that it is passing to the lower branch. If the lower sheath is taken en masse there is no danger to this aberrant artery (a) and (b).

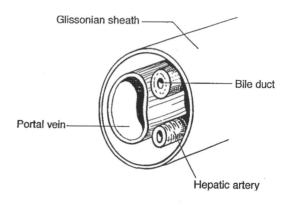

FIGURE 2.12   Typical relationships of portal trinity structures within the Glissonian sheath.

rules of importance for the surgeon embarking on biliary enteric anastomoses. First, the portal vein tends to lie posterior to the bile duct and hepatic artery. Second, the bile duct tends to lie superior to the artery (Fig. 2.12) and is always close to it.

The intrahepatic portal vein

The distribution of the left portal vein is relatively constant. It is usually about 3–5 cm in length and at the left end of the portal fissure it changes direction by curving forwards in the umbilical fissure. At the level of this curvature it gives off the vein to segment II and as it passes forwards it gives off the vein to segment III on the left and the vein to segment IV on the right. The ligamentum teres is attached to the vein in the umbilical fissure (Fig. 2.1).

The right portal vein appears to be the continuation of the main trunk of the portal vein and is usually only 1–3 cm in length. It divides into two main divisions. The division to the right lateral sector of the liver describes a gentle curve towards the right posterior aspect of the liver. The branch to segment VI then arises from the curve and the continuation of the vein supplies segment VII.

The trunk to the right medial sector can arise at an angle from the general direction of the right division from its superior surface or sometimes anteriorly. However, when viewed from below, intraoperatively, the medial sector sheath with its contained vein often appears to be the continuation of the main right sheath. It describes a gentle curve with its concavity being towards the centre of the liver. It terminates by branching into anterior branches for segment V and posterior branches for segment VIII.

Variations in the region of the hilum occur in about 20% of cases and are of surgical importance if the surgeon uses the extrahepatic approach to liver resection. For instance, the right lateral vein or right medial vein can arise directly from the main portal vein or occasionally even from the left branch of the portal vein.

Variations in segmental supply also occur, with the commonest being the absence of a common trunk for the right lateral sector. The portal veins for segment VI and segment VII then arise separately from the main trunk. Couinaud suggests this is less common than a single right lateral trunk. Our operative experience tends to suggest the opposite. Occasionally there are two right medial veins with one arising normally and the other arising from one of the other veins in the region. These variations are of importance in the intrahepatic approach to the Glissonian sheaths.

Intrahepatic bile ducts

The segmental ducts of the left liver are relatively constant and follow the sheaths. In the right liver, the right hepatic duct is formed by the junction of the right lateral and right medial ducts. It is usually a simple matter to recognize the right lateral duct on a cholangiogram because it curves

around the right medial duct – so-called Hjortsjo's crook (Fig. 2.13). The right lateral duct therefore joins the left side of the right medial duct and curves behind the other right medial sheath structures. It is this crook which places the right lateral sector bile duct at risk when the right medial sector sheath is divided. An example would be an extended left hepatectomy when the right lateral sector is being retained. Stricture formation is a well known complication of the operation.

Another major variation of surgical significance is that in about 30% of cases some of the segments of the right side drain into the main left hepatic duct. This is usually the right lateral duct (segments VI and VII) but occasionally it is the right medial duct (segments V and VIII). This means that drainage of the left liver with an enteric anastomosis to the left hepatic duct when the confluence is occluded may be associated with some biliary decompression of the right side of the liver. It also means in left hepatectomy there is a risk of causing obstruction to the drainage of these respective right segments. As they usually drain into the left hepatic duct near the confluence, it should encourage the surgeon to tie the left hepatic duct as far to the left as practicable. Similarly, a left sided bile duct can drain into the right hepatic duct. As the right main sheath is often quite short, damage to such an aberrant left duct is best avoided by dividing the right lateral and right medial sheaths separately, if possible, rather than the main right sheath itself.

Intrahepatic arteries

Variations in the intrahepatic arteries are common but most of the variations do not have surgical significance. One variation which occurs in about 20% of cases is an origin of the artery, or an artery, to segment IV which arises from the right hepatic artery or from the main hepatic artery. However this artery runs behind and to the left of the left hepatic artery and never arises to the right of the common bile duct. Therefore if the right hepatic artery is divided to the right of the common bile duct during a right hepatectomy, this aberrant supply to segment IV is not endangered. The right hepatic artery is relatively constant in following the Glissonian sheaths within the liver.

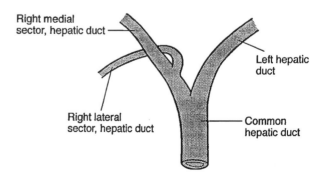

FIGURE 2.13 Hjortsjo's crook – the right lateral sector duct hooks around the right medial sector duct.

THE FISSURES OF THE LIVER

Although a couple of the less important fissures exist as definable openings, the more important ones do not exist as such, but have to be made by the surgeon. And yet a knowledge of these non-existent fissures can be of critical importance in liver resections.

The Shorter Oxford Dictionary describes a fissure as 'An opening, usually long and narrow, made by cracking, splitting or separation of parts'. The terms 'scissure' or 'scissura' can be used interchangeably with the term fissure – but the latter is more idiomatic and is most commonly used. The doyen of liver anatomy, Claude Couinaud, defines a portal fissure as follows:

> A portal fissure is the limit between the territories supplied by two adjacent pedicles: the blood flow from one pedicle cannot trespass the fissure, though a continuity is secured by the sinusoids.

The importance of the fissures of the liver is that they mark the boundaries of portal units of the liver, and as they can be more or less accurately defined, they help greatly in removing the anatomically defined portions of the liver. And equally important is that the main hepatic veins run in the main fissures of the liver.

The main fissure

The main fissure separates the right side of the liver from the left side of the liver, and unlike some of the other fissures its plane is fairly constant (Fig. 2.14). The plane is more or less vertical and separates segments V and VIII (the right medial sector) from segment IV. On the anterior and superior surface of the liver its plane is in a line which joins the tip of the gall bladder bed back to about the midpoint of the inferior vena cava. On the inferior surface the line runs down the middle of the gall bladder bed across the caudate process and then up along the middle of the inferior vena cava. The main trunk of the middle hepatic vein lies within this fissure.

The left fissure

This fissure separates the left posterior sector (segment II) from the left anterior sector (segments III and IV; Fig. 2.14). The main trunk of the left hepatic vein lies in this fissure. No great variability has been reported in this fissure, which can be marked approximately on the liver surface by joining two points. The first point is midway along the anterior edge of the liver between the falciform ligament and the left extremity. The second point is at the left side of the base of the triangular insertion of the falciform ligament in front of the inferior vena cava (Fig. 2.2). The plane of the fissure is approximately midway between horizontal and vertical in its obliquity back to the inferior vena cava (Fig. 2.14).

The umbilical fissure

This fissure separates segment III from segment IV and it is marked morphologically on the inferior liver surface at the point where the falciform ligament reaches the anterior border of the liver. There usually is a bridge of liver tissue over the ligamentum teres as it lies in the depths of this fissure. On the superior surface of the liver the fissure lies deep to the line of attachment of the falciform ligament

There is often a vein of some surgical importance which lies in this fissure – best called the vein of the umbilical fissure to avoid confusing it with the umbilical vein running with the round ligament.

The fissure venosum

This fissure is also marked morphologically on the liver surface and it is the continuation of the umbilical fissure on the posterior surface of the liver. The lesser omentum passes into this fissure and in its depths lies a fibrous cord which connects the left branch of the portal vein with the left hepatic vein – this was the ductus venosum in fetal life. The caudate process lies behind this fissure separated from it only by the lesser omentum. The fissure lies more or less in a coronal plane and the continuation of this plane leads to the plane of the dorsal fissure.

The dorsal fissure

Perhaps the least definable of all the fissures, this separates the posterior aspect of segment IV from segment I (Fig. 2.15). It is in the same plane as the fissure venosum, so that when the surgeon places the fingers in this fissure they point to the division between segment I behind and segment IV in front.

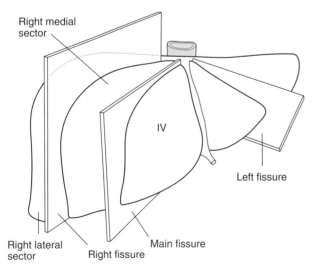

Right medial sector

IV

Left fissure

Right lateral sector

Right fissure

Main fissure

FIGURE 2.14 The planes of the fissures of the liver.

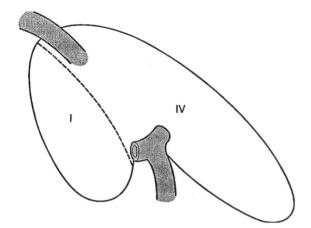

FIGURE 2.15 Lateral view showing the plane of the dorsal fissure.

Couinaud calls that portion of the caudate lobe lying posterior to segments VIII and IV, segment IX (Fig. 2.16).

The right fissure

The right fissure of the liver runs between the right medial sector (segments V and VIII) and the right lateral sector (segments VI and VII; Fig 2.17a). The right hepatic vein runs in this fissure. The plane of this fissure tends more to the coronal than anything else, but it is very variable in its anterior extent (Fig. 2.17c).

It is usually described as running from the point midway between the gall bladder bed and the right extremity of the liver. However this situation occurs in only about 50% of cases. In about 40% of cases the fissure lies much closer to the right margin of the gall bladder bed and in some cases it actually becomes confluent with the main fissure (Fig. 2.17b). In such cases segment V does not appear at all on the anterior margin or inferior surface of the liver, and thus segment VI is large. In about 10% of cases the other extreme occurs and the right fissure extends out to the right anterior

extremity of the liver. Then it is segment V which is large and segment VI is small (Fig. 2.17c).

In a number of individuals a vestigial fissure is seen on the undersurface of the liver to the right of the gall bladder and this probably corresponds with the right fissure. It is called the fissure of Gans by Couinaud.

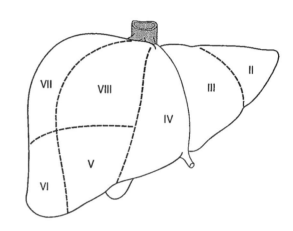

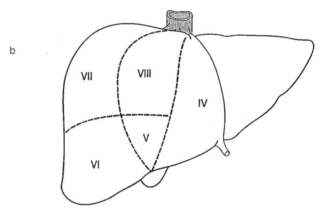

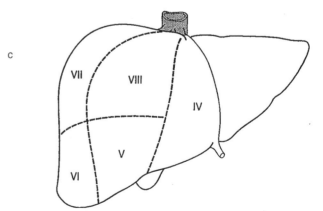

FIGURE 2.17 The right fissure and its extremes. (a) Usual position; (b) the fissure joining the main fissure; (c) the fissure displaced laterally.

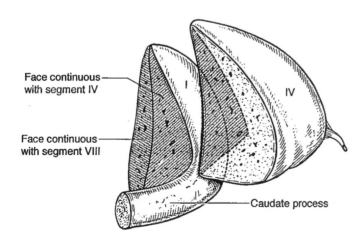

Face continuous with segment IV

Face continuous with segment VIII

Caudate process

FIGURE 2.16 The face continuous with segment IV is the dorsal fissure.

THE HEPATIC VEINS

There are three major hepatic veins (Fig. 2.18) and they do not correspond with the portal segmentation. In fact the major hepatic veins lie between the four major sectors of the liver. Thus the right hepatic vein lies between the right medial and right lateral sectors, the middle hepatic vein lies between the right and left livers (between segments V and VIII and segment IV) and the left vein lies between the anterior (IV and III) and posterior (II) sectors of the left side of the liver. Because of their situation between the sectors of the liver, during resection the surgeon should at all times be aware that the vein is being approached and at all times be searching for the vein so that dissection can proceed on one or other side of it.

The left hepatic vein

The left hepatic vein drains segments II and III only. It emerges from the plane of the left fissure between segment III (anterior and superior) and segment II (posterior and inferior) and runs across the posterior part of the fissure for the ligamentum venosum. The vein is situated in the posterior 2 cm of this fissure and makes up part of the posterior edge of the liver. At this level, the vein is covered only by the connective tissue of the left triangular ligament.

The vein then travels transversely and posteriorly to the right in the direction of the vena cava, following the superior edge of segment I. It terminates in the inferior vena cava, usually receiving the middle hepatic vein before it does so (see next section). The left hepatic vein receives two main branches within the liver. A posterior branch drains the posterior part of the left liver, including segment II and a part of segment III. It runs to the right and upwards to the posterior part of the fissure of the ligamentum teres. An anterior branch drains the anterior part of this area and it receives the vein of the umbilical fissure which lies beneath the falciform ligament. This vein also receives venules, or even a more major vein from segment IV. The vein of the umbilical fissure is

inconstant however (less than 60% of cases). This has surgical importance because if the middle hepatic vein is divided without removing segment IV, this segment may then rely on venous drainage via the vein of the umbilical fissure.

The middle hepatic vein

This ends as a single trunk in the inferior vena cava in only 3–15% of cases. In the great majority of cases it forms a common trunk with the left hepatic vein, this trunk usually being 5 mm or less in length.

Therefore it should be a surgical maxim that there are only two major hepatic veins entering the inferior vena cava – the right and the confluent middle and left vein. The reason for stressing this point is that the surgeon is less likely to ligate inadvertently the right hepatic vein if it is assumed that there are only two major veins entering the cava.

The middle hepatic vein arises from the confluence of two veins anteriorly and passes backwards receiving veins from the parts of the right and left sides of the liver which lie contiguous with the main fissure. Two branches require special mention. The vein from segment IV is long, tenuous, sagittal and enters the middle vein on its left side. Usually much larger is the vein of segment VIII. This is posterior and usually runs transversely, into the right side of the middle vein. It is sometimes large enough to be mistaken for the middle vein itself and sometimes even enters the vena cava separately. The middle hepatic vein can receive a substantial amount of the venous drainage from segment VI in about 25% of cases.

The right hepatic vein (Fig. 2.18)

Although usually the largest of the hepatic veins, it is also the most variable, depending partly on the size of the middle hepatic vein and also accessory veins (see below). It lies between the right lateral and medial sectors and it drains some of segments V and VIII and usually all of segments VI and VII.

It commences near the anteroinferior angle of the liver on the right and has a long course, largely in a *coronal plane* in the living. Near its termination it lies almost horizontally. It enters the inferior vena cava at about the same level as the upper pole of the caudate lobe, and this level is a few millimetres lower than the entry of the left trunk into the vena cava. It may receive (usually very small) branches from the upper part of the caudate lobe. In extrahepatic mobilization of this vein, the ligament of the inferior vena cava should first be divided.

Other hepatic veins

The hepatic veins can be regarded as having superior, middle and inferior groupings, and the three veins considered above are the superior group and much the most major of the veins. However, on the right side the middle and inferior

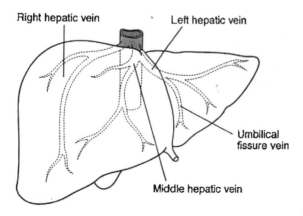

FIGURE 2.18 The major hepatic veins.

Right hepatic vein

Left hepatic vein

Umbilical fissure vein

Middle hepatic vein

hepatic veins can assume some importance. In about 25% of cases the middle (sometimes) or the middle and inferior (sometimes) or the inferior vein (usually) can be quite large (Fig. 2.19). Enlargement of these veins has surgical significance. First, during right hepatectomy the veins should always be ligated before commencing parenchymatous dissection. And second, when large, they may drain either segment VI or segment VII (usually the former) so that in resections for malignant disease it is sometimes possible to ligate the main right hepatic vein and yet maintain drainage of segment VI.

The veins of the caudate lobe

These drain the caudate lobe and caudate process into the inferior vena cava and usually number one to three. In about 70% of cases there is only one caudate hepatic vein. It can emerge from the lower or middle third of the caudate lobe but virtually never from the upper third. Very small branches from the upper third sometimes drain into the right hepatic vein or inferior vena cava – but these are nearly always too small to be of surgical significance.

THE ANATOMY OF THE SEGMENTS OF THE LIVER

Segment II

Segment II is the left posterior sector of the liver, which is the only sector made up of a single segment. It lies posterolateral

to the left fissure of the liver and the left hepatic vein runs between it and segment III (Fig. 2.20).

There is usually only a single Glissonian sheath to segment II and it arises from the main sheath as this bends forwards in the umbilical fissure (Fig. 2.21). Because of the relative smallness of the peripheral part of the left hepatic vein, it was long ignored as an hepatic fissural vein. Because the umbilical fissure was more obvious, and sometimes had an hepatic vein running in it (the vein of the umbilical fissure), it was regarded wrongly as the left fissure. However, studies of comparative anatomy and awareness of the inconstant nature of the vein of the umbilical fissure led to a realization that segment II was the true posterior sector of the left liver. Nevertheless the segment is often small, and it is unusual to remove this segment alone. It is only when it is critical to retain as much functioning liver as possible that its removal alone is justified.

Segment III

Segment III lies between the base of the falciform ligament and umbilical fissure on the right and the left fissure and segment II on the left (Figs 2.20 and 2.22). The left hepatic vein lies between segment II and segment III and a vein of the umbilical fissure lies between segment III and segment IV in about two-thirds of cases.

Segment III commonly joins segment IV by a bridge of liver tissue which lies superficial to the ligamentum teres in the umbilical fissure. This bridge of tissue is easily broken down by coagulating diathermy as it contains no important structures.

There are usually one or two Glissonian sheaths to segment III and occasionally three.

The venous drainage is predominantly via the left hepatic vein, but the vein of the umbilical fissure can occasionally provide adequate drainage for all of segment III if the distal part of the left hepatic vein is removed.

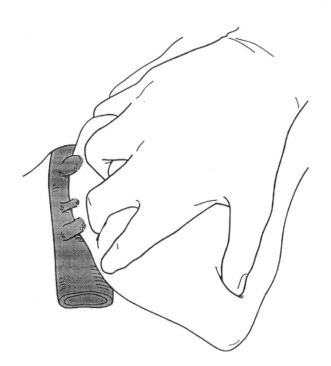

FIGURE 2.19   Large inferior right hepatic vein and smaller middle right hepatic vein.

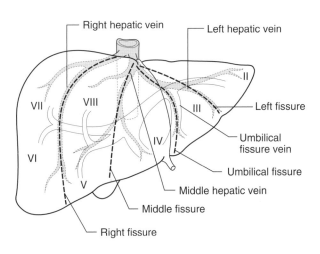

FIGURE 2.20   Segmental anatomy.

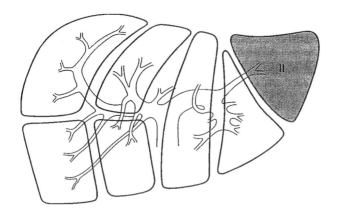

FIGURE 2.21 Segment II.

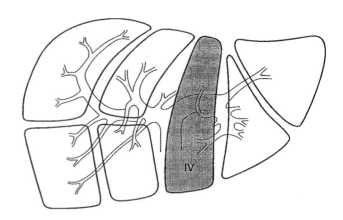

FIGURE 2.23 Segment IV.

Segment IV

Segment IV lies between the main fissure on the right and the umbilical fissure on the left (Figs 2.20 and 2.23). The middle hepatic vein lies between segment IV and the right medial sector of the liver (segments V and VIII), and the vein of the umbilical fissure, when present, lies between segment IV and segment III.

Posteriorly segment IV extends back and is separated from segment I by the dorsal fissure (Figs 2.15 and 2.16).

Some authors suggest that the quadrate lobe is only the anterior part of segment IV, calling it segment IVb, although there is no particular reason why the whole segment should not be called the quadrate lobe. However there is a practical point here. If the area of the quadrate lobe on the inferior surface of the liver is resected vertically then not all of segment IV is taken (Fig. 2.24). On the superior surface of the liver, segment IV extends back to the inferior vena cava. The initial studies of Couinaud in 1957 suggested there was no useful purpose in removing the posterior part of segment IV (segment IVa). In fact there arc several reasons why this posterior part of segment IV often is not resected. First, and no doubt foremost, is that the posterior part represents less than 20% of segment IV (Fig. 2.24) and it is much the most

difficult part to resect. This is because draining into the middle hepatic vein there are several moderate-sized veins which traverse this area. As well, posteroinferiorly in the region behind the confluence there is no clear demarcation between segment I and segment IV (Fig. 2.16). Furthermore, in resection for metastatic disease in which segment IV is being resected along with a large amount of other liver substance, e.g. right hepatectomy plus segment IV, then conservation of functioning liver tissue may be important. And, if the segment is being resected in order to gain access to the confluence then it is clearly not necessary to resect the posterior portion.

The pedicles to segment IV have more variations than any other segment in the liver. Thus the portal pedicles commonly are between three and 10 in number and there may be many more. The arterial and biliary pedicles are even more variable and when the structures are dissected individually for the removal of segment IV, the surgeon is putting the blood supply and/or biliary drainage of segments II and III at considerable risk.

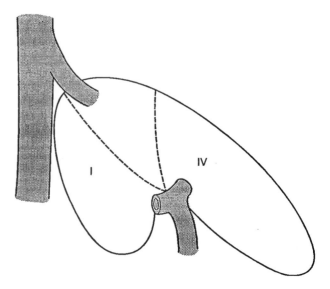

FIGURE 2.24 The anterior and posterior parts of segment IV.

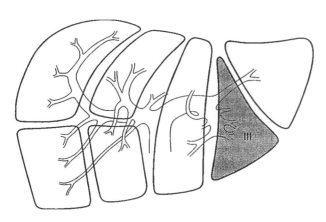

FIGURE 2.22 Segment III.

In no other part of liver surgery is the advantage of dissecting outside the Glissonian sheaths more clearly demonstrated than in removal of segment IV. This point has recently been re-emphasized in the split and reduced liver graft techniques in liver transplantation. Therefore it cannot be emphasized too strongly that the surgeon should avoid entering within Glisson's capsule for dissection of the portal trinity structures to segment IV.

The surgeon can be certain of remaining outside the sheath by dissecting outside the hilar plate in the porta hepatis and incising 5 mm to the right of the umbilical fissure within liver parenchyma. The reason for this being much safer is that *within* segment IV itself there are no anomalies, so this plane of dissection does not put any other part of the liver at risk.

The major sheaths to segment IV come from the right side of the sheath lying in the umbilical fissure and they are also directed towards the right. There are usually two or three such sheaths. However additional sheaths, sometimes quite small, arise from the main left sheath as it traverses the base of the quadrate lobe – these arise from the anterior superior surface of the left main sheath, both before and after giving off the sheath to segment II.

These sheaths supply the posterior part of segment IV, which is the reason why the posterior part can be safely left undisturbed, even though the main sheaths to segment IV have been divided.

Although the major venous drainage of segment IV is via the middle hepatic vein, occasionally the vein of the umbilical fissure provides enough drainage to allow the quadrate lobe to survive if the middle hepatic vein is removed.

Segment V

Segment V is the anterior segment of the right medial sector and it lies between the main fissure and the right fissure (Figs 2.20 and 2.25). The anterior part of the middle hepatic vein lies between it and segment IV. Its posterior boundary lies approximately in the coronal plane of the porta hepatis, behind which lies segment VIII.

The right fissure is very variable in its anterior extremity and so the size of segment V is also variable. In the small percentage of cases when the main fissure and the right fissure become confluent anteriorly, segment V is much reduced in size and may not appear at all on the anterior and inferior part of the liver. On the other hand, when the right fissure passes to the right extremity of the liver segment V is a large segment (Fig. 2.17). The Glissonian sheaths to segment V may be single but are usually multiple and its venous drainage is by the right hepatic and middle hepatic veins.

Segment VIII

This is situated mainly on the superior aspect of the liver and there is little to define its borders on the surface of the liver. Its left border is the main fissure, its right border is the right fissure, its posterior border approximates the superior leaf of the right coronary ligament and its anterior margin approximates the coronal plane of the hepatic hilum (Figs 2.20 and 2.26).

Intrahepatically it lies between the posterior parts of the right hepatic vein on the right and the middle hepatic vein on the left (Fig. 2.20). It therefore has no part of itself showing on the inferior face of the liver. Its situation between the two veins, particularly posteriorly, helps to define lesions in the area with the use of intraoperative ultrasound.

After the right medial sheath has given off the anterior divisions to segment V, the remaining sheath is destined for segment VIII and it sometimes breaks up into several divisions.

The segment drains via the right and middle hepatic veins. There is often a transversely running vein situated posteriorly in segment VIII which is quite large and it usually drains into the middle hepatic vein. Occasionally it drains directly into the inferior vena cava.

Segment VI

Segment VI forms the right inferior extremity of the liver and it lies to the right and behind the right fissure, with

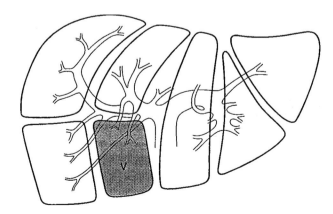

FIGURE 2.25 Segment V.

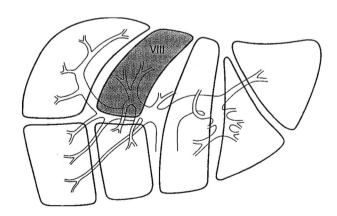

FIGURE 2.26 Segment VIII.

segment V lying largely in front and the originating portion of the right hepatic vein lying between the two segments (Figs 2.20 and 2.27).

The number of cases in which a single Glissonian sheath supplies segment VI is probably less than half. There are often two or even three sheaths with the first sheath arising from the right main sheath (Fig. 2.27).

The venous drainage is mainly to the right hepatic vein. However in a substantial minority of cases segment VI drains via a dominant middle hepatic vein.

The size of segment VI tends to vary inversely with the size of segment V. When the right fissure is far to the left segment V is small and segment VI is large. When the fissure is far to the right then segment V is large and segment VI is small (Fig. 2.17).

Segment VII

This segment forms the major portion of the posterior part of the right liver, lying to the right and behind the right fissure of the liver and separated from segment VIII by the right hepatic vein (Figs 2.20 and 2.28).

The sheath to segment VII is directed posteriorly and is sometimes difficult to dissect out because of its depth. It is however usually single. The venous drainage of this segment is by the right hepatic vein and to a lesser degree the lesser right hepatic veins which drain into the inferior vena cava. In about 10% of cases one of the lesser right hepatic veins can drain significantly more of the posterior part of the liver. In these circumstances removal of the right hepatic vein does not necessarily mean that segment VII will lose its venous drainage, as would usually be the case.

The variations in the right fissure have already been discussed.

Segment I (caudate lobe)

The caudate lobe used to be regarded as difficult to excise, even by such an inveterate liver anatomist as Claude Couinaud. Ton That Tung is usually regarded as having

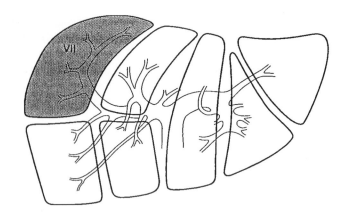

FIGURE 2.28 Segment VII.

provided the first description of its removal. The importance of segment I has increased in recent years since it has been appreciated that many high bile duct cancers also involve the ducts of segment I.

The segment lies largely to the left side of the midline and has a lateral half which lies relatively free and a medial half which is confined by various (mainly vascular) structures (Fig. 2.29).

Thus the lateral half has the fissure for the ligamentum venosum in front and also the lesser omentum which, although filmy, separates this free-lying part from segments II and III. Behind, segment I overlies the aorta.

The medial half lies on the left side of the inferior vena cava and is contained between the termination of the left and middle hepatic veins above and the confluence below. Its anterior face is continuous with segment IV (Fig. 2.29) and its right extremity blends with segment VIII. The main fissure of the liver is the dividing line posteriorly between segment VIII and segment I and the coronal plane between I and IV is the dorsal fissure. The portion lying behind VIII and IV is called segment IX by Couinaud.

Beneath the confluence the caudate lobe extends to the right in front of the inferior cava as the caudate process and the tissue blends with segment V.

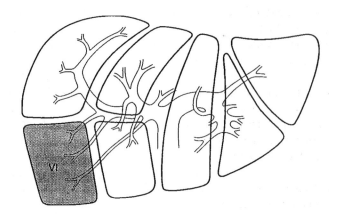

FIGURE 2.27 Segment VI.

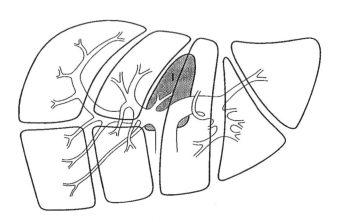

FIGURE 2.29 Segment I.

The Glissonian sheaths to the caudate lobe are several in number and are derived from both right and left main sheaths (Fig. 2.30). The left sheaths usually supply most of the caudate lobe and the right sheaths supply a small portion of the caudate lobe and also the caudate process. These branches arise from the posterior surfaces of the right and left main sheaths. The veins of the caudate process drain directly into the inferior vena cava. There are often several veins but usually only one or two of any size. These nearly always emerge from the posterior surface of the lower third or less often the middle third of the caudate lobe, but there are almost never any veins of surgical significance higher than this.

THE PORTA HEPATIS AND HEPATIC PEDICLE

The porta hepatis is the fissure in the liver between the quadrate lobe in front and the caudate process and the caudate lobe behind. It receives the structures of the hepatic pedicle, i.e. hepatic duct, hepatic artery and portal vein and also the two ligaments at its left end (teres and venosum) and the gall bladder neck lies at its right end. The structures of the hepatic pedicle can usually be simply occluded by opening the lesser sac to the left of them and passing a tape around them from left to right through the opening of the epiploic foramen. If rapid occlusion is required then a clamp or the fingers can occlude the free edge of the lesser omentum with the posterior jaws of the clamp passed from right to left through the epiploic foramen and the anterior jaw lying in front of the free edge.

The usual arrangement of the structures in the free edge of the lesser omentum is shown in Figure 2.31. Thus while both the common hepatic/bile duct and the hepatic artery

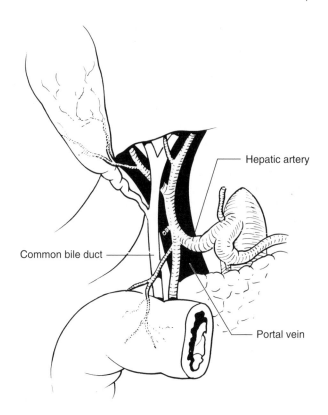

FIGURE 2.31 Porta hepatis and structures in the free edge of the lesser omentum.

lie in the same plane in front of the portal vein, the duct tends to be to the right of it and the hepatic artery more directly overlies the portal vein. As the structures reach the porta their division leads to increased complexity of relations to each other but the portal vein and its divisions almost always remain most posterior. The 'normal' relationships shown in the diagram only occurs in about a third of cases; variations in ductal and arterial anatomy are numerous and are described subsequently.

In dissecting the structures in the free edge of the lesser omentum little difficulty is encountered with the common duct because of its accessibility. However the supra-duodenal artery crossing transversely anterior to the duct immediately above the duodenum is often divided when the peritoneum over the duct is opened and the vessel needs to be cauterized. The major difficulty encountered with the hepatic artery is the fact that it is surrounded by nerve and lymphatic plexuses which require division before the vessel proper is dissected free. The portal vein is often mobilized when portal hypertension is present so great care is needed. Fortunately the middle portion of the vein between its branching and the duodenum usually does not have any tributaries. Fortunately, also, the wall of the vein is quite thick.

As the vein is dissected towards the duodenum several tributaries may be found. These cause troublesome, even catastrophic bleeding if they are damaged by injudicious blunt dissection. The first of these veins is the superior

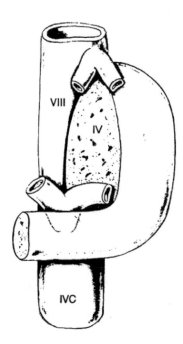

FIGURE 2.30 Segment I. IVC = Inferior vena cava.

pancreaticoduodenal vein or veins which enter the right side of the portal vein behind or immediately above the duodenum. The right and sometimes left gastric veins also enter the portal system somewhat variably. If they join the portal vein they do so on its left side usually behind the duodenum but occasionally higher, where they will be in the field of dissection. As the vein is dissected towards the porta it is usually possible to dissect individually the right and left branches of it. On the right a small vein from the gall bladder may be encountered and on the left a tributary from the quadrate lobe may enter close to the branching of the portal vein.

THE INFERIOR VENA CAVA

The inferior vena cava

The inferior vena cava is formed by the confluence of the right and left common iliac veins in front of the fifth lumbar vertebra. It ascends retroperitoneally to the right of the aorta and passes in a groove in the liver or occasionally it is actually embedded in liver substance by hepatic tissue bridging it posteriorly. The inferior vena cava perforates the tendinous portion of the diaphragm and the pericardium to enter the inferoposterior part of the right atrium. There are no valves in the cava distal to a somewhat vestigial valve at its entry into the right atrium.

The inferior vena cava is crossed at its origin by the right common iliac artery, although the crossing is perhaps more often at the left common iliac vein. In its ascent the inferior vena cava is crossed by the root of the mesentery and the right gonadal artery both from left above to right below and it lies behind the duodenal C with its contained head of pancreas. It lies posterior to the epiploic foramen where it is covered only be peritoneum. It then lies behind the liver to the right of the caudate lobe, although an extension from that lobe, the caudate process, lies anterior to it. The two lowermost right lumbar arteries cross behind it lower down, as does the right renal artery higher up. The small inferior phrenic and right suprarenal arteries cross behind it where it lies posterior to the liver. The right adrenal gland lies to its right and partly behind the cava as it becomes retrohepatic. The other important posterior structure, surgically speaking, is the right sympathetic chain which is overlain by the inferior vena cava in its abdominal course.

The inferior vena cava is most directly accessible where it lies behind the epiploic foramen covered only by a glistening layer of peritoneum. After division of the peritoneum via a vertical incision over the inferior vena cava it is usually a relatively simple matter to place a tape around it as this point is above the entry of the renal veins and below the higher tributaries. If the renal veins are being sought the duodenum and pancreas should be Kocherized and the retropancreatic cava is thereby exposed. There are numerous anomalies, particularly of the infrarenal inferior vena cava, but fortunately these are not very common. Perhaps the most common is a double system up to the renal veins. The variations can produce problems for the surgeon who is setting out either to introduce a venous filter into the inferior vena cava or to ligate the cava to prevent pulmonary embolic disease.

TRIBUTARIES OF THE INFERIOR VENA CAVA

Lumbar veins

There are usually four pairs of lumbar veins, but it is only the caudal third and fourth pairs which regularly drain into the posterior aspect of the inferior vena cava. Their major surgical significance is that the two left veins pass behind the aorta and are therefore at risk during mobilization of that structure. The right veins are easily damaged when the inferior vena cava is retracted anteriorly during lumbar sympathectomy. The second pair of lumbar veins may drain into the cava at the level of the renal veins but, like the first pair of lumbar veins, they often drain into ascending lumbar or lumbar azygos veins.

The gonadal veins (testicular, ovarian)

It is only on the right side that the gonadal veins drain into the inferior vena cava just below the right renal vein. The left vein drains into the left renal vein. Older texts suggest that a varicocele is due to varicosity of the testicular veins. However it is rare indeed for this to be the case, with a varicocele being due to varicosity of the cremasteric plexus of veins.

The renal veins

The renal veins usually enter the cava at an angle of about 45° to the vertical and the left vein is usually higher than the right by 1–2 cm. The right vein is usually short and about 2 cm in length. The left vein, on the other hand, is long and its major surgical significance is its relationship to the aorta. It is often described as being draped across the front of the aorta, usually immediately distal to the superior mesenteric artery origin. It receives a large left adrenal vein from above and left gonadal vein from below, both entering the vein to the left of the aorta. Although described in anatomy texts as being posterior to the splenic vein and pancreas, this relationship is quite variable and the left renal vein is often more inferior than the splenic vein. In patients with portal hypertension there is usually a much thickened layer of fibrovascular tissue between the two veins so that the renal vein lies at several centimetres posterior to the splenic vein. The left renal vein can nearly always be found by mobilizing along the front of the abdominal aorta. Nearly always, because occasionally a renal vein crosses posterior to the aorta or is double and crosses both anteriorly and posteriorly.

The supra renal veins

These both exit from the adrenal hilum. The left passes down the medial border of the gland to join the left renal veins; the right is very short and drains into the posterior aspect of the inferior vena cava just before it becomes retrohepatic in position.

The inferior phrenic vein

The right inferior phrenic vein drains the undersurface of the diaphragm and drains into the vena cava usually above the entrance of the right hepatic vein. The left inferior phrenic vein is often double, with a posterior branch draining into the left adrenal or left renal vein but the anterior branch passes in front of the oesophageal hiatus to drain into the inferior vena cava or the left hepatic vein.

The hepatic veins

There are several hepatic veins. The lower group are small-sized veins which are variable in number, usually from one to three on both right and left sides, with the right draining segment VIII of the right side of the liver and the left draining segment I (caudate lobe). In about 15% of cases a vein in the right group may be moderately large and it is then called an accessory right hepatic vein. These veins usually have a short 1–2 cm extrahepatic course and they can be approached for ligation by dividing the peritoneal attachments of the liver and retracting the appropriate lobe to the right or left. Alternatively, when the liver is being removed for trans-plantation, but the inferior vena cava is being retained, division of the lower veins can be carried out after division of the upper (major) hepatic veins. There is a tributary-free plane anterior to the retrohepatic cava and a finger can be gently inserted into this plane from above, below the major veins. The liver can then be divided through the main portal fissure down to the finger and the sides of the liver are opened out like a book. The tributaries entering the anterolateral surfaces of the cava can then be dissected free and ligated.

The upper group of hepatic veins are the major veins draining the liver. Their intrahepatic course has already been considered. The left and middle hepatic veins usually join together to enter the vena cava as a common trunk. The main trunks of all the veins have a short extrahepatic course and can be dissected free after division of the peritoneal attachments of the liver. As the retrohepatic vena cava is usually included with the liver in a liver transplant, the variations in hepatic drainage are not usually of importance for this procedure. Variations usually involve one of the segments such as VI, VII or VIII draining directly into the inferior vena cava.

FURTHER READING

Champeau M, Pineau P, Leger P 1966 Chirurgie du-foie et des voies biliares. Ernest Flammarion, Paris
Couinaud C 1957 Le foie – études anatomiques et chirurgicales. Masson, Paris
Ton That Tung 1962 Chirurgie d'exerese du foie. Masson, Paris.
Trinh Van Minh, Galizia G 1990 La segmentation du foie et les variations anatomiques du systeme porte. Ann Chir 44:561–569.

3 Resectional surgery of the bile ducts; biliary-enteric anastomosis: the anatomy of extrahepatic biliary ducts

Glyn Jamieson and Leslie Blumgart

Biliary exposure and precise dissection are the most important steps in any biliary operative procedure. A thorough anatomical knowledge is essential for optimal results.

The right and left liver are drained by the right and left hepatic ducts whereas the caudate lobe is drained by several ducts joining both ducts. The hepatic ducts formed by the confluence of the intrahepatic ducts exit from the liver in a common sheath together with the branches of the portal vein and the hepatic artery (as the portal triads). Two major hepatic ducts are confluent to form the common hepatic duct (Fig. 3.1). By convention this changes its name to the common bile duct at the point of entry of the cystic duct. The common bile duct runs down anterior to the portal vein and to the right of the hepatic artery in the free edge of the lesser omentum and passes behind the first part of the duodenum to the right of gastroduodenal artery and behind or in the pancreas. At its lower end, it curves to the right where it is joined by the pancreatic duct and enters the second part of the duodenum at the ampulla of Vater. Biliary anomalies are common (vide infra).

The biliary ducts are composed of fibroareolar tissue and contain no muscle within their walls apart from the occasional myocytic cell. They are lined by columnar epithelium which contains mucus-secretory glands.

RIGHT AND LEFT HEPATIC DUCTS

In a surgical sense, only the termination of the right hepatic duct is accessible, outwith the liver parenchyma. On the other hand, the left hepatic duct describes quite a long course at the base of the quadrate lobe surrounded only by the fibrous tissue of the Glisson's sheath which is often referred to as the hilar plate.

The right hepatic duct draining segments V, VI, VII and VIII of the right liver arises from the junction of the two main right sectoral tributaries. The right posterior sectoral tributary has an almost horizontal course and is constituted by the confluence of the ducts of segments VI and VII. This duct runs to join the right anterior sectoral duct as it descends in a vertical manner. The right anterior sectoral duct drains segments V and VIII. The main right hepatic duct is short in its extrahepatic length before joining the left hepatic duct to constitute the confluence lying in front of the portal vein (Fig. 3.1).

Depending on the width of the quadrate lobe, the left hepatic duct may be oblique and short or transverse and long. It is exposed by dividing the peritoneum at the base of the quadrate lobe and opening the hilar plate. This allows the left hepatic duct and portal vein to be delivered from the hilum. The left hepatic artery lies more laterally at the base of the umbilical fissure but nevertheless enters the same fibrous tissue sheath. The left hepatic duct is usually the highest of the three structures encountered and lies above the left branch of the portal vein. As it is traced to the left, it enters the umbilical fissure of the liver at the upper end of which the ligamentum teres terminates in the re-curved portion of the left portal vein. The tributaries from segments II, III, and IV join the left hepatic duct within or at the base of the umbilical fissure. The segment III duct lies just above the segment III branch of the portal vein and is a useful and accessible duct for biliary enteric anastomosis if it is impossible to use the main left hepatic duct (Fig. 3.2).

The right and left hepatic ducts unite outside the liver within the hilar plate main trunk in about 60% of cases and usually within 2 cm of the exit of the right hepatic duct from the liver parenchyma. In the remaining 40% of cases, there is a variant anatomy, the right anterior and posterior sectoral ducts entering separately into the left hepatic ducts/common hepatic duct/common bile duct. The most common variations of the right hepatic duct are important to mention. First, the right posterior sectoral duct may not unite with the right duct and may indeed join the common hepatic duct low down at an acute angle and almost at the point of entry of the cystic duct. Indeed, the cystic duct may enter the right sectoral duct at this point (Fig. 3.3). Second, the right posterior sectoral duct quite frequently is independent of the right anterior sectoral duct and may curve posteriorly to the anterior right sectoral duct and join the left hepatic ducts some short distance proximal to the confluence (Fig. 3.4). The latter circumstance occurs frequently but is a source of operative confusion and may lead to biliary injury or biliary fistula during liver resections.

It should be noted that the left hepatic duct is consistent in its anatomy except in about 3% of patients in whom segments II, III or IV ducts enter the confluence separately. The

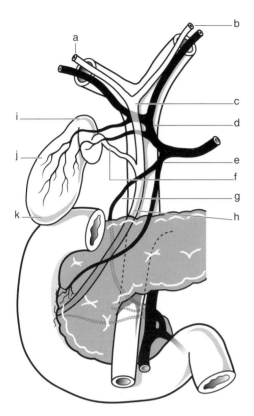

FIGURE 3.1 Anterior aspect of the biliary anatomy: a, right hepatic duct; b, left hepatic duct; c, common hepatic duct; d, hepatic artery; e, gastroduodenal artery; f, cystic duct; g, retroduodenal artery; h, common bile duct; i, neck of the gall bladder; j, body of the gall bladder; k, fundus of the gall bladder. Note particularly the situation of the hepatic bile duct confluence anterior to the right branch of the portal vein, the posterior course of the cystic artery behind the common hepatic duct and the relationship of the neck of the gall bladder to the right branch of the hepatic artery. (Reprinted from Blumgart L H, Fong Y (eds) 2000 Surgery of the liver and biliary tract, 3rd edn. WB Saunders, London by permission of the publisher.)

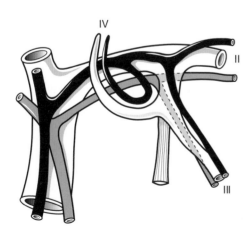

FIGURE 3.2 Biliary and vascular anatomy of the left liver. Note the location of the segment III duct (black) above the corresponding vein (white). The anterior branch of the segment IV duct is not represented. (Reprinted from Blumgart L H, Fong Y (eds) 2000 Surgery of the liver and biliary tract, 3rd edn. WB Saunders, London by permission of the publisher.)

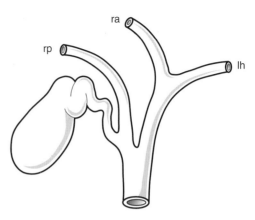

FIGURE 3.3 Variation of the hepatic duct confluence (Couinaud 1957) showing absence of right hepatic duct and low entry of the right posterior sectoral duct into the common bile duct. Note that the cystic duct drains onto the right posterior sectoral duct close to its point of entry into the common bile duct. rp=right posterior sectoral duct; ra=right anterior sectoral duct; lh=left hepatic duct. (Reprinted from Blumgart L H, Fong Y (eds) 2000 Surgery of the liver and biliary tract, 3rd edn. WB Saunders, London by permission of the publisher.)

caudate lobe also drains by one or more branches into the left hepatic duct.

The common bile duct

This runs either behind or embedded within a groove on the posterior surface on the head of the pancreas (Fig 3.1). This groove is usually palpable from behind. The length of the common bile duct is variable mainly because of the entry of the cystic duct (see Ch. 5). The average outer diameter of the duct varies from about 6 to 9 mm with a tendency for a greater diameter in older patients. It is commonly held that the duct dilates after cholecystectomy, although evidence for this is lacking.

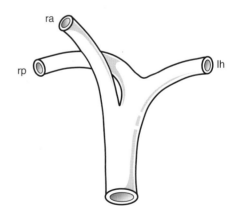

FIGURE 3.4 Main variation of the hepatic duct confluence (Couinaud 1957) showing the right anterior sectoral duct joining the common hepatic duct separately from the right posterior sectoral duct, which curves posterior to it and enters the left hepatic duct. rp=right posterior sectoral duct; ra=right anterior sectoral duct; lh=left hepatic duct. (Reprinted from Blumgart L H, Fong Y (eds) 2000 Surgery of the liver and biliary tract, 3rd edn. WB Saunders, London by permission of the publisher.)

The blood supply to the bile duct typically comes from the posterior superior pancreaticoduodenal artery below and from the cystic artery above. Occasionally the supply to the lower bile duct is from the gastroduodenal artery or the hepatic artery itself. The arterial supply forms a plexus around the duct. Some have stated that the major supply is from below and so it would seem prudent, if dividing the duct, to divide it as high as practical. It is also important in hepatic transplantation to tie the cystic artery away from the bile duct in order not to obstruct the blood supply from the cystic artery to the bile ducts.

As noted in Chapter 4, the right hepatic artery sometimes crosses in front of the common bile duct and, in a less common variation, the right anterior and posterior sectoral arteries separate, one running in front of the portal vein and the other behind it.

The posterior branch of the superior pancreaticoduodenal artery nearly always crosses in front of the bile duct just above, at the level of, or behind the duodenum. It is often divided with a vertical incision of the common bile duct taken down to the level of the duodenum, as in the performance of choledochoduodenostomy, and then it can cause annoying bleeding from the distal part of the incision. The common bile duct lies initially superior and then posterior to the pancreatic duct and the two join within the sphincter of Oddi usually 1.5–2 cm proximal to the ampulla of Vater at which point they enter the duodenum. The sphincter of Oddi with its smooth muscle walls usually embraces the common biliary/pancreatic duct.

Occasionally, the two do not join and open separately into the ampulla of Vater. The ampulla is medially placed, tending to be posterior on the wall of the duodenum at about the junction of the upper two-thirds and the lower third of the second part of the duodenum although variations in its position do occur.

When carrying out operative or endoscopic sphincterotomy, it is important to keep the incision in the superior portion of the ampulla in order to avoid damage to the pancreatic duct. The incision should not extend more than 1.5 cm proximal to the papillary orifice since an anterior branch of the pancreaticoduodenal artery crosses the duct at this point and bleeding may ensue should this be damaged.

Other abnormalities such as a double common bile duct and entry of the common bile duct directly into the stomach have been described but are exceedingly rare.

THE INNERVATION OF THE BILIARY SYSTEM

This is from the celiac plexus and contains efferents, sympathetic and parasympathetic fibers and afferent fibers which runs with the sympathetic efferents. The nerves run with the hepatic artery to form an hepatic plexus in the hilum. It has been stated that fibres from the right phrenic nerve sometimes enter the hepatic plexus and this may explain the rarely seen right shoulder tip pain encountered with liver or gallbladder disease. Pain in the right hypochondrium may be elicited by rapid swelling of the liver stimulating pain fibres coming from Glisson's capsule. Forceful contraction of the muscle of the sphincter muscle may also cause pain.

The relationship between gallbladder disease and coronary artery contraction is well known clinically but the anatomical basis for this remains speculative.

LYMPHATIC DRAINAGE OF THE BILE DUCTS

The upper ducts drain into nodes at the hilum of the liver around the hepatic artery. The lower part of the duct drains into the nodes along the hepatic artery and also along the superior pancreaticoduodenal nodes and behind the pancreas into the retroduodenal nodes. All these nodes drain back towards the celiac axis.

FURTHER READING

Blumgart L H, Hann L E 2000 Surgical and radiologic anatomy of the liver and biliary tree. In: Blumgart L H, Fong Y, Surgery of the liver and biliary tract, 3rd edn. WB Saunders London, p 3–34.

Couinaud C 1957 Le foie – etude anatomiques et Chirurgicales. Masson, Paris.

4

Ligation and/or cannulation of the hepatic artery: the anatomy of the hepatic artery

Glyn Jamieson and Derek Alderson

In embryonic life the liver receives three hepatic arteries: a right, a middle and a left. Usually the right and left arteries disappear, leaving the middle as the source of supply.

Persistence of the middle primordial artery

The most usual anatomy for the common hepatic artery is for it to arise from the coeliac trunk and pass superior to the pancreas and to the right towards the duodenum. It gives off the right gastric artery (which is usually only small) and the gastroduodenal artery and then ascends as the hepatic artery proper in front of the portal vein and to the left of the bile duct. In the region of the porta hepatis the artery divides into right and left branches with the right branch crossing in front of the portal vein and behind the common bile duct, often coming into proximity with the cystic duct. The left branch ascends to the left of the common hepatic duct.

In two-dimensional anatomical drawings the common hepatic artery appears to run close and parallel to the superior border of the gastric antrum. In reality it is much deeper, lying behind the posterior wall of the lesser sac immediately superior to the body and neck of the pancreas. There is consistently a large flat ovoid lymph node which lies anterior to the hepatic artery close to the junction with the gastroduodenal artery and smaller nodes which lie in the groove between the artery and the upper border of the pancreas. Removal of this large lymph node is the easiest way of accessing the hepatic artery proper.

Origins have been described from a trunk with the splenic artery only, a trunk with the left gastric artery only, directly from the aorta and from the superior mesenteric artery. Variability of its origin however does not alter its usual relationships (Fig. 4.1), with the exception of the origin from the superior mesenteric artery when the hepatic artery runs behind the portal vein.

The point of division of the hepatic artery into its right and left branches is also variable (Fig. 4.2). A low division occurs in about 20% of cases and this takes several forms. In about 15% of cases there are two vessels arising from the region of the gastroduodenal artery. In the remainder of cases (5%) the division occurs even earlier and the importance of this group is that the right hepatic arises *first* and crosses *behind* the portal vein to achieve its normal position (Fig. 4.2).

The left branch of the hepatic artery

In about 75% of cases the left branch of the hepatic artery lies in front of the left branch of the portal vein and in most of the remainder of cases it lies to the left of it. A retroportal position has been described, but is unusual. The left branch of the artery usually lies to the left of the hepatic duct. In other words, the left branch, is usually the most anterior and left-lying structure in the porta hepatis.

The right branch of the hepatic artery

In about 80% of cases the right hepatic artery crosses behind the common hepatic duct to enter the liver with a low division, the artery crosses behind the common bile duct and in remaining cases it crosses in front of the biliary system. The artery usually lies to the left of the cystic duct and in about 50% of cases it lies in close proximity to the left of the duct. Occasionally it is found in front of or behind the cystic duct. As with the left branch, the right branch usually lies in front of the portal vein, although in a small number of cases it has been found to the right, and even behind the right branch of the portal vein.

Persistence of the left primordial artery

It is very rare for this artery to persist as the *sole* blood supply to the liver. Much more common, however, occurring in approximately 10% of cases, is persistence of the left artery as well as a normal common hepatic artery. This persistent left hepatic artery usually arises from the left gastric artery or the aorta, lies in the lesser omentum and enters the liver through the fissure venosum (Fig. 4.3). The area of the liver supplied by this artery varies from supplemental supply to the left liver to being the sole arterial supply to the left liver.

Persistence of the right primordial artery

Persistence of this vessel as the *sole* source of supply to the liver is also rare but it is not uncommon for it to persist along with the common hepatic artery (approximately 10% of cases). It usually arises from the superior mesenteric artery and ascends behind the head of the pancreas and the duodenum

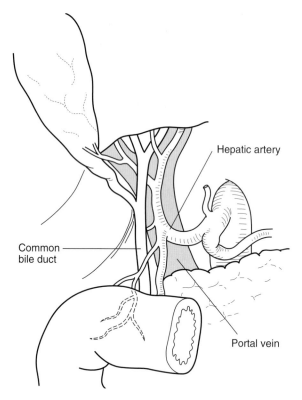

FIGURE 4.1 Usual relationships of the hepatic artery in the region of the free edge of the lesser omentum and the porta hepatis.

passing behind (rarely in front of) the portal vein in the free edge of lesser omentum (Fig. 4.4). Other origins are shown in Figure 4.5. As with the left artery, the area of liver supplied varies from supplementary supply to sole arterial supply to the right liver.

Persistence of all three arteries

Although rare the liver can have a persistent left, a persistent 'normal' common hepatic and a persistent right artery, or only persistent right and left arteries arising from the superior mesenteric artery and left gastric artery respectively. In one case known to us, all three vessels arose directly from the aorta.

THE BRANCHES OF THE COMMON HEPATIC ARTERY

The right gastric artery

The right gastric artery usually arises before the gastroduodenal artery and descends towards the pylorus. It may give off the small artery which runs above the pylorus, called the supraduodenal artery. The right gastric artery is usually small in size but can be important when the stomach is used as an alimentary conduit for oesophageal replacement. In fact when the stomach is transposed to the neck, the right gastric pedicle can be the limiting factor. It should be preserved if possible, as occasionally the right gastro-omental (epiploic) artery alone may not be enough to supply the transposed stomach.

The gastroduodenal artery

This arises from the common hepatic artery behind or above the duodenum. The origin relative to the duodenum is variable and if it is several centimetres superior to the duodenum it is easy for the inexperienced surgeon to mistake the gastroduodenal artery for the hepatic artery itself. The portal vein lies immediately posterior to the descending portion of the gastroduodenal artery. Occasionally the gastroduodenal artery arises from the superior mesenteric artery, or accessory right hepatic or other arteries in the region.

Although variable in origin, the artery's course behind the first part of the duodenum in front of the neck of the pancreas is fairly constant and lies in a groove closely applied to the anterior pancreatic capsule. The main trunk or its supraduodenal branch is commonly involved in bleeding

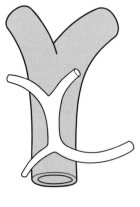

'Normal' 80%

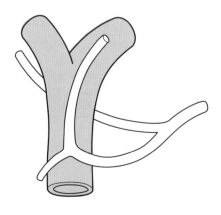

Low division 15%   Early division 5%

FIGURE 4.2 Modes of division of the hepatic artery.

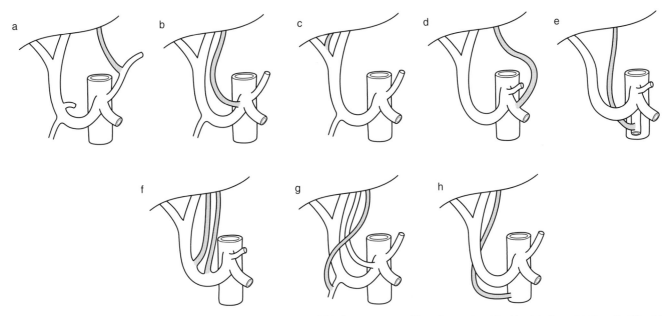

FIGURE 4.3 Varying modes of origin for an accessory left hepatic artery. (a) Left gastric origin; (b) coeliac trunk origin; (c) origin from right hepatic; (d) origin from splenic; (e) superior mesenteric origin; (f) double origin from right gastric and common hepatic; (g) from gastroduodenal; (h) from aorta. The most common variation by far is (a) with (b) also sometimes occurring. The other variations are rare.

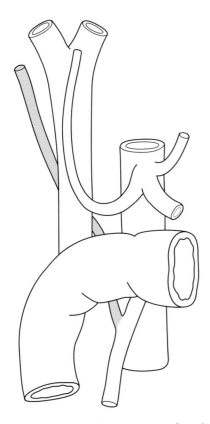

FIGURE 4.4 Origin of accessory right hepatic artery from the superior mesenteric artery.

duodenal ulcer. The gastroduodenal artery terminates by dividing into the right gastro-omental artery (gastroepiploic) which descends in front of the neck of the pancreas before turning to the left as the gastro-omental (gastroepiploic) arch, and usually two superior pancreaticoduodenal arteries. These anterior and posterior branches descend between the duodenum and head of pancreas anastomosing with corresponding branches of the inferior pancreaticoduodenal artery. These marginal vessels give off branches to the duodenal wall and head of pancreas and in the case of the posterior branch, to the distal bile duct.

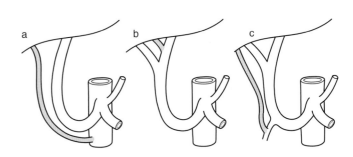

FIGURE 4.5 Rarer origins of an accessory right hepatic artery; (a) from the aorta; (b) from the left branch of the hepatic artery; (c) from the gastroduodenal artery.

FURTHER READING

Hiaff J R, Gabbay J, Busuttil R W 1994 Surgical anatomy of the hepatic arteries in 1000 cases. Ann Surg 220:50–52.

Van Damme J-P, Bonte J 1990 Vascular anatomy in abdominal surgery. Thieme Medical, New York.

5

Cholecystectomy: laparoscopic and open: the anatomy of the gall bladder and related structures

Glyn Jamieson and Nathaniel Soper

THE GALL BLADDER

In the uninflamed state the gall bladder has a slate-blue appearance through its peritoneum. The green colour of the contained bile is more obvious when the peritoneum is removed. Repeated episodes of inflammation result in thickening of the wall and deposition of fat, with the wall becoming whitish-yellow in appearance. Its wall is composed of fibromuscular tissue with non-striated muscle cells arranged in circular, oblique and longitudinal fashion. Its mucosa is a single layer of cuboidal epithelium.

The gall bladder lies in its own fossa on the under-surface of the liver at the junction of the right and left sides of the liver, to which it is attached by loose fibro-areolar tissue. Its fundus usually lies below the inferior margin of the liver and it is completely covered by peritoneum. About 5% of the time the fundus does not protrude inferior to the liver edge and is visible only after elevating the right lobe of the liver. The fundus and body are covered by peritoneum continuous with that on the undersurface of the liver. The body of the gall bladder ascends towards the hilum of the liver to reach the neck of the gall bladder, where the body narrows down to form the cystic duct which turns downward to enter the common hepatic duct. The statement that the fundus lies against the abdominal wall at the point where the outer edge of the rectus sheath crosses the costal margin is often made, but even in health the position of the fundus is very variable. In diseases such as a mucocele or long-standing obstruction, the fundus can reach down to the iliac crest.

Surgeons do not visualize the gall bladder in its normal position as they are used to seeing it with the liver retracted upwards so that the gall bladder appears to descend towards its cystic duct (Fig. 5.1). At laparotomy, exposure of the gall bladder can be improved by displacing the liver inferiorly by a pack above the liver, between the liver and diaphragm or simply by introducing a hand between the liver and diaphragm to allow air into this potential space. During laparoscopic cholecystectomy, the gallbladder itself is grasped and pushed cephalad and laterally to elevate the entire right hemiliver, thus exposing the gallbladder and porta hepatis.

The neck of the gall bladder and the cystic duct contain spiral folds of mucosa within and this gives a twisted appearance to the outside of the duct. This is called the spiral valve and it can prevent the passage of a catheter during operative cholangiography. The folds are easily broken down by the passage of a metal probe however.

The expansion at the proximal extent of the gall bladder, known as Hartmann's pouch, is probably a pathological occurrence related to stones. The cystic duct then appears to exit from the left hand edge of the gall bladder distant from its apex (Fig. 5.1). This relationship of the cystic duct to Hartmann's pouch often is seen best during laparoscopic cholecystectomy. In many individuals there is no pouch, but the body of the gallbladder tapers gradually down to the cystic duct.

The gall bladder lies in close relationship to the duodenum and the hepatic flexure of the colon and adhesions between the gall bladder and these structures are often found even when disease of the gall bladder is not evident. The close relationship between the neck of the gall bladder and the duodenum is exemplified by the fact that a gallstone may ulcerate its way through this region into the duodenum, producing the condition known as gallstone ileus.

Developmental abnormalities such as double gall bladder, absence of the gall bladder, intrahepatic gall bladder and left-sided gall bladder have been described, but they are extremely rare. Much more common, and of surgical importance, are the variations in the anatomy involving the cystic duct and cystic artery.

The cystic duct

The cystic duct joins the common hepatic duct to form the common bile duct, usually passing downwards and backwards to do so. The length of the cystic duct varies from about 2 to 8 cm; yet its apparent length at operation is more of a range from 2 to 4 cm. This discrepancy is due to the manner in which the cystic duct enters the common hepatic duct under a layer of soft tissue surrounding the porta hepatis. The three major modes of entry have been described as parallel, angular and spiral (Fig. 5.2). The length which the cystic duct runs either in parallel or in spiral is variable and can be over several centimetres. This may be seen on an operative cholangiogram, with the ducts not actually uniting until just before the bile duct enters the duodenum. Thus

a

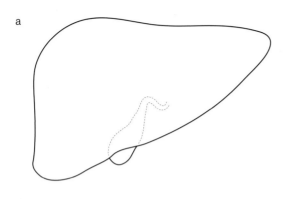

b

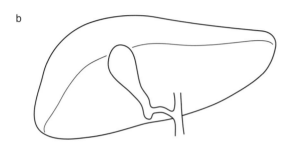

FIGURE 5.1 (a) The normal position of the gall bladder; (b) the surgeon's view.

division of the cystic duct at its apparent point of entry into the hepatic duct probably only achieves a short cystic duct stump in about 70% of cases. This may not be of great importance in cholecystectomy providing no calculi are left in the cystic duct stump, as the long cystic duct stump as a cause of symptoms has probably been exaggerated. However in conditions where the biliary system is dilated and the common bile duct is opened, as for choledochoduodenostomy for instance, the method of termination of the cystic duct is important and the surgeon should make sure that it is the common bile duct/common hepatic duct which has been opened and not a dilated cystic duct stump. Furthermore, a large stone contained within a parallel-lying

cystic duct may cause obstruction of the common bile duct (so-called Mirizzi's syndrome).

The method of entry is also of importance in liver transplantation where the cystic duct remnant can be tied at both ends, the gall bladder end by intention and the bile duct end unintentionally during the bile duct to bile duct anastomosis. Continuing mucus secretion in the closed segment can then cause an obstruction mucocele.

Although uncommon, the cystic duct occasionally joins the right hepatic duct. In one study, this occurred in just over one case in 100. The study also found the cystic duct crossing an anomalous low lying right hepatic duct in about one in every 1000 cases. The anomalies are of clinical importance as injury to these aberrant ducts can occur because they appear to be in continuity with the cystic duct itself.

The cystic artery

The cystic artery is quite variable in its relationship to the cystic duct. The most usual arrangement is for the artery to arise from the right hepatic artery on the right side of the right hepatic duct and pass laterally to reach the gall bladder. It usually divides into two branches – an anterior and a posterior, the latter running a course between the gall bladder and the liver.

The cystic artery is not infrequently double with the branches unequal in size. In about 25% of cases the artery arises to the left of the duct system and it then usually crosses in front of the ducts to reach the gall bladder. Sometimes the cystic artery is very short with the right hepatic artery being in close proximity to or even adherent to the cystic duct or Hartmann's pouch. In 2 or 3% of patients the artery divides early into multiple small branches, and a significant cystic artery is never discovered during dissection.

Calot's triangle (Hepatocystic triangle) (Fig. 5.3)

Calot described a triangle bounded by the cystic artery, cystic duct and common hepatic duct, but a more useful triangle takes the undersurface of the liver and not the cystic

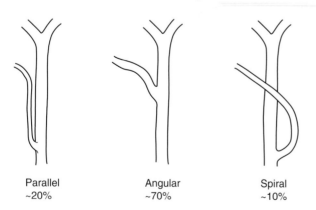

Parallel
~20%

Angular
~70%

Spiral
~10%

FIGURE 5.2 Three common methods of termination of the cystic duct.

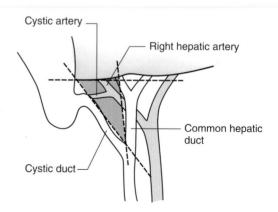

Cystic artery

Right hepatic artery

Common hepatic duct

Cystic duct

FIGURE 5.3 Calot's triangle (shaded) is shown by the interrupted lines.

artery as its base. Therefore, perhaps it is better to refer to the hepatocystic triangle, this being an upside-down triangle with the base being the undersurface of the liver, the two sides the cystic duct and the common hepatic duct, and the apex the junction between the two. It is quite a useful concept as it is formed by and contains the most important structures related to cholecystectomy. In particular the right hepatic artery and its variations nearly always cross through the floor of this triangle and of course the cystic artery crosses also. A large Hartmann's pouch can obscure the structures in the hepatocystic triangle and make exposure of the cystic duct and artery difficult.

The cystic veins are several in number but the one which occasionally causes annoying bleeding (particularly during cannulation of the duct for operative cholangiography) runs with the cystic duct, often on its superior aspect.

The lymphatic drainage of the gall bladder

There is usually a prominent lymph node overlying the anterior branch of the cystic artery near its insertion onto the gallbladder. Because of its location it is often termed the sentinel node, but is also called the cystic node or Calot's node. There are two chains of lymph nodes lying along the portal vein. The first chain lies between the common bile duct and the portal vein and most of the external surface of the gall bladder drains (via a node at the junction of the gall bladder and cystic duct) into this chain, which joins with pancreaticoduodenal nodes and drains to aortic nodes. The second chain lies between the hepatic artery and the portal vein and this receives lymph from the hepatic surface of the gall bladder, and drains into coeliac nodes. Thus a lymphadenectomy for gall bladder cancer should involve skeletonization of the hepatic vessels, bile duct and portal vein, as well as removing nodes along the upper border of the duodenum.

In about 10% of cases lymphatic channels from the external surface of the gall bladder traverse segment V of the liver before eventually draining into the portal vein–bile duct chain and in another 10% of cases the internal surface has lymphatic channels which traverse segment IV to drain to the portal vein–hepatic artery chain.

It is because of these lymphatics that some surgeons advocate the removal of segments IV and V of the liver with cancer of the gall bladder.

LAPAROSCOPIC CHOLECYSTECTOMY

Points of anatomy worth making are:

- A large branch of the middle hepatic vein lies close to the liver surface in the gall bladder bed in about 8% of cases.
- The cystic duct is best dissected and clipped close to its entry into the gall bladder in order to avoid any of the variations of ductal, arterial or venous anatomy in this region.
- In approximately 10% of patients there is no capsule between the gall bladder and its liver bed ('intrahepatic'), rendering the dissection more difficult and bloody.
- The most common cause for major bile duct injury is mistaking the common bile duct for the cystic duct. This is usually due either to significant adhesions tethering the infundibulum to the side of the common hepatic duct or due to improper traction placed on the gall bladder – directly cephalad, aligning the cystic and common bile ducts, rather than pulling the gall bladder lateral to accentuate the angle between cystic and common bile ducts.

FURTHER READING

Strasberg SM, Hertl M, Soper NJ 1995 An analysis of the problem of biliary injury during laparoscopic cholecystectomy. J Am Coll Surg 180:101–125.

Takeyuki M, Masato K, Katsumaro S et al 1999 Ultrasonographic assessment of the risk of injury to branches of the middle hepatic vein during laparoscopic cholecystectomy. Am J Surg 178:418–421.

Yoshida J, Chijiiwa K, Yamaguchi K et al 1996 Practical classification of the branching types of the biliary tree: analysis of 1094 consecutive direct cholangiograms. J Am Coll Surg 182:37–40.

6

Pancreatic operations; portosystemic shunts: the anatomy of the pancreas and duodenum and associated veins

Glyn Jamieson and Michael Sarr

Although perhaps seeming at first glance a strange combination of operations to consider with this anatomy, further consideration shows why: the anatomy of the portal venous system is intimately associated with both procedures. As well, for certain portosystemic shunts, the anatomy of the pancreas assumes some importance.

THE PANCREAS

The pancreas consists of the head of the gland lying within the duodenal C loop, a short thin portion (the neck) which joins the head to the body that passes upwards, backwards and to the left, and the distal aspect of the gland called the tail. In addition, the uncinate process, which is variable in relative size, may be considered part of the head of the pancreas but will assume a prominent position in relationship to the superior mesenteric artery and vein.

The head (and uncinate process)

It is reasonable to consider the pancreatic head, including the uncinate process, in its entirety separately from the rest of the gland as it is this region alone which is removed during pancreaticoduodenectomy, the most common pancreatic resection today. The head lies within the concavity of the duodenum and tends to overlap the duodenum a bit anteriorly and posteriorly, so that the duodenum makes a gutter within the substance of the pancreas. The head region is relatively flat and normally only about 3–4 cm thick. The pancreatic neck is much thinner (1–2 cm) than the head of the gland. The head sends a projection (or process) of variable length from the left inferior margin behind the superior mesenteric vessels: this is the uncinate process.

The ductal system of the pancreas as it passes through the head usually consists of two ducts: the major duct (of Wirsung), which usually (70% of the time) joins with the intraduodenal common bile duct to open onto the major papilla, and the accessory duct (of Santorini), which opens onto the minor duodenal papilla which lies about 2 cm proximal to the major duodenal papilla and more anteriorly.

The major papilla is situated about 7 cm distal to the pylorus and often located just superior to the crossing of the duodenum by the overlying right transverse colon. It is usually located in the middle of the second part of the duodenum but may be situated at the junction of the second and third parts of the duodenum or even in the third part itself. The length of the intrapancreatic portion of the common bile duct therefore varies between 2.5 and 6 cm. If the bile duct is seen to overlie the vertebral column on operative cholangiography, it should alert the surgeon to the possibility of an abnormally distal major papilla.

Before the common bile duct and pancreatic ducts enter the duodenal wall, they run parallel for 2–10 mm. They may join completely during their intraduodenal course (forming a 'common channel' draining into the ampulla of Vater; 70%), they may join at the ampulla of Vater, or they may enter the duodenal lumen completely separately (5%), in which case there is no formal ampulla. Should an ampulla exist, it is usually only 2–3 mm long. The length of the narrowed distal bile duct in its intramural course varies from 7 to 38 mm. When the terminal bile duct and pancreatic duct fuse, the pancreatic duct almost always has a posteromedial relation to the bile duct. Only very rarely does the main pancreatic duct open anteriorly into the common bile duct, in which case it is at risk during division of the sphincter of Oddi.

The main pancreatic duct begins as an identifiable structure about 2.5 cm from the tip of the tail, where its diameter is 0.5 mm. Beginning about 10 cm from the tail, its diameter ranges from 1.5 to 3 mm and increases to an average of 3.5 mm in the head; the size of the duct may increase somewhat as age increases. Also, the pancreatic duct may bifurcate into two ducts in the mid to distal body of the pancreas as it progresses toward the pancreatic tail.

The common variations in entry of the accessory and main pancreatic ducts are shown in Figure 6.1. About 6–9% of the time, the primitive accessory duct persists with no connection with the main duct (pancreas divisum). The accessory duct may atrophy and lose its communication with the duodenum (44%) or end even blindly at the duodenum (8%) or have only a negligibly small opening into the duodenum (9%). Thus, in about 30% of individuals, the accessory duct may be able to provide adequate drainage for a proximally obstructed main pancreatic duct.

The head of the pancreas has several important anatomic relations. It lies in front of the inferior vena cava and renal

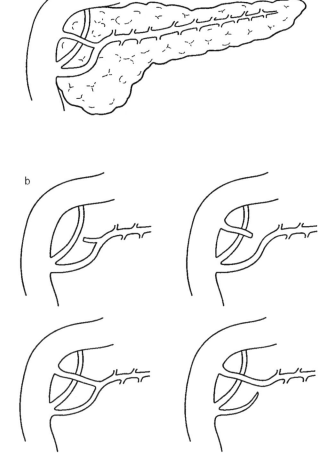

FIGURE 6.1 (a) Arrangement of main and accessory pancreatic ducts found in about 30–40% of cases; (b) other arrangements found less frequently.

veins, while the common bile duct runs in a groove behind and sometimes within the posteriomedial parenchyma of the pancreatic head. The posterior superior pancreaticoduodenal artery crosses the pancreatic head posteriorly. To its left anteriorly lie the portal vein and its formation from the junction of the superior mesenteric and splenic veins, while inferoposteriorly on the left the uncinate process passes behind the superior mesenteric vein and on occasion extends even behind the superior mesenteric artery.

The anterior relations of the head of the pancreas are straightforward in concept, but when the structures must be dissected off the head of the gland, those relations become more complex because of the variability of the peritoneal attachments. The hepatic flexure of the colon lies in front of the pancreatic head, most prominently in the region in which it is acquiring its mesentery (the right transverse mesocolon). During pancreaticoduodenectomy, most surgeons mobilize the duodenum widely and extend the dissection downward to mobilize also the right side of the upper ascending colon. While this manoeuvre is important,

it must be remembered that returning to the hepatic flexure, the plane of dissection/mobilization must continue in front of the duodenum. As the colon is mobilized off the pancreatic head, it begins to acquire a mesentery so the inferior layer of the transverse mesocolon may have to be divided. A right colic vein often joins the superior mesenteric vein after passing in front of the pancreatic head. One or more of these veins are sometimes quite large and can be damaged easily while mobilizing the colon off the head of the gland.

The blood vessels of the head of the pancreas and duodenum

The arteries (Fig. 6.2)

The blood supply to the head of the pancreas and to the duodenum arises primarily from the coeliac axis and to a lesser degree from the superior mesenteric artery. As all of the major vessels approach the duodenum from the open end of its C shape, the duodenum, with the head of the pancreas, may be mobilized off the inferior vena cava and aorta and rotated medially (the Kocher manoeuvre) without interrupting any of the blood supply.

The supraduodenal artery. This little vessel, when present, usually arises from the proximal gastroduodenal artery and crosses above or behind the first part of the duodenum, in front of the bile duct to enter the posterior aspect of the duodenum.

The gastroduodenal artery. As already described (Ch. 4), the gastroduodenal artery takes origin from the common hepatic artery at a variable distance above the duodenum and descends immediately behind the pylorus but in front of the portal vein. It often gives off the posterior superior pancreaticoduodenal artery behind the duodenum just before it emerges in front of the pancreas where it divides into the right gastro-omental (epiploic) artery, which runs to the left along the greater curvature of the stomach in the gastrocolic omentum and the anterior superior pancreaticoduodenal artery, which angles downwards toward the junction of the second and third parts of the duodenum where it runs for a variable distance across the anterior face of the

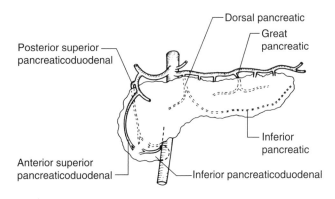

FIGURE 6.2 The arteries of the pancreas.

head of the pancreas. It is unusual for the anterior superior pancreaticoduodenal artery to be other than typical in origin.

The inferior pancreaticoduodenal arteries. These arteries arise most commonly from a single branch of the superior mesenteric artery, which runs behind the superior mesenteric vein before giving off an anterior and posterior division within the more posterior aspect of the parenchyma of the uncinate process. This arcade courses to supply the pancreatic head (and duodenum) by also anastomosing with the corresponding superior pancreaticoduodenal arteries in the pancreatoduodenal groove.

The concept of anterior and posterior pancreaticoduodenal arcades rather than separate arteries is a useful one as it is probably more accurate than regarding them as separate vessels. Thus the head of the pancreas is encircled by an anterior and a posterior arterial arcade, the vessels of which are continuous with each other in front of and behind the pancreas, respectively. These arcades give off branches to supply the duodenum and the pancreatic head. Therefore it is important to avoid extensive dissection in the plane between the pancreas and the duodenum for fear of devascularizing the duodenum.

Variations. There are many important arterial variations. The right hepatic artery arises from the superior mesenteric artery in about 10% of subjects after which it usually passes upwards *behind* the head of the pancreas, to reach a position to the right and posterior to the common bile duct, where the vigilant surgeon can palpate its presence during pancreaticoduodenectomy. Rarely this 'replaced' right hepatic artery passes anterior to the head of the pancreas.

The origin of the middle colic artery usually lies below the pancreas. But in two situations it is at risk in resections of the area. The first and commonest is a high origin. The vessel then tends to exit with the main trunk of the superior mesenteric artery, in which case there is no particular problem. However, occasionally it emerges directly from the substance of the pancreas. It may also arise rarely from the gastroduodenal artery, in which case it descends across the anterior surface of the head of the pancreas.

The veins (Fig. 6.3)

Although typically the visceral veins run with their corresponding arteries, their course is often different. For example, the anterior superior pancreaticoduodenal vein usually drains into the right gastro-omental (epiploic) vein and the posterior superior vein drains into the portal vein. Perhaps of most concern to the surgeon resecting the pancreatic head are the inferior pancreaticoduodenal veins. These are variable in number and mode of drainage. The inferior pancreaticoduodenal veins drain into the right side of the superior mesenteric vein. There is often a middle pancreaticoduodenal vein as well as one or more unnamed branches, which also drain directly into the right side of the superior mesenteric and/or portal vein. These veins are brought into view

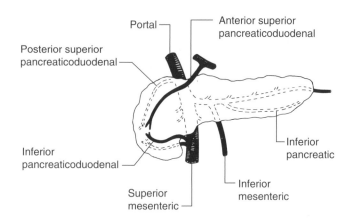

FIGURE 6.3 The veins of the pancreas.

and are often troublesome when dissecting the uncinate process free from the superior mesenteric vein, because they may bifurcate immediately before joining the superior mesenteric vein. Furthermore, in about 20% of subjects there is a short vein draining the pancreatic neck and entering the anterolateral aspect of the superior mesenteric from the left. Some of these veins can be exposed early during the pancreaticoduodenectomy as the transverse mesocolon is dissected off the pancreatic head from right to left.

The middle colic vein drains into the superior mesenteric vein at about the point that the superior mesenteric vein passes behind the neck of the pancreas. The middle colic vein can thus be used as a very reliable guide to the superior mesenteric vein.

The body and tail of the pancreas

The narrow, thin neck of the gland typically overlies the confluens of the superior mesenteric and splenic veins which form the portal vein. The neck inclines upwards and to the left as well as anteriorly from the head region; the body of the pancreas not only inclines backwards but also usually a bit upwards and to the left. The body is described as being somewhat triangular in cross-section with anterior, posterior and inferior surfaces. In an operative sense, however, it seems much more to have just anterior (or anteroinferior) and posterior (posterosuperior) surfaces. It crosses anterior to the aorta where its posterior surface overlies the origin of the superior mesenteric artery. The pancreatic duct is nearer to the posterior than the anterior surface as it traverses the gland. The splenic vein lies variably behind the pancreas, often within a fibrous tunnel, which on occasion, except for its posterior surface, is almost completely surrounded by the pancreatic tissue. It may also be found along the inferoposterior surface of the gland on occasion. The vein's position can most readily be found by tracing the entrance of the inferior mesenteric vein into it. In the region of its origin in the splenic hilum, the splenic vein usually runs superior to the tail of the pancreas before gradually assuming the position behind the gland. The splenic artery can be very tortuous, especially in the elderly, and runs along the superior border of the pancreas. Its anterior surface is covered with the peritoneum of the floor of the lesser sac.

The body and tail region also have important anatomic considerations. The posterior aspect of the stomach overlies the body of the gland. By transecting the gastrocolic omentum (ligament), the stomach can be mobilized upwards and anteriorly, thereby exposing the anterior surface of the body of the pancreas. There are often 'adhesions' joining the pancreas to the posterior wall of the stomach; these so-called 'congenital' adhesions are usually bloodless and can be divided without bleeding. The tail of the pancreas is on occasion tucked up into the hilum of the spleen and can be injured if the surgeon is not careful when ligating the splenic artery and vein during a splenectomy. The left adrenal gland typically lies posterior to the inferior aspect of the mid body of the pancreas.

The arterial supply to the body and tail of the pancreas (Fig. 6.2)

The dorsal pancreatic artery usually arises either from the coeliac trunk, the proximal common hepatic artery, or the splenic artery just after its origin. It descends into the neck of the gland or to the left, sometimes behind the splenic vein, and divides into two main branches. The right branch supplies some of the head and uncinate process to ultimately connect with the pancreaticoduodenal arcade, while the left branch runs along the inferior border of the gland (but slightly posteriorly) as the transverse pancreatic artery.

The splenic artery gives off from two to 10 unnamed small pancreatic branches, but one entering at the junction of the middle and distal third is often larger and is called, somewhat grandly, the great pancreatic artery, despite being smaller than the dorsal pancreatic artery.

The venous drainage of the body and tail of the pancreas (Fig. 6.3)

Previously regarded as unimportant surgically, these veins have assumed some importance since the advent of the Warren shunt in particular, and also with pancreas-preserving splenectomy. The inferior pancreatic vein accompanies the artery of the same name along the lower border of the pancreas posteriorly. It empties either into the portal vein or the superior mesenteric vein. There are a variable number of unnamed smaller pancreatic veins, which drain into the splenic vein. They have been described as being from three to 13 in number, and their course is invariably short. They are easily torn when dissecting the splenic vein away from the pancreas and, thus, they must be handled with great gentleness, especially when portal hypertension exists. These veins nearly always enter the superior or anterior aspect of the splenic vein so that the posterior and inferior aspects are usually free of tributaries – other than the inferior mesenteric vein (Fig. 6.4).

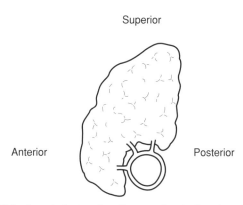

FIGURE 6.4 Aspect of entry of small pancreatic veins into the splenic vein.

The lymphatic drainage

The tail of the pancreas drains towards nodes in the splenic hilum, while the body drains to nodes along the splenic artery and more proximally either along the common hepatic artery (superior pancreatic nodes) or the superior mesenteric nodes. Lymphatic drainage of the head/uncinate region is more complex. The more anterior rostral area drains along the gastroduodenal artery to the hepatoduodenal ligament as well as in the duodenopancreatic groove via the pancreaticoduodenal arcade (both anterior and posterior). The more inferior pancreatic head and uncinate drain via the inferior pancreatoduodenal artery to the superior mesenteric nodal basin. For instance, carcinoma of the head of the pancreas is most often associated with nodal metastases along the superior mesenteric artery.

Pancreatic pain fibres

Afferent pathways from the gland exist to the central nervous system, but little is known of them. It is thought that the afferent fibres conducting pain run with the sympathetic nerve supply to the pancreas. The fibres carrying pain from the pancreas interconnect through the coeliac and superior mesenteric plexuses. Denervation of the pancreas thus means it has to be separated from these plexuses. Denervation of more central pathways involves division of the greater, lesser, and least splanchnic nerves (splanchnicectomy) and removal of the sympathetic trunks from T9 to LI segments. The lack of success of such central denervation procedures in alleviating pain from chronic pancreatitis or pancreatic cancer, however, suggests that other pathways are involved as well.

Annular pancreas (Fig. 6.5)

This uncommon congenital anomaly usually consists of a complete ring of pancreatic tissue around the duodenum. The duct system encircles from right to left around the duodenum to join the main pancreatic duct. For this reason, if the ring is to be interrupted by removal of tissue, dissection

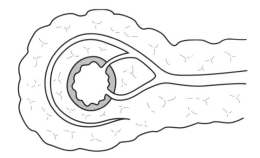

FIGURE 6.5 Annular pancreas.

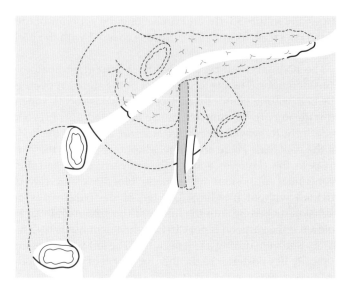

FIGURE 6.6 Relations of the duodenum.

should commence behind the duodenum. If the reason for operation is that the annular pancreas is compressing the duodenum mechanically, a duodenoduodenostomy is a better choice than excision of the annular pancreas.

THE DUODENUM

The proximal 2–4 cm of the first part of the duodenum (on occasion referred to as D1) is not intimately associated with the pancreas like the rest of the duodenum. This part lies, if anything, in front of the left side of the head of the pancreas. This fact, and the fact that this portion of the duodenum has its own separate blood supply from the supraduodenal and gastroduodenal arteries, means that almost all of the first part of the duodenum can be dissected away from the pancreas with relative ease when undertaking gastrectomy and for pylorus-preserving pancreatectomy The other important anterior relationship of the first part of the duodenum is the neck of the gall bladder, to which it is often adherent. This close relationship explains why gallstones can ulcerate into the duodenum in this region leading to a cholecystoduodenal fistula.

The second part of the duodenum (D2) is retroperitoneal and can be mobilized by incising the peritoneum along its right border, allowing the duodenum (and head of the pancreas) to be elevated anteriorly and to the left – the Kocher manoeuvre. The blood supply to the second portion of the duodenum comes from the head of the pancreas and is not disrupted with this mobilization. The third part of the duodenum (D3) passes anterior to the aorta and vena cava back to the left side of the abdomen, but notably behind the base of the small bowel mesentery containing the superior mesenteric artery and vein. This part of the duodenum is the least easily mobilized because of these anterior relationships. To the right it is covered by the parietal peritoneum extending downward from the root of the mesocolon, before which it is crossed by the superior mesenteric vessels and the root of the mesentery (Fig. 6.6). The mobilization of this portion and the proximal fourth part of the duodenum (D4), where it turns up to the right of the mesenteric vessels, is most difficult. The blood supply to the third portion of the duodenum comes from the pancreatic uncinate process,

while that to the fourth portion of the duodenum comes from branches off the superior mesenteric artery within the mesentery to the proximal jejunum.

The suspensory ligament of the fourth part of the duodenum (ligament of Treitz) is a fibrous band, sometimes containing muscle fibres, which suspends the superior and left aspect of the duodenojejunal flexure to the right crus of the diaphragm. The ligament requires division when the fourth portion of the duodenum must be mobilized for pancreaticoduodenectomy or when repairing an abdominal aortic aneurysm. The third and fourth parts of the duodenum are associated with the recesses of the peritoneum known as the paraduodenal fossae; anatomy books often describe these paraduodenal fossae as being of surgical significance, but internal herniation into these small fossae is exceedingly rare.

THE SPLENIC VEIN (Fig. 6.3)

The splenic vein arises from the splenic hilum and usually courses for a few centimetres superior to the pancreas before taking a fairly straight course behind the body of the pancreas. This vein is typically contained at least partially within a fibrous tunnel (Fig. 6.4). The splenic vein receives from three to 13 small pancreatic veins usually entering on its anterior and superior surface before it joins the superior mesenteric vein behind the neck of the pancreas to form the portal vein. In about 70% of subjects, the inferior mesenteric vein joins the splenic vein within 2 cm of its termination; in about 30% of subjects the inferior mesenteric vein joins the confluence of the splenic and the superior mesenteric vein, and the remainder of the time it joins the superior mesenteric vein. Sometimes one or two veins enter the superior surface of the splenic vein near the portal vein, usually aberrant tributaries, for example from the right gastroepiploic vein. The coronary (left gastric) vein drains into the superior surface of the splenic vein in about 20% of subjects and into the portal vein in the remaining majority.

These facts have an important significance for operations which involve dissecting the vein from the pancreas. First, the splenic vein can be difficult to find in its tunnel, particularly when it lies more superiorly than is shown in Figure 6.3 or when there is extensive chronic pancreatitis or peripancreatic inflammation. Second, the inferior mesenteric vein is usually found easily in its retroperitoneal, paraduodenal (fourth portion) position and, if traced upwards, it will lead to the splenic vein in 70% of subjects, while in the remainder it leads to the superior mesenteric vein. The left anterior border of the superior mesenteric vein can then be dissected upwards until the entry of the splenic vein is found. Even though great care is required in mobilizing the splenic vein, the tunnel within which it lies is a real one and actually aids considerably in the mobilization. Third, also worth noting is that, apart from the inferior mesenteric vein, there are usually no venous tributaries entering the splenic vein from posteriorly or from below (Fig. 6.4). If the splenic vein is being dissected for construction of a portosystemic shunt for portal hypertension and the left gastric vein drains into the splenic vein, the left gastric vein can usually be mobilized enough as it enters the splenic vein to allow its ligation, as part of a Warren shunt.

THE SUPERIOR MESENTERIC VEIN (Fig. 6.7)

The superior mesenteric vein drains the small intestine and the large intestine to the level of the distal transverse colon. The vein takes origin in the distal small bowel mesentery where ileal and caecal branches join; as it ascends in the mesentery of the small bowel, it receives ileocolic, ileal, and jejunal branches, as well as the right colic and middle colic veins. There may be more than one middle colic vein, and the length of the main trunk of the superior mesenteric vein below the pancreas is also variable. The more rostrally these veins are when they drain into the superior mesenteric vein, the less the length of the trunk of the superior mesenteric vein available, for instance, for an anastomosis as in a mesocaval shunt. In about two-thirds of subjects, there is a 2–3 cm trunk just proximal to the main branches. At the lower margin of the pancreas, the right gastrocolic vein and a bit more rostrally the inferior pancreatic duodenal veins enter from the right. In practice, the part of the superior mesenteric vein most accessible for use in shunting procedures is a segment between the entry of the ileocolic vein and the right colic vein. This part of the vein, sometimes called the surgical trunk, is 2 cm or more in length in about two-thirds of subjects. However, this trunk is not always of sufficient calibre to accept an anastomosis, in which case dissection of the main trunk more cephalad is required. Although the commonest finding is for the ileocolic artery to pass behind the superior mesenteric vein, the surgeon should be aware that

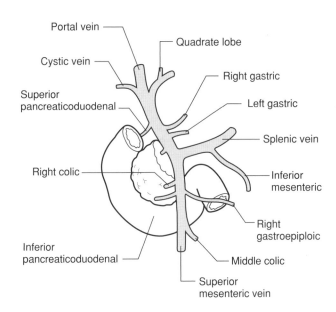

FIGURE 6.7 The veins of the portal system.

in perhaps a third of subjects, the ileocolic artery passes in front of the vein.

As the vein passes in front of the uncinate process of the pancreas to then pass under the neck of the gland, it receives several small tributaries from the right and from behind as well as small, unnamed branches from the head of the pancreas, usually from the right side. Some of these can be seen (and ligated if resection is planned) once the colon and its mesocolon have been dissected off the head of the gland. Several other possible named veins entering the superior mesenteric vein should be mentioned. In about 20% of subjects, a short wide vein draining the neck of the pancreas enters the superior mesenteric vein superiorly from the left. In about 30% of subjects, the inferior mesenteric vein joins the left side of the superior mesenteric vein. The right gastric vein may enter the anterior or left edge of the portal vein or the termination of the superior mesenteric vein; this anomaly can interfere with blind passage of the finger or clamp between the gastroduodenal artery and the anterior surface of the portal vein during supraduodenal dissection of the portal vein when beginning the mobilization for pancreaticoduodenectomy.

THE PORTAL VEIN (Fig. 6.7)

The portal vein is formed behind the neck of the pancreas by the union of the superior mesenteric and splenic veins. It then ascends to the liver in the free margin of the epiploic foramen lying behind the bile duct and hepatic artery – usually the bile duct lies to the right and the proper hepatic artery overlies it and a bit to the left. The direction of the portal vein varies from an almost vertical to the more usual horizontal lie with its typical direction being about 30–45° to the vertical.

Behind the first part of the duodenum, the gastroduodenal artery lies in front of and a bit to the right of the portal vein. Gentle blunt dissection behind the artery and inferiorly will open up a plane between the portal vein and the neck of the pancreas. This manoeuvre is usually possible, because all venous tributaries to the superior mesenteric/portal vein tend to enter from the right, posteriorly and the left, but not anteriorly. On very rare occasions, a small venous tributary may enter the anterior surface of the portal or superior mesenteric vein, so care must be exercised in performing this manoeuvre.

The inferior vena cava is the direct posterior relation of the portal vein as the portal vein passes toward the liver in the free edge of the lesser omentum (apart from the epiploic foramen itself). Because of this association, it might be thought that bringing the portal vein and inferior vena cava together for a side-to-side portocaval shunt would be easy. However, this is not always the case due to several factors. First, the length of the portal vein in its free margin is variable and, if short, it allows much less mobility without extensive mobilization. Second, the portal vein may cross the vena cava almost at a right angle making it more difficult to carry out an anastomosis than if two veins run in parallel to one another. Third, and most important, when portal hypertension is present, segment I of the liver (especially the left aspect of the caudate lobe) is hypertrophied as it passes to the right in front of the inferior vena cava. This hypertrophy can lead to a physical separation of several centimetres between the portal vein and the inferior cava.

Usually the portal vein has no venous tributaries draining into it as it lies in the free margin of the lesser omentum; its tributaries occur more proximally or distally. Proximally, the posterior superior pancreaticoduodenal vein enters the right posterolateral margin behind the first part of the duodenum. On the left of the portal vein, the right and the left gastric veins usually join the left lateral portal vein (although the left gastric vein most often drains into the splenic vein).

In the porta hepatis, the portal vein divides into a short, wide, right branch (which may receive a cystic vein) and a longer but smaller diameter left branch which may receive a branch from the quadrate lobe.

In portal hypertension, the areas of communication (decompression) with systemic veins are many in number. The most important ones from a clinical point of view are the submucosal veins of the upper stomach and oesophagus, which drain cephalad into the azygos system; these veins become dilated and are referred to as gastroesophageal varices. These veins are considered in Chapter 20.

Varices of the inferior rectal (haemorrhoidal) veins in the wall of the rectum sometimes occur with portal hypertension, as suggested in some older texts, because there are no venous valves in the splanchnic venous system allowing generalized broad distribution of portal pressure throughout the splanchnic venous system. However, these texts also suggest that these are the same as haemorrhoids, which is not true. The varices are true veins and occur craniad to the haemorrhoidal venous plexuses.

Another area of collateral development of surgical importance is the ligamentum teres. Occasionally the lumen of the umbilical vein opens up and becomes quite large. More often, however, small paraumbilical veins, which run with the ligamentum teres, enlarge and allow dilatation of contiguous veins in the umbilicus and abdominal wall. The importance of these venous enlargements is not in the production of the rare but picturesquely named caput medusa, but rather because abdominal incisions can prove to be difficult secondary to impressive venous bleeding. The other area of development of portosystemic collateral venous communications is the retroperitoneum. Multiple, usually small, veins from the splenic venous system can enlarge and communicate with diaphragmatic, adrenal, or renal veins.

FURTHER READING

Drapanas T 1972 Interposition meso-caval shunt for treatment of portal hypertension. Ann Surg 176:435–445.

Hiraoka T, Watanabe E, Katoh T et al 1986 A new surgical approach for control of pain in chronic pancreatitis: complete denervation of the pancreas. Am J Surg 152:549–551.

Holyoke E A, Clayton Davis W, Harry R D 1975 Surgical anatomy of the mesocaval shunt. Surgery 78:526–530.

7 Splenectomy and partial splenectomy, laparoscopic and open approaches: the anatomy of the spleen and its blood vessels

Glyn Jamieson and David Watson

THE SPLEEN

The spleen lies posteriorly in the left upper quadrant of the abdomen with its convexity against the diaphragm and its concavity in relation to the stomach, pancreas and kidney (Fig. 7.1). Its longest axis lies in the line of the 10th rib and it lies approximately deep to the 9th–11th ribs. In health its anterior margin does not reach beyond the mid axillary line and so it is not palpable. The concavity of the spleen adopts one of two configurations. Approximately half are gently curved, with the remainder more 'horse shoe' shaped.

It forms originally in the dorsal mesentery of the stomach and divides that mesentery into two portions (Fig. 7.2), i.e. the gastrosplenic (gastrolienal) ligament and the splenorenal (lienorenal) ligament. In life the spleno-renal ligament is short and carries the splenic artery and vein and their branches to the hilum. In about 50% of cases the tail of the pancreas passes in it as well, abutting or close to the spleen. The gastrosplenic ligament carries the short gastric and left gastroepiploic vessels (the Nomina Anatomica has changed the name to the gastro-omental vessels) to the stomach. Immediately below the lowermost pole of the spleen the colon is attached to the diaphragm by the phrenocolic ligament. The pole of the spleen 'sits' on this ligament so that if the spleen enlarges it pushes the splenic flexure of the colon ahead of it. The practical significance of this is that there is almost never any colon found anterior to even the largest spleen, so that percussion over it is dull (unlike an enlarged kidney, for instance, which has colonic resonance in front of it).

The uppermost portion of the gastrosplenic ligament is usually very short so that the greater curvature of the stomach and the spleen are often very close here and rarely more than 1 cm apart. Care must therefore be exercised in ligating short gastric vessels here so that stomach wall is not included in the ligature.

All of the peritoneal attachments of the spleen are relatively bloodless in normal circumstances. However this assumption cannot be made in patients with portal hypertension where collateral channels may open up and normally bloodless incisions in the peritoneum can lead to excessive blood loss.

From a practical point of view it should be assumed that there will be adhesions between the inferior medial aspect of the spleen and the greater omentum. These are not true adhesions, but rather ligamentous connections which contain accessory vessels to the spleen. They do not exist in every patient, but are sufficiently common to be a potential problem during gastric or colonic mobilization.

The variable entry of the arteries and veins into the spleen is described in the next section. These vessels may be large or small and assume practical significance in any operation in the upper abdomen. Traction downwards on the splenic flexure of the colon or on the stomach can tear at least the smaller of these vessels as they enter the spleen and troublesome bleeding ensues. This can lead to an otherwise unwarranted splenectomy, so it is worth seeking the smaller of these vessels, and dividing them prior to exerting traction. A clue as to whether such vessels exist comes from an examination of the anterior margin of the spleen. In about two-thirds of cases this contains one to several notches. When there are no notches and the margin is smooth then the morphology of the vessels in the hilum tends to be typical without 'wild' branches entering at sites far removed from the hilum. When it is notched however the likelihood for 'wild' vessels is much greater.

Accessory spleens (splenunculus, spleniculus) occur in about 10% of individuals and probably represent a splenic segment which has developed separately from the main bulk of the splenic tissue. They usually occur in the hilus or along the vessels of the splenic pedicle but occasionally have been reported elsewhere, particularly in the greater omentum.

The segments of the spleen are based on its arterial supply and are described below.

THE SPLENIC ARTERY

The coeliac axis typically terminates as two major trunks, the common hepatic artery and the splenic artery. This latter travels along the superior border of the pancreas (occasionally at lower levels behind or in the gland). It is almost always very tortuous in adults. It usually gives off the dorsal pancreatic artery as its first branch to the region of the neck of the pancreas and then from two to 10 pancreatic branches,

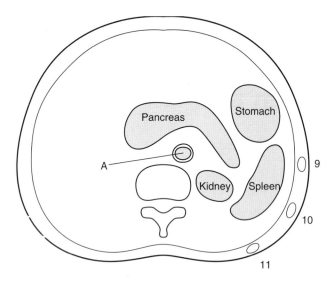

FIGURE 7.1 Diagrammatic representation of CT scan view of the spleen and its relationships. The numbers 9–11 refer to the ribs associated with the spleen. A = aorta.

including the great pancreatic artery (if present) – a slightly larger branch at about the junction of the middle and distal thirds of the pancreas (Fig. 6.2). Its point of division into its terminal branches is variable from this point so that the short gastric arteries and left gastroepiploic artery may arise from the main trunk or from the superior or inferior divisions into which the splenic artery usually divides. The left gastroepiploic artery arises from a common trunk with the lower division of the splenic artery in about two-thirds of cases.

In about 75% of individuals the division of the splenic artery is several centimetres proximal to the spleen and it usually is a Y-shaped division. In the remaining individuals the division occurs close to the splenic hilum, in which case it is more a T-shaped division (in both instances with the Y

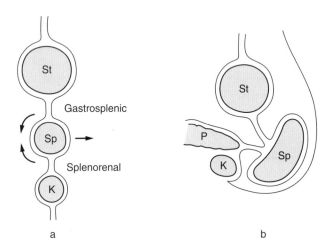

FIGURE 7.2 The ligaments of the spleen, seen in coronal section. (a) In embryonic life; (b) when full development has occurred. St = stomach, Sp = spleen, K = kidney, P = pancreas.

and the T lying horizontally). The branches to the spleen come off the inside of the Y or the outside of the bar of the T.

Often omitted from both anatomical and surgical texts is a branch of the splenic artery arising from about its midpoint and passing upwards behind the lesser sac and forwards to about the junction posteriorly of the fundus and body of the stomach. This is the posterior gastric artery and it passes forwards just superior to the lower leaf of the peritoneum below the bare area of the stomach. It is present in about two-thirds of individuals.

The spleen has been shown to be divisible into well delineated segments based on its blood supply. There are upper and lower polar segments and from one to five central segments. In about 40% of cases the artery to the upper polar segment arises well proximally from the main splenic or its upper division. An even greater number of inferior polar arteries arise proximally (about 75%) and about half of these arise from the left gastro epiploic artery. These branches were not previously seen as having much surgical significance. However, since splenic preservation is now an accepted goal, division of segmental arteries can be carried out in the performance of partial splenectomies.

Other small arteries can enter at any point on the spleen's visceral surface and this may bear some relationship to the morphology of the spleen (see above).

THE SPLENIC VEIN

The formation of the splenic vein has similar variability to the branches of the splenic artery but a confluence of two to six tributaries usually occurs in the splenorenal ligament. As with the arteries an upper or lower polar vein often exits separately to join the splenic vein at a considerable distance away from the spleen. The splenic vein or one of its major tributaries receives the left gastroepiploic vein. The short gastric veins drain by penetrating the splenic substance rather than draining into the splenic vein outside the spleen.

The splenic vein takes a fairly straight course behind the body of the pancreas, typically contained at least partially within a fibrous tunnel. It receives from three to 13 pancreatic veins usually entering on its anterior and superior surface and joins the superior mesenteric vein behind the neck of the pancreas to form the portal vein.

The more centrally situated part of the splenic vein is considered in Chapter 6.

APPROACHES FOR SPLENECTOMY

Open approach

With a normal sized spleen it can be approached in one of two ways. The most anatomical and possibly the best approach is an anterior approach through the gastro colic omentum. The pancreas and the tortuous splenic artery are usually easily found by this approach and the splenic artery can be mobilized and tied in continuity. It is worth noting that the splenic artery often seems to be a reasonably thin walled vessel and great care is needed in mobilizing it for ligature. The splenic vein is then sought further laterally in the splenic hilum or the surgeon can revert to the next approach, which is a posterior approach. With the posterior approach the posterior leaf of the splenorenal ligament (peritoneum) is divided and this allows the spleen to be gently mobilized medially recreating the midline abdominal position of embyronic life. Although the spleen can often be relatively easily held out of a midline wound it should be remembered that the pancreatic tail often lies in the posterior attachment to the abdomen. It is usually a straightforward matter to divide attaching structures with the spleen held forward.

With very large spleens it can be difficult approaching the splenic artery by the anterior approach and the very size of the organ can make any operation difficult. Consideration should then be given to embolizing the splenic artery under radiological control on the way to the operating theatre. This can lead to a much smaller and more pliable spleen.

Laparoscopic approach

The usual approach is to place the patient in a left lateral position. This encourages the stomach, omentum and colon to fall away from the splenic hilum. On entering the peritoneal cavity, any attachments or adhesions between the colon and the spleen, or the omentum and the spleen are divided. Surgeons should be aware that the omental attachments to the lower pole of the spleen often contain one or two vessels which supply the lowermost segment of the spleen, so care is required when dividing these attachments.

There are two common approaches to laparoscopic splenectomy:

❶ initial dissection of the hilar vessels followed by splenic mobilization, or
❷ division of the posterior leaf of the splenorenal ligament first.

The latter approach allows the spleen to fall medially under its own weight, facilitating further posterior dissection. This progresses until the spleen is fully mobilized, revealing a 'mesentery' which contains the pancreatic tail and the splenic vessels. Although the splenic vessels can be dissected and ligated individually, many surgeons use a linear cutting stapler across the hilum and its structures. With this approach the stapler should abut the hilum of the spleen, to minimize the risk of damage to the pancreatic tail. This step can be more difficult if the concavity of the spleen has a more pronounced horse shoe shape.

FURTHER READING

Nomina Anatomica 1983 5th edn. Williams and Williams, Baltimore.
Redmond H P, Redmond J M, Rooney B P, Duignan J P, Bouchier-Hayes D J 1989 Surgical anatomy of the human spleen. Br J Surg 76:198–201.

Gastrectomy; gastric tubes; pyloroplasty: the anatomy of the stomach and pylorus

Glyn Jamieson and Jean Marie Collard

THE STOMACH

The stomach is divided somewhat arbitrarily into several sections. That which lies above the level of entry of the left side of the oesophagus is called the fundus; below the fundus is the longest part of the stomach, the body. This ends on the lesser curvature at the incisura which is a point of indentation on the lesser curve seen radiologically. Anatomically it is the region where the vessels and nerves of the lesser omentum are seen to fan out as the 'crow's foot'. A line drawn from this point at about 45° from the vertical strikes the greater curvature at the arbitrary termination of the body and distally is the antrum terminating at the pylorus. The antrum is sometimes divided into a proximal and distal section, the pyloric antrum and the pyloric channel. Most of these definitions come from radiological studies of the empty stomach. Studies with radionuclides in the fed stomach often show the stomach divided by a mid gastric band into proximal and distal sections. This band corresponds more with the midpoint of the stomach.

The division between body and antrum corresponds with a histological division of the stomach, with parietal cells and chief cells occurring predominantly in the fundus and body and gastrin-producing cells occurring predominantly in the antrum. However, the level to which a band of antral mucosa rises along the lesser curvature of the stomach is variable and it can reach as high as the gastro-oesophageal junction.

The point at which the tubular oesophagus joins the stomach is known as the cardia. This distinction is made because the mucosa of the stomach in this region contains mainly mucus cells and glands. It is called junctional mucosa and usually covers an area 2 cm or less in length. The mucosa usually persists for 1–2 cm into the oesophagus where it joins the squamous mucosa at an irregular interface called the Z line. There is increasing evidence that the junctional mucosa of the cardia is not normal mucosa, but metaplastic epithelium as a result of the action of gastric juice on the lowermost squamous mucosa of the oesophagus. The junctional mucosa has assumed importance out of proportion to its area in recent years because of the increasing incidence of cancer arising from the mucosa – adenocarcinoma of the cardia. At present it is controversial as to whether there is ever 'normal' cardia mucosa – or whether it represents the earliest metaplastic change which occurs as a result of reflux damage.

The stomach is contained in a ventral and dorsal mesentery in fetal life (Fig. 8.1) and differential rotation leads to the ventral mesentery forming the lesser omentum. This splits to enclose the stomach. It exits from over the stomach as the dorsal mesentery. That part of the dorsal mesentery which passes to the spleen is called the gastrosplenic ligament and that part which passes in front of the colon is called the gastrocolic omentum. The dorsal mesentery is redundant and hangs down over the colon as the greater omentum. Its posterior layer fuses with the peritoneally enclosed colon and forms the anterosuperior part of the transverse mesocolon (Fig. 8.1). Thus, to remove all draining lymph nodes of the stomach, the greater omentum has to be removed, but not the colon. Clearly the stomach lies in front of much of the lesser sac but posteriorly the peritoneum leaves the stomach, at a variable point, leaving the posterior aspect of the fundus bare of peritoneum (Fig. 8.1). It is through here that the posterior gastric artery passes to the stomach and also the left gastric vessels, although they are often at a more inferior point and are contained in their own peritoneal fold – the superior gastro-pancreatic fold.

THE MUSCULATURE OF THE STOMACH

The musculature consists of an outer longitudinal coat and inner circular and oblique fibres. These latter are of greatest importance in the region of the cardia and lesser curve. They sweep around the fundus at the point of entry of the oesophagus and probably play a role in maintaining the acute angle of entry of the oesophagus – the angle of His.

They may also be responsible by their contraction for directing some oral intake down the lesser curvature of the stomach (the magenstrasse). Circular muscle fibres have been described as holding the limbs of these inverted U fibres together – so-called clasp fibres. In the region of the cardia these fibres probably play a role in the formation of the anatomical lower oesophageal sphincter (Fig. 8.2).

When the muscle fibres reach the pylorus they tend to end in a fibrous septum – at least on the anterior inferior and

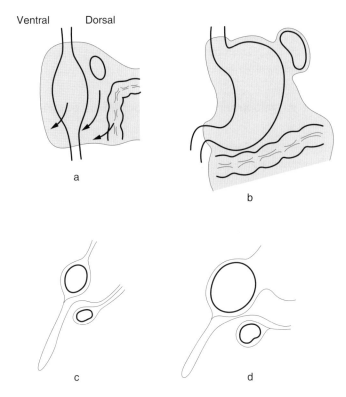

FIGURE 8.1 The mesenteries of the stomach. (a) Fetal life; (b) adult life; (c) the formation of the greater omentum and transverse mesocolon; (d) the bare area of the posterior part of the stomach.

posterior surfaces. On the lesser curve aspect they are more likely to be continuous with duodenal muscle fibres.

The muscle coat and in particular the circular muscle coat is thickest in the antrum.

The pylorus

The pyloric region has been shown to have a complex anatomical structure. On the greater curve of the stomach,

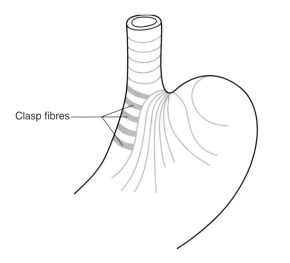

FIGURE 8.2 Clasp fibres of the stomach.

the circular muscle thickens to form two discrete muscle loops: the proximal and the distal pyloric sphincters. These loops define the anatomical borders of the pylorus, and they enclose a sheet of circular muscle between them. The distal sphincter or loop exists for only a short distance at the narrowest point of the gastroduodenal junction and is thus quite distinct. The proximal sphincter is less prominent, occurring over a longer segment of the greater curvature.

The two sphincters are clearly separated only on the greater curve aspect, while on the lesser curve they fuse with the circular muscle of the pyloric channel to form a muscular knob known as the pyloric torus. The distal sphincter and the torus form the thickest portion of the gastroduodenal junction and are generally regarded as the main pyloric sphincter. It ends abruptly with a clear-cut change to the much thinner duodenal musculature.

The lumen can be widened greatly by dividing the pyloric region longitudinally and sewing it up transversely – a pyloroplasty.

Its function can also be attenuated by removing part of its muscle anteriorly (pyloromyomectomy) or dividing the muscle longitudinally (pyloromyotomy). With both techniques care and patience are required in dividing the muscle as it is easy to perforate the duodenal mucosa.

THE GASTRIC BLOOD SUPPLY

From an operative point of view the blood supply of the stomach is of fundamental importance. Typically it arises from the three major branches of the coeliac axis – the hepatic, splenic and left gastric arteries. However, a small supply to the proximal stomach can come through oesophageal arteries directly from the aorta. A very important feature of the blood supply is the rich anastomosing networks which exist in the gastric wall at three levels, mucosally, submucosally and intramuscularly. These networks are everywhere well developed except along the lesser curvature of the stomach where anastomosing channels are of finer calibre and more of the arteries of supply appear to be end arteries.

Left gastric artery

This usually arises from the main trunk of the coeliac artery, but occasionally it arises directly from the aorta. It passes upwards and to the left and then forwards to about the gastro-oesophageal junction or a little below on the lesser curvature of the stomach. It tends to raise a fold of peritoneum called the gastropancreatic fold and this is best seen through the lesser sac when approached from below the stomach. The artery gives off oesophageal branches and turns downwards and usually divides into anterior and posterior branches which supply appropriate walls of the stomach.

In about 20–30% of cases a left hepatic artery arises from the left gastric artery and this courses through the lesser omentum, to the left side of the liver.

An accessory left gastric artery is present in about 10% of patients. It arises from the splenic artery and travels in the bare area to the stomach. It is like a posterior gastric artery but is more to the right and travels to the lesser curve of the stomach.

Right gastric artery

This is much more variable in both size and origin than the left gastric artery, but most typically arises from the hepatic artery before or after it has given off the gastroduodenal artery. It descends to the lesser curvature of the stomach contained in the leaves of the lesser omentum and passes to the left, anastomosing with branches of the left gastric artery. Its variability in origin and size is of little surgical importance.

The left gastro-omental (gastroepiploic) artery

The official name for this artery in the Nomina Anatomica is the left gastro-omental artery (in its anglicized form). This artery typically arises from the main trunk or one of the branches of the splenic artery and passes forwards in the short splenorenal ligament and then gastrosplenic ligament to reach the greater curvature of the stomach at about the level of the lower pole of the spleen. It then runs in the greater omentum approximately 1 cm from the greater curvature of the stomach, as the gastro-omental arcade, which is formed at the right end by the right gastro-omental artery. The left artery gives off some short gastric arteries to the fundus of the stomach as it passes forwards and anterior and posterior gastric branches from the arcade. It also gives off branches to the omentum, one of which is larger and is called the left omental artery. This descends in the omentum and anastomoses with a similar vessel from the right gastro-omental artery.

The right and left sides of the gastro-omental arcade occasionally fail to anastomose and so if the omentum is kept attached to the stomach, continuity of blood supply through the arcade can be maintained via the right and left omental arteries and their anastomoses.

Surgeons sometimes seem to expect the gastro-omental arcade to extend higher than is actually the case. Usually it extends along only about two-thirds of the greater curvature, and it is not found once the spleen is reached, because it is at this point that the left gastro-omental artery comes forwards to form the gastro-omental arcade.

The right gastro-omental (gastroepiploic) artery

This artery typically arises as one of the two terminal branches of the gastroduodenal artery, after that artery has passed behind the first part of the duodenum. The right gastro-omental artery passes to the left in the greater omentum and is a sort of mirror image to the left gastro-omental artery, giving off similar branches and forming the right end of the gastro-omental arcade.

Short gastric arteries and the posterior gastric artery

The short gastric arteries arise either from the splenic artery or its branches and pass forwards in the gastrosplenic omentum to supply the fundus of the stomach. The posterior gastric artery is rather like the most proximal short gastric and is present in a majority of patients. It arises from the splenic artery and arches forwards over the top of the lesser sac to reach the stomach through the bare area. It approximately parallels the left gastric artery but is about 3–6 cm further to the left.

Venous drainage

The venous drainage of the stomach parallels the arterial supply although the mode of termination is not through major trunks.

The left gastric vein tends to lie in the angle between the hepatic artery and the splenic artery and it is usually encountered before the left gastric artery when approached from below.

The veins have no particular surgical importance in the context of gastrectomy operations. They are of importance however in portal hypertension. The terminations of these veins is considered in Chapter 6. Collateral posterior veins sometimes drain the stomach via the left inferior phrenic vein and left adrenal vein into the left renal vein.

GASTRIC DEVASCULARIZATION PROCEDURES

There has been an appreciable experience in interrupting the blood supply to the stomach, in an effort to lower acid secretion but more importantly as a means of preventing bleeding from varices in portal hypertension. One such of these procedures still used extensively, in certain parts of the world mobilizes (that is, divides the blood supply) to the oesophagus and stomach from the level of the inferior pulmonary vein in the thorax to the level of the pylorus in the abdomen. All vascular connections between these points are divided and yet gastric necrosis has not been a problem. Therefore when the stomach is left in its normal position and there are no anastomoses performed it is extremely resistant to ischaemia.

Proximal gastric vagotomy is also a devascularization operation of the lesser curvature of the stomach and again the incidence of ischaemic phenomena after the procedure is very small. That it occurs at all may be related to the fact that the lesser curvature of the stomach does not share quite so readily with the rest of the stomach in the rich vascular anastomotic network.

GASTRECTOMY PROCEDURES AND BLOOD SUPPLY

For distal gastrectomy procedures there is obviously an abundant blood supply to the remaining stomach from the left gastric, posterior gastric and short gastric arteries. However, as the amount of stomach taken starts to increase some care is necessary. Thus for a high partial gastrectomy the left gastric artery and some of the short gastric arteries are usually divided. If all of the short gastric arteries and the posterior gastric artery are divided then the remaining stomach has to live on supply from the oesophagus and very occasionally from the left phrenic artery. This degree of devascularization does not automatically mean that the stomach remnant will necrose, but it is prudent for the surgeon to make sure that the wall looks a normal colour and that the edges are bleeding. If there is any doubt then a total gastrectomy should be performed. If the procedure is being performed for benign disease then the left gastric should be transected close to the stomach in order to retain the ascending branches to the cardia and oesophagus. For proximal partial gastrectomy there is again no problem because of the blood supply from the right gastric and right gastro-omental arteries.

GASTRIC TRANSPOSITION PROCEDURES AND THE FORMATION OF GASTRIC TUBES

The use of the stomach to replace the oesophagus has increased in popularity in recent years. The stomach is mobilized from all vascular structures except the right gastric and right gastro-omental (right gastroepiploic) pedicles. The mobilization of the greater curvature is undertaken with great care in order to maintain the gastro-omental arch. If the arch is deficient then the blood supply can sometimes be maintained by preserving the greater omentum with its right and left omental arteries providing vascular continuity. Initially it was thought that it might be important to ligate the left gastric artery close to its origin in order to maintain a sort of right/left gastric arch. However, experience has shown that such is not the case and it may even be preferable to resect most of the lesser curvature (which makes the stomach into a tube) as the lesser curve is more susceptible to ischaemia than other areas of the stomach. With the formation of isoperistaltic gastric tubes the greater curvature and fundus are reliant on the blood supply from the right gastro-omental artery alone. While it is true that most often this blood supply is sufficient there is no doubt that the procedure of stretching the stomach up to the neck for an anastomosis puts added strain on an adequate blood supply and it has been suggested that the distal-most 20% of the tube

(i.e. approximately the fundus) should be discarded on the grounds that its blood supply is often marginal.

Reversed gastric tubes have been used less frequently, with their blood supply being based on the left gastric artery and splenic artery.

LYMPHATIC DRAINAGE OF THE STOMACH AND D2 GASTRECTOMY

In most fields of surgery radical operations attempting to remove all of an organ's draining lymph nodes have lost popularity. However, at the present time some surgeons, and in particular Japanese surgeons, continue to favour total gastrectomy and removal of the stomach's draining lymph nodes – a so-called D2 gastrectomy. This refers to the regional nodes draining the stomach, Dl being the region of the cancer only, D2 the region and draining lymph nodes and D3 removal of secondary nodal groups (e.g. gastrectomy plus pancreatectomy, colectomy, block dissection of superior mesenteric nodes, coeliac nodes etc.).

The stomach has four major sets of nodes draining roughly to the areas, as shown in Figure 8.3. A large portion of the upper stomach drains to left gastric nodes. Some also drains to pancreaticosplenic nodes. The lower stomach drains to gastro-omental nodes and pyloric nodes and the pylorus and distal antrum drain to hepatic nodes.

The gastro-omental nodes often occur several centimetres out into the omentum. Thus in order to undertake a gastrectomy which removes all nodal areas it is necessary to undertake a total gastrectomy and splenectomy and omentectomy and remove all tissue from the hilum of the liver back to the pylorus, the nodes on the pancreatic head adjacent to the pylorus, nodes along the splenic artery and along the left gastric artery back to its origin. The advantages of this radical approach in the treatment of gastric cancer remain to be established.

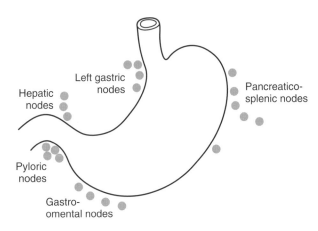

FIGURE 8.3 Gastric lymph nodes.

FURTHER READING

Maruyama K 1988 The R2 gastrectomy. Surgery: The Medicine Group (UK) 1297–1299.

Maruyama K, Gunven P, Okabayashi K, Sasako M, Kinoshita T 1989 Lymph node metastases of gastric cancer. Ann Surg 210:596–601.

Nomina Anatomica 1983 5th edn Williams and Wilkins, Baltimore

Schein M, Saadia R 1989 Post-operative gastric ischaemia. Br J Surg 76:844–848.

Thomas D M, Langford R M, Russell R C G, LeQuesne L P 1979 The anatomical basis for gastric mobilization in total oesophagectomy. Br J Surg 66:230–233.

Yu W, Wang I 1990 Surgical implications of the posterior gastric artery. Am J Surg 159:420–423.

9

Truncal, selective and proximal gastric vagotomy: the anatomy of the abdominal vagi

Glyn Jamieson and Haile Debas

The history of division of the vagus nerves therapeutically is interesting, and one which has aided our understanding of the physiology of the stomach. With the advent of effective medical therapy for duodenal and gastric ulcers the place of vagotomy operations has faded somewhat. Occasionally special circumstances may still lead to a vagotomy being undertaken however.

The vagus nerves to the abdomen derive from the oesophageal plexuses in the thorax and they exhibit considerable variability, some of which is relevant to the surgery of peptic ulcer disease and other gastric operations.

THE ANTERIOR VAGAL TRUNK

The anterior vagal trunk forms from the oesophageal plexus and contains fibres mainly from the left vagus nerve. Most commonly it forms a single trunk as it passes through the hiatus but occasionally two or even three trunks are found. It divides into two divisions, the larger of which continues as the greater anterior gastric nerve. In surgical parlance this is the anterior nerve of Latarjet, an eponym which pays just tribute to a pioneer French surgeon in vagotomy procedures. This nerve continues parallel to the lesser curvature of the stomach about 1 cm or more into the lesser omentum. It gives off two to 12 branches to the anterior gastric wall and usually terminates at a variable point on the antrum, without reaching the pylorus. In about 5% of cases the nerve may reach as far as the pylorus.

The other division of the anterior trunk is the hepatic nerve which arises just above, in or most typically just below the oesophageal hiatus and passes in the lesser omentum to the hilum of the liver. It gives off a branch which descends to the left of the hepatic artery to supply the pylorus and first part of the duodenum.

The anterior vagal trunk in the thorax tends to lie on the left side, anterior to the oesophagus, and then it progressively comes to lie to the right as it passes through the hiatus. Therefore, at the level of the hiatus, it varies in position from a little to the left of the midline of the oesophagus to the right side of the oesophagus. The anterior trunk lies very close to the oesophagus and when the peritoneum over the oesophagus has been divided and the oesophagus is placed under tension the trunk tends to lie deep in the oesophageal muscle. It can be felt as a taut bowstring in this region. In carrying out an anterior myotomy of the oesophageal muscle in achalasia, it is important to mobilize the vagus away from the oesophagus. Because of the oblique direction of the vagus, the myotomy usually commences at the gastro-oesophageal junction on the left of the anterior trunk and crosses beneath the trunk to lie on its right side.

The variations in the anatomy of the anterior trunk are numerous but most do not have surgical relevance. Those having surgical importance are outlined below (Fig. 9.1).

The hepatic division is often double or triple and sometimes a second and smaller branch passes parallel to the anterior nerve of Latarjet and supplies the distal antrum and pylorus directly (Fig. 9.1). Also in some instances the hepatic division receives contributions from both the anterior and posterior vagal trunks. Occasionally the anterior nerve of Latarjet is absent, with all anterior branches coming from the anterior vagal trunk or the hepatic division. Under these circumstances the pyloric branch assumes some importance as all anterior branches are at risk of being divided during proximal gastric vagotomy (Fig. 9.1). Also occasionally the oesophageal plexus is low on the oesophagus and the formation of the anterior trunk and its division is low, such that they are susceptible to inadvertent division (Fig. 9.1). This may not matter if the hepatic branch is left intact but if the hepatic branch is taken as well then a clinically important problem with gastric emptying may ensue.

Occasionally an antral branch reaches the greater curvature and passes to the left with the gastro-omental arch, as a recurrent branch supplying some of the greater curvature of the body of the stomach.

THE POSTERIOR VAGAL TRUNK

The posterior vagal trunk is subject to less variation than the anterior trunk and is formed mainly from right-sided vagal fibres of the oesophageal plexus. The trunk tends to parallel the anterior trunk but lies further to the right. This means that by the time it has passed through the oesophageal hiatus it usually lies behind and away from the oesophagus on its right side close to the aorta. It divides below the

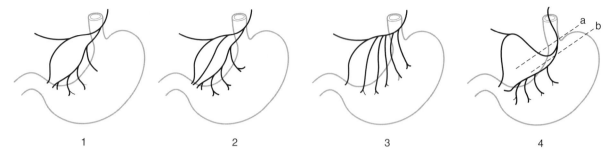

FIGURE 9.1 Variations in the anterior vagus nerve. (1) The typical situation; (2) additional antral/pyloric branch; (3) absence of anterior nerve of Latarjet; (4) low division of the anterior trunk. Dissection in plane (a) will divide the hepatic (and therefore pyloric) division. Dissection in plane (b), spares the hepatic division.

diaphragm with one division, carrying the major portion of its fibres, which travels backwards along the left gastric artery – the coeliac division. In almost all cases the division is single and passes to the coeliac plexus. The other division – the posterior gastric nerve or posterior nerve of Latarjet – parallels the anterior gastric nerve but supplies fewer fibres to the antrum (Fig. 9.2).

When, on the rare occasion, the posterior nerve of Latarjet is absent, gastric nerves to the fundus and body arise directly from the posterior trunk and its coeliac branch (Fig. 9.2). Occasionally the first gastric branch arises in the hiatus or above and crosses behind the oesophagus to the left to reach the fundus. This nerve is often referred to, perhaps somewhat melodramatically, as the 'criminal nerve' of Grassi. It is noteworthy that the posterior vagal trunk is not a major nerve of supply to the antrum (this comes from the anterior trunk) and it has never been described as supplying innervation to the pylorus.

VAGOTOMY OPERATIONS

Truncal vagotomy (total abdominal vagotomy)

This was initially carried out through a thoracotomy approach but today it is almost always performed through the abdomen. When performed through the thorax despite the variations in the formation of the anterior and posterior

vagal trunks, providing all trunks around the oesophagus in the region of the hiatus are divided, a complete truncal vagotomy is likely to be achieved. This is also true when the procedure is carried out through the abdomen. More than two trunks occur in less than 10% of cases for the anterior nerve, and even less commonly with the posterior nerve.

Something which seems to escape mention in general anatomy texts is the variation in size between the anterior and posterior trunks. Usually the posterior trunk is larger than the anterior trunk and the two trunks appear to be each other's converse. Thus if the posterior trunk is found to be small the anterior trunk is usually large and vice versa. The posterior trunk occasionally appears to be missing altogether, in which case the anterior trunk is usually double its normal size. This situation should only be accepted however when all the tissue between the oesophagus and aorta has been dissected and divided to the right, posteriorly and to the left of the oesophagus.

Note that a truncal vagotomy is essentially a total abdominal vagotomy. When first introduced in Europe and the USA, the effect on gastric motility was found to be unpredictable. In general terms it seems that about one-third of patients had a continuing problem with gastric emptying (and required a drainage procedure), one-third had a gastric emptying problem which improved with time and one-third had no problem at all. Whether these differences were related to failure always to achieve total vagotomy or to some other explanation is unknown.

Selective vagotomy (total gastric vagotomy)

The aim of a selective vagotomy was to denervate the stomach whilst leaving intact the innervation to the rest of the abdominal cavity. This was achieved by dividing the anterior trunk immediately below the hepatic division and the posterior trunk immediately below the coeliac division. Providing all of the tissue was divided around the gastro-oesophageal junction below the hepatic division anteriorly and below the left gastric artery (and its coeliac branch) posteriorly, the anatomical variations do not have a great deal of

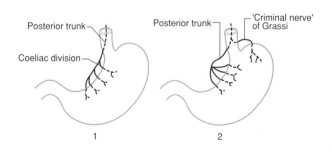

FIGURE 9.2 Variations in the posterior vagus nerve. (1) The typical situation; (2) absence of the posterior nerve of Latarjet.

significance as a total gastric vagotomy was achieved under all circumstances.

This operation retained pyloric innervation from the right hepatic division but denervated the antrum, body and fundus of the stomach. The incidence of gastric emptying problems was apparently much less than after truncal vagotomy – around 10%. This figure may represent the proportion of cases where the pyloric nerve supply is through the anterior nerve of Latarjet rather than through the hepatic branch or it may relate to dysfunction of the denervated antrum.

Proximal gastric vagotomy (highly selective vagotomy)

The aim of this operation was to denervate the major portion of the acid-producing parietal cell mass of the stomach, i.e. the fundus and body of the stomach. Although usually this would be achieved by dissecting out and dividing the individual branches to the stomach, in practice such an approach would be very time-consuming and an equal effect is produced by separating the anterior and posterior vagal trunks and the anterior and posterior nerves of Latarjet away from the lesser curve of the stomach, from the lower oesophagus to the antrum. Over the distal antrum, the nerve of Latarjet fans out into several terminal branches creating a 'crow's foot' appearance. Thus the proximal stomach and lower oesophagus were denervated and the antrum and pylorus retained their innervation from the anterior trunk (predominantly for the antrum, solely for the pylorus).

In view of the relatively small role played by the posterior vagus in innervation of the antrum, some surgeons advocated that an anterior proximal vagotomy and a posterior selective vagotomy achieved an essentially similar result.

Variations which need to be noted in carrying out a proximal gastric vagotomy are the already mentioned criminal nerve of Grassi and a recurrent branch or branches along the gastro-omental arcade. The former is taken care of by making it a routine to dissect free the fundus to the left of the oesophagus and the latter by dividing the gastro-omental arcade at the estimated junction between the antrum and the body of the stomach. Also some of the variations shown in Figure 9.1 will put the nerve supply to the antrum at risk as it is likely to be divided by a routine proximal gastric vagotomy. This is probably less important when the situation is such as is shown in Figure 9.1(3) where the pyloric nerve supply is retained, but, when the situation is such as is shown in Figure 9.1(4), the vagotomy is at risk of dividing the antral and pyloric supply. In most large series of proximal gastric vagotomy operations there is about a 5% incidence of gastric emptying problems and this may be partly explained by anatomical variations such as these.

The lesser curvature of the stomach is the only area of the stomach where the blood supply is not particularly rich in vascular anastomoses (see Chapter 8). This may in part account for ischaemic complications after proximal gastric vagotomy which may uncommonly lead to lesser curve gastric ulceration. The rare complications of ischemic necrosis and gastric perforation at the lesser curve, however, are thought to result from inadvertent incorporation of the gastric wall in a ligature.

As mentioned previously the introduction of successful drug treatment for peptic ulcer disease has meant that these operations are infrequently performed today. Their contribution to understanding gastric physiology, however, was considerable.

FURTHER READING

Dragstedt L R, Owen FM Jr 1943 Supradiaphragmatic section of vagus nerves in treatment of duodenal ulcer. Proc Soc Exp Biol Med 53:152.

Latarjet C R 1921 Seanc Hebd Soc Biol 84:985.

Jamieson G G 1983 Operations available for duodenal ulcer: an overview. In Carter D C (ed) Peptic ulcer disease. Clinical Surgery International: Churchill Livingstone, London.

Peptic ulcer disease. Clinical Surgery International: Churchill Livingstone, London.

Harkins H N, Stavney L S, Griffith C A, Savage L E, Kaj T, Nyhus L M 1963 Selective gastric vagotomy. Ann Surg 158:448.

Goligher J C 1974 A Technique for highly selective (parietal cell or proximal gastric) vagotomy for duodenal ulcer. Br J Surg 61:337.

10 Antireflux surgery, open and laparoscopic: the anatomy of the distal oesophagus and associated structures

Glyn Jamieson and John Hunter

Anatomical relations of the distal oesophagus and fundus

In the lower thorax, the oesophagus first lies anteriorly and then anteriorly and to the left of the aorta before it passes further to the left as it traverses the oesophageal hiatus and then enters the stomach. The segment of oesophagus which lies in the abdomen during repose is about 3 cm long. However there is appreciable shortening during swallowing, belching and vomiting. The abdominal oesophagus is more or less retroperitoneal with peritoneum covering its anterior and left side only. Posteriorly the oesophagus lies on the left pillar of the oesophageal hiatus which separates it from the aorta. Anterior to the abdominal oesophagus lies the left lobe of the liver and to its right, the caudate lobe. The physical presence of these structures means that the most direct access to the abdominal oesophagus is anteriorly and from the left. Visualization can be improved by retracting the left lobe of the liver cranially and to the right. If necessary, access can be improved further by dividing the left triangular ligament and folding the left lobe inferiorly on itself before retracting it to the right. This manoeuvre is not usually necessary however.

The angle of entry of the oesophagus into the stomach, termed the angle of His, varies between 30° and 70° in health. The gastro-oesophageal junction is often referred to as the cardia, however this term is frequently used loosely. The fundus is arbitrarily defined as the segment of stomach above an imaginary line drawn horizontally through the point of the angle of His. The height of the fundus above the angle varies between about 2 and 5 cm. Anteriorly the fundus of the stomach is covered with peritoneum. Posteriorly it is incompletely covered. The area above the upper reaches of the lesser sac not covered by peritoneum is known as the bare area of the stomach. Posteriorly the fundus lies directly on the diaphragm.

Musculature

As with the gastrointestinal tract in general, there is an outer longitudinal layer and an inner circular layer of muscle, with the latter layer being the thicker of the two. The muscle is smooth muscle in type. Opinion is divided as to whether a morphological lower oesophageal sphincter exists or not. In the distal 1–2 cm of the oesophagus and particularly on its left side some thickening of the musculature has been described and this may represent the uppermost gastric sling fibres – oblique muscle fibres which sling around the oesophago-gastric junction from the lesser curve side of the stomach. It is accepted that the thickening does not correspond with the whole 2–3 cm of the manometrically measurable lower oesophageal sphincter.

The submucosa deep to the muscularis propria is composed of loose areolar tissue. Consequently the mucosa can be easily dissected away from the muscle. This laxity is surgically useful in the operation of oesophagomyotomy for achalasia. Once a small incision has been made through the oesophageal muscle into the submucosa a fine clamp can be inserted and gently opened and closed in order to separate the muscle from the mucosa. Division of the muscle overlying the jaws of the clamp is then a simple procedure.

Transection of the oesophagus at the level of the hiatus can be followed by retraction of the proximal cut end into the posterior mediastinum as result of contraction of the longitudinal muscle layer which is fixed superiorly. The retraction also results in pouting of the cut oesophageal mucosa tube beyond the muscular tube by up to 1 cm.

Contraction of the longitudinal muscle may also contribute to the development of sliding hiatus hernia.

Blood supply

The cardia of the stomach and the lower oesophagus, just above it, are supplied predominantly by ascending branches from below. The anterior and right sides are supplied by one or more ascending branches of the left gastric artery and the posterior and left sides by branches of the posterior gastric or fundal branches of the splenic artery. The left inferior phrenic artery infrequently plays any role in the blood supply, in spite of its proximity to the area. The lower thoracic oesophagus may also receive one or more small direct branches from the aorta. The oesophagus has a rich intramural arterial anastomosis in its submucosal layer which is continuous with a network in the submucosa of the stomach. This no doubt explains how an upper gastric remnant retains viability when its external blood supply has been completely excluded, as occurs during near total gastrectomy.

Nerve supply

The distal oesophagus is autonomically innervated. Vagal inhibitory, non-cholinergic, non-adrenergic fibres are responsible for sphincteric relaxation associated with swallowing, belching, vomiting and at least some episodes of gastro-oesophageal reflux. There are also excitatory vagal cholinergic fibres responsible in part for basal sphincteric tone. The physiological role of the inhibitory sympathetic adrenergic innervation, which has been identified pharmacologically, remains to be determined. Vagal nerves innervating the distal oesophagus after leaving the vagal trunks run a long downward course which is largely intramural. This explains why skeletonization of up to 5 cm of the distal oesophagus, as practised in proximal gastric vagotomy, does not result in permanent dysfunction of the lower oesophageal sphincter.

The phreno-oesophageal ligament

This structure tends to be given greater prominence in surgical texts than in anatomy texts. It is the structure which attaches the oesophagus anteriorly to the peritoneum and endo-abdominal fascia. It is in fact a condensation of the endo-abdominal fascia from the undersurface of the diaphragm, with the fascia splitting into two layers – a filmy layer which passes downwards to the gastro-oesophageal junction and a stronger superior layer which passes through the hiatus to blend with areolar tissue surrounding the oesophagus. When viewed from above it is the layer of tissue which binds the oesophagus to the edges of the oesophageal hiatus. It is most easily demonstrated as a ligament or membrane from below. When the peritoneum in front of the hiatus is put on the stretch by downward traction, it can be seen to form a white line similar to the white line seen alongside the ascending and descending colon. Division of the peritoneum along the inferior aspect of the white line and the tissue immediately deep to it takes the surgeon through into the mediastinum in front of the oesophagus. With the clarity of exposure now obtained in laparoscopic surgery some surgeons are re-attaching the phreno-oesophageal ligament after antireflux surgery – trying to prevent recurrence of hiatal herniation.

MOBILIZATION OF THE DISTAL OESOPHAGUS – OPEN APPROACH

Mobilization of the distal oesophagus is achieved most simply by entering the lower mediastinum through the phreno-oesophageal ligament, as described above. This allows entry to the loose areolar tissue in front of the oesophagus. The normal oesophagus can then be encircled with the forefinger

passing from left to right behind the oesophagus. There is always fibroareolar tissue posteriorly which must be broken through. The higher in the mediastinum the encirclement is undertaken, the weaker the posterior layer becomes. Mobilization posterior to the distal oesophagus should be undertaken with great care when previous transmural peptic oesophagitis has resulted in perioesophageal inflammation and scarring. Under these circumstances it is advisable to perform the mobilization sharply under direct vision as the oesophageal wall, which is not robust, might otherwise be split by the mobilizing finger passing too anteriorly through the plane of least resistance.

When mobilized in this way by blunt dissection the encircling finger nearly always contains the anterior trunk of the vagus nerve and excludes the posterior trunk which tends to lie between the oesophageal hiatal pillars, posteriorly and to the right of the oesophagus. The amount of the oesophagus which can be mobilized upwards through the hiatus is limited by the dimensions of the oesophageal hiatus. Exposure can be improved, if further mobilization is required, either by dividing the right and left pillars of the hiatus or by dividing the hiatal opening vertically, anterior to the oesophagus, coming forwards until the pericardium is reached. Care must be taken with this median phrenicotomy as the anterior branch of the left inferior phrenic vein usually crosses in front of the oesophageal hiatus on its way to the inferior vena cava or left hepatic vein.

The mobilization of the oesophagus distally is limited at the cardia, or just below, by the left gastric trinity which attaches here (the left gastric vein, the left gastric artery and the coeliac branch of the posterior vagal trunk). If it is required to mobilize distal to the cardia then the mobilization should commence to the right of the lesser curve about 3 cm below the gastro-oesophageal junction and cross obliquely below the cardia towards the angle of His. This is done both anteriorly and posteriorly. Care must be taken not to damage the anterior vagal trunk in this dissection. The anterior vagal trunk, which is palpable as thin cord when the region is put on the stretch from below, is closely applied to the anterior surface of the oesophagus 5 cm above the cardia. As it passes inferiorly it passes to the right. At the level of the phreno-oesophageal ligament it is still close to the right side of the oesophagus. In the lesser omentum it is about 1 cm from the lesser curve. Such distal mobilization is required during proximal gastric vagotomy and ensures that both vagal trunks are displaced to the right away from the oesophagus.

MOBILIZATION OF THE DISTAL OESOPHAGUS LAPAROSCOPICALLY

The structure most easily seen in the region of the hiatus, on initial entry into the abdomen and after retraction of the left lobe of the liver, is the lesser omentum passing to the right in front of the caudate lobe of the liver. The hepatic division or divisions of the anterior trunk of the vagus nerve (and occasionally an accessory left hepatic artery) can be seen passing to the right in the lesser omentum. If a window is created in the lesser omentum immediately above the hepatic division of the vagus it takes the operator immediately to the right pillar of the hiatus – a helpful point of orientation. In obese patients there is often a triangular fat pad (apex towards the diaphragm) lying on the right pillar which should be excised. There are two grooves which are perhaps produced by the surgeon, but which are useful concepts. These are the right and left oesophago-hiatal grooves. If a blunt instrument is gently pushed against the tissue immediately to the left of the right pillar (this tissue is the phreno-oesophageal ligament), a groove occurs between the pillar and the oesophagus – and it is this groove which is opened to enter the mediastinum. The left oesophago-hiatal groove is more difficult to demonstrate, although it is undoubtedly present when a similar manoeuvre just to the right of the left pillar is undertaken. When mobilization is carried out posterior to the oesophagus, unlike in open surgery, the posterior vagus nerve trunk tends to stay with the oesophagus. Interestingly, with laparoscopy, the posterior vagus nerve seems to be more of a direct posterior relation of the oesophagus than is the situation in open surgery.

MOBILIZATION OF THE FUNDUS AND UPPER BODY OF THE STOMACH PRIOR TO FUNDOPLICATION AT EITHER OPEN OPERATION OR LAPAROSCOPICALLY

The operation of fundoplication is performed differently by different surgeons. Because the anterior wall of the stomach is lax, it is possible to pick it up and push it behind the mobilized oesophagus and then bring it around in front of the oesophagus and stitch it to itself. However, some surgeons prefer formally to mobilize the fundus and upper greater curvature of the body of the stomach. There are several anatomical points worth noting when this is carried out. First, several of the upper short gastric vessels are very short and travel adjacent to the anterior leaf of the gastrosplenic ligament. At this point there is often no adjacent posterior leaf, which is 1–3 cm inferior where the posterior peritoneum falls short, leaving the bare area of the stomach. Thus one or more vessels travelling to the stomach adjacent to the posterior leaf of the gastrosplenic ligament may be significantly caudad and to the right of the anteriorly visible short gastric vessels. As the surgeon mobilizes the greater curve from caudad to craniad the short gastrics, in the more superficial anterior plane, should be ligated and divided before attention is directed to the posterior plane in which the posterior gastric vessels are to be found.

The caudad limit for this dissection is arbitrary. There is an unnamed triangular fold of peritoneum which corresponds with the point where the gastrosplenic ligament becomes the gastrocolic ligament and this serves as a useful landmark to limit the distal dissection.

The mobilization superiorly is limited by the left pillar of the diaphragm and medially is usually limited by the left gastric artery, which is of course left intact.

THE OESOPHAGEAL HIATUS

This is the opening in the diaphragm through which the oesophagus passes. It is at the level of the 10th thoracic vertebra and it lies to the left of the midline, with its anterior margin about 1 cm posterior to the central tendon of the diaphragm. It is formed by the left and right crura of the diaphragm, but in a somewhat variable fashion. It is not only a somewhat longitudinal opening but also an oblique opening. Its anterior and superior margin may lie 1–2 cm in front of its posterior and inferior margin. This obliquity adds to the difficulty of the radiologist when trying to define the level of the gastro-oesophageal junction relative to the hiatus. The tissue which forms the inferior margin of the oesophageal hiatus also forms the median arcuate ligament across the front of the aorta (Fig. 10.1).

The crura of the diaphragm arise from the anterior surfaces and discs of the first to the third lumbar vertebrae as well as from the anterior longitudinal ligament of the spine. The right crus tends to reach slightly lower in its origin from the first three lumbar vertebrae, the left tending to arise from the first two lumbar vertebrae. Fibres arising from the right side of the lumbar vertebrae most commonly diverge and then converge to form the boundaries of the oesophageal hiatus. Fibres on the right side of the hiatus are innervated by branches of the right phrenic nerve and those on its left side by branches of the left phrenic nerve.

The way in which the fibres of the crura cross each other is quite variable. The considerable debate over such variations is of little surgical importance at the present time.

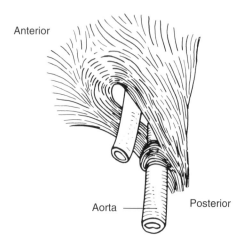

FIGURE 10.1 The oesophageal hiatus showing its obliquity.

Because the commonest arrangement is for the right crus to form the hiatus, it is more accurate to name the right and left sides of the hiatus as the right and left pillars of the hiatus, which makes no assumption as to which of the crura are involved. Three points however are relevant to antireflux surgery. First, the tendinous tissue binding the right and left limbs of the hiatus together inferiorly, of which the median arcuate ligament is a part, is not easy to delineate. Surgeons who use this structure to place anchoring sutures in reality use a variety of tissues lying in front of the aorta, including some of the neural tissue of the coeliac plexus. Nevertheless these tissues hold sutures well.

Second, the limbs of the crura are musculotendinous structures embryologically distinct from the remainder of the diaphragm and their tendinous portions tend to lie posterior to the muscular portions. Operating from the chest the tendinous portions are the most accessible portion of the crura, but for the surgeon operating from the abdomen they are the least accessible portions. From the abdomen, in open surgery the inferior limbs of the crura which are more tendinous than muscular can often be identified by palpation. When narrowing the hiatus, it is obviously important to stitch the tendinous portions. Thus the hiatus is best narrowed behind and inferior to the oesophagus. This approach also maximizes the intra-abdominal length of the oesophagus.

Third, it is fortunate for the laparoscopic surgeon that however the oesophageal hiatus is formed the muscles cross the midline before forming the hiatus. If the right crus formed the right pillar and the left crus the left pillar it would be impossible to narrow the hiatus posterior to the oesophagus. As it is, the posterior part of the pillars come together in a V shape in front of the vertebrae enabling the surgeon to narrow the hiatus by bringing the pillars into apposition posteriorly.

The hiatus and the phreno-oesophageal ligament, previously thought to be so important in maintaining gastro-oesophageal competence, probably play their major role during sharp increases in intra-abdominal pressure.

Small bowel resection; ileostomy; ileal pouches and the use of ileal conduits to replace the oesophagus: the anatomy of the small bowel

Glyn Jamieson and John Wong

JEJUNUM AND ILEUM

In life, the length of the small bowel is very much less than the 6 or 7 m which is measured in the cadaver, with 3–5 m being a more realistic measurement. There is no anatomical division between the jejunum and ileum and the arbitrary convention is that the jejunum is the proximal two-fifths and the ileum the distal three-fifths of the small bowel.

Nevertheless, if one takes the proximal part of the jejunum and compares it with the distal part of the ileum there are clear differences between the two. These are outlined in Table 11.1.

Most often the surgeon defines a particular loop by proceeding forwards from the duodenojejunal flexure or backwards from the ileocaecal junction. However, in certain circumstances the incision may not permit this certain identification. Therefore if the bowel is small, has mesenteric fat up to the wall and no circular mucosal folds can be palpated through the wall, then it is ileum which is being held. If it is important to know the direction of the loop then the fingers can be slid inwards keeping against the mesentery until the posterior abdominal wall is reached. If there is no twist felt then the upper portion of the loop is the proximal portion of the loop.

The difference in colour between the two areas is related to blood supply which is much more abundant proximally in the small bowel. The vascular patterns to the small bowel are considered below.

The small bowel has a well formed serosal coat from the peritoneum and an outer longitudinal and inner circular muscle coat in common with the rest of the gastro-intestinal tract. In keeping with the larger size of the jejunum, the small bowel is thicker proximally than distally. The submucosal layer is lax and allows considerable movement between the mucosa and the muscle layer, so that when the jejunum is rolled between finger and thumb the mucosa can be felt through the muscle coat like a shirt sleeve through a coat sleeve.

The circular mucosal folds (valves of Kerkring, plicae circularis, plicae semilunaris) are easily palpable in the jejunum and, unlike gastric rugae, they are not obliterated by distension of the bowel lumen. In the ileum the folds become less and less evident until they tend to disappear altogether by the time the terminal ileum is reached.

When small bowel is divided the muscle retracts to a small degree but, particularly proximally, the redundancy of the mucosal folds becomes evident by the mucosa pouting out as a separate layer from the muscle. Because it is actually *redundant* mucosa there is no likelihood of narrowing the lumen if the redundancy is excised prior to making an end-to-end anastomosis.

The small bowel mesentery

The small bowel mesentery is formed by the posterior peritoneum sweeping forwards to enclose the small bowel in a peritoneal covering. The vessels, nerves and lymphatics run in the mesentery which also contains a variable amount of fat. The root of the mesentery begins to the left of the first or second lumbar vertebra and crosses obliquely downwards and to the right to overlie the right sacroiliac joint. It is about 15 cm in length and crosses successively such structures as the third (usually) or fourth part of the duodenum, the aorta, the inferior vena cava and the right ureter. In a surgical sense the important one of these is the third and fourth parts of the duodenum, as in surgical resections of the duodenum and pancreas the root of the mesentery makes dissection in the area difficult.

The superior mesenteric artery and vein enter the mesentery at the level it crosses the duodenum and initially run in

Table 11.1 Comparison of the proximal part of the jejunum with the distal part of the ileum

	Jejunum	Ileum
Size (diameter in cm)	3–4	2.5–3.5
Circular mucosal folds	Prominent	Absent in terminal ileum
Length of straight arteries (vasa recta)	Long	Short
Vascular arcades	1–2	4–5
Colour	Pink	White
Fat in mesentery	Does not reach bowel wall	Reaches bowel wall

its base. However they usually pass into the mesentery towards the left and only the ileocolic vessels continue to run in the base towards the caecum.

Quite obviously, because of the disparity in length between the small bowel and the root of the mesentery, the mesentery has to form into a series of convolutions, usually described as being like a fan.

THE ARTERIAL SUPPLY TO THE SMALL BOWEL AND SMALL BOWEL RESECTIONS

The whole of the small bowel is supplied by the superior mesenteric artery. This arises behind the neck of the pancreas and at this point it usually gives off the inferior pancreaticoduodenal artery and middle colic artery and then passes in front of the duodenum to enter the root of the mesentery. Quite high up it gives off a right colic and ileocolic branch from its right side (sometimes coming off as a single trunk). The main stem then passes into the mesentery itself whilst the ileocolic continues on in the root of the mesentery to pass towards the caecum.

On its left side in the mesentery the superior mesenteric artery gives off about 15 intestinal branches, with five being proximal and large and the rest distal and small.

In the mesentery each intestinal branch divides into a superior and inferior branch which anastomoses with its similar fellow above and below to form a series of arcades. These are shown in Figure 11.1. In the proximal small bowel there is usually only one or two arcades but their number increases until by about the mid small bowel and beyond, their number may be five or six. Then the number progressively falls again until the terminal ileum is reached, where only one or two are found again. These arcades can be deficient, particularly between the first, second and third jejunal arteries.

The vasa rectae (arteriae rectae) arise from the arcade farthest from the superior mesenteric artery and pass straight to the bowel wall. They are essentially end arteries. This is an important point because the small bowel does not have an abundant intramural plexus like the oesophagus or stomach. Injection experiments in humans have suggested that intramural anastomoses might be able to sustain lengths of 7–15 cm of small bowel to which the arteria recta have been divided. However, at operation, it is rare for even 5 cm to be isolated from its vasa rectae without a severe colour change occurring. Therefore in practice only about 2–4 cm can be excluded from its blood supply with confidence of the bowel's viability. For practical purposes an anastomosis should only be carried out using small bowel of normal colour.

It is clear from the foregoing that division of the small bowel mesentery is most simply accomplished either at the level of the vasa recta or at the level of the intestinal arteries. Because of the fat in the mesentery the latter option is not easy, and if it is thought necessary, as in some unusual cancer operation of the small bowel, it is best formally to identify the superior mesenteric artery in order to avoid its inadvertent ligation.

THE VENOUS DRAINAGE

This usually follows the arterial supply although the veins tend to be fewer in number. This means that the artery and vein do not always lie close together and in dissection the vein should be treated separately from the corresponding artery.

CONSTRUCTION OF SMALL BOWEL CONDUITS

The principles of construction of small bowel conduits for the restoration of gastrointestinal continuity are similar no matter what their length, perhaps with the exception of a free jejunal graft. Differences usually revolve around the length of jejunum which it is necessary to prepare. Most often the length is not great, but occasionally more often-used substitutes (stomach, colon) are not available and a length to reach the cervical oesophagus is required.

It has been mentioned already that only a few of the vasa rectae can be divided without causing ischaemia to the bowel, so that in order to produce a conduit it is the major supplying arteries which must be divided – the jejunal branches.

The first jejunal artery overlies the fourth part of the duodenum and is relatively short. The fourth jejunal artery is usually the largest and the longest of the jejunal arteries and it is often necessary to divide it if a long conduit is required. Division of the mesentery begins just beyond the duodenal jejunal flexure and continues towards the fourth jejunal artery. For shorter conduits the length is much less critical. A point on the jejunum about 20–25 cm distal to the duodeno jejunal flexure usually corresponds to the third or fourth artery and there is normally reasonable length in the mesentery by this point. The usually single arcade with its long vasa recta can be well demonstrated using transillumination of the mesentery with a bright light. It is important to make sure there are no arterial gaps between the arcades. If

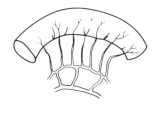

1 Vascular arcade

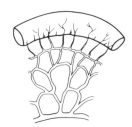

3 Vascular arcades

FIGURE 11.1 Vascular arcades in the mesentery of the small bowel.

present, the surgeon should choose the gap as the starting point. The technique is most often used in the construction of a Roux-en-Y anastomosis after a gastrectomy, in which case division of one jejunal artery, or at most two, is all that is required to be able to take the jejunum up to the oesophageal hiatus or even higher into the chest (Fig. 11.2).

With ligature and division of the jejunal arteries of supply it is important not to compromise the point where the artery branches to form the arcade and so ligature of the vessel should be at least 1 cm, preferably 2 cm proximal to the point of branching. It is as well to dissect out all areas to be divided before dividing them and to occlude the vessels and the bowel with non-crushing clamps to check on colour change. If the proximal part of the jejunum (the part furthest from the blood supply) becomes discoloured (ischaemic) then it may be worth dissecting out a further jejunal branch and clamping it also. This mobilizes an even greater length of small bowel to be taken upwards. Of course the ischaemic end is likely to increase in length also, but the increased length of ischaemic bowel may be less than the increase in length from the extra mobilization (Fig. 11.3).

As the base of the mesentery is so much shorter than the bowel which it eventually envelops, there may be considerable redundancy of bowel in long segments which are mobilized. This can be overcome by resecting a central segment of bowel (Fig. 11.4). Providing the dissection ligates only the vasa recta to the segment to be resected, this does not appreciably affect the blood supply to the mobilized segment.

It is worth repeating that the jejunal arteries and veins do not always lie side by side and they should be dissected out and ligated separately.

Some specific situations are worth mentioning. First if a Polya (Bilroth II) gastrectomy has been constructed previously, the jejunum is not usually suitable to use for a long conduit. Second if the small bowel conduit is being used after a total gastrectomy the most popular reconstruction is a Roux-en-Y configuration. However, the duodenum can be used. The oesophagojejunal anastomosis is carried out as for a Roux-en-Y. Then the conduit is placed close to the duodenum and an appropriate site is chosen for distal jejunal division. The distal portion of the conduit is then anastomosed to the

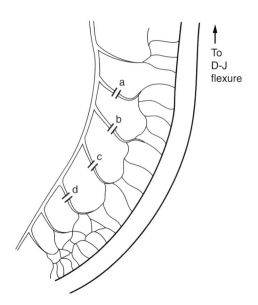

FIGURE 11.2 Division of vasa rectae for construction of a Roux-en-Y loop. Division at point a or a–b will usually provide enough length to reach into the lower chest. Division of points c and d in addition will often provide enough length to reach to the neck. D-J = duodenojejunal.

duodenum, following which jejunal continuity is restored between the remaining bowel ends.

Free jejunal grafts

The piece of jejunum (or ileum) chosen perhaps matters less here as what is required is a reasonable-sized artery and vein. However, as mentioned the largest arteries occur proximally and the fewer arcades and larger-diameter bowel all mean that it is best to use a segment of proximal jejunum for a free graft.

ILEAL POUCHES

The use of ileal pouches as an ileoanal reservoir after mucous proctectomy and total colectomy has developed quickly in recent years. Occasionally the apex of the pouch

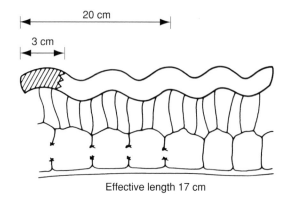

Effective length 17 cm

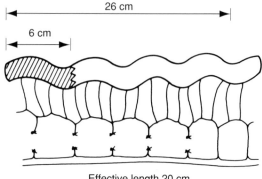

Effective length 20 cm

FIGURE 11.3 Division of further vasa rectae increases the length of the ischaemic bowel, but also increases the length of mobilized, well vascularized bowel.

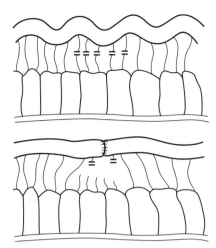

FIGURE 11.4 Overcoming redundancy in small bowel loops by resection of a central segment of bowel. routinely and extra length can be achieved by making relaxing incisions in the peritoneum of the mesentery. If the apex of the pouch can be brought to 6 cm below the inferior margin of the symphysis pubis, then a tension-free anastomosis can be constructed. If there is any doubt.

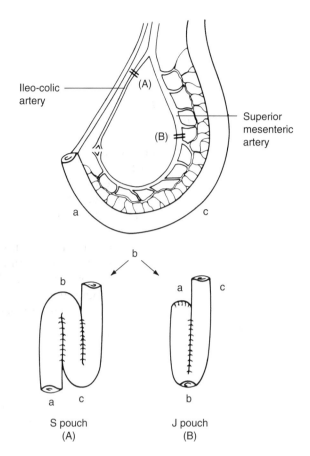

FIGURE 11.5 Construction of an ileal pouch. One or other of the terminal portion of the ileocolic or superior mesenteric artery usually has to be divided. The blood supply to the bowel then comes from the undivided artery of the arcade. For construction of an S pouch the point of division is usually the ileocolic artery (A) and for a J pouch it is division of the terminal superior mesenteric artery at (B).

(i.e. that part which is to be anastomosed to the anus) may not reach to the anus without tension. Freeing the mesentery up to the duodenum should be undertaken routinely and extra length can be achieved by making relaxing incisions in the peritoneum of the mesentery. If the apex of the pouch can be brought to 6 cm below the inferior margin of the symphysis pubis, then a tension-free anastomosis can usually be constructed. If there is any doubt then a trial descent should be performed before anastomosis is attempted.

Sometimes it is necessary to divide one of the main arteries of supply, i.e. the ileocolic or the superior mesenteric artery (Fig. 11.5). The point of division may vary but division should always be preceded by a trial of vascular occlusion with appropriate clamps. The pouch configuration may dictate which vessel is divided but in general terms it will be the ileocolic artery for an S pouch and the major continuation of the superior mesenteric artery for the J pouch.

The ileocolic artery should always be preserved at an initial operation where the potential exists for a subsequent ileoanal pouch procedure.

It is worth pointing out that if an end-to-end anastomosis to the upper anal canal is performed without an endoanal mucosal proctectomy, the apex of the pouch will reach the point of anastomosis more easily.

For construction of continent pouches within the abdomen pressure rises are minimized by cross-folding of the pouch. The posterior wall is made by suturing the vertical limbs together and the anterior wall is sutured transversely (Fig. 11.6). The pouch can then be invaginated between the mesenteries of the two limbs to produce a spherical configuration. This type of pouch has also been used for ileoanal anastomoses but an anastomosis may be under more tension.

MECKEL'S DIVERTICULUM AND OTHER CONGENITAL ANOMALIES

A Meckel's diverticulum is a diverticulum of the distal small bowel and represents a partial persistence of the vitelline duct from fetal life. It always arises on the antimesenteric border of the ileum and the great majority are found within 100 cm of the ileocaecal valve.

It is not an uncommon occurrence, being found in about 2% of individuals. It consists of an outpouching of ileum of variable length but usually less than 5 cm. Its wall is normal ileum except there is an incidence of heterotopic gastric mucosa occurring in about 10% of cases. Less often, heterotopic pancreatic tissue may occur. The diverticulum has a rudimentary mesentery and is supplied by its own ileal branch from the superior mesenteric artery.

Occasionally it retains a fibrous connection from its tip to the umbilicus and very rarely it remains patent to the umbilicus, or opens up in later life as an enteric fistula.

Very rarely a vitelline artery, or arteries, from the superior mesenteric artery to the umbilicus persist into adult life. If

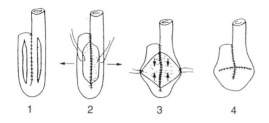

FIGURE 11.6 Construction of a pressure-less pouch. (1) The limbs are sewn together and vertical incisions are made in each limb. (2) The two internal walls are sewn together as the posterior wall of the anastomosis. (3) The outside walls are distracted laterally (a sort of pyloroplasty manoeuvre). (4) The pouch is closed transversely.

present they are usually associated with a Meckel's diverticulum.

Enterogenous cysts (duplications) are usually completely separate from the lumen of the normal bowel and arise in the small bowel mesentery alongside the normal bowel. They are made up of the normal bowel wall. They are similar to diverticula, but whereas these have retained their connection with the lumen, a small bowel duplication has lost its connection. Diverticula occur most frequently in the proximal small bowel and are often multiple. Some authors regard them as developmental rather than congenital, with a similar pathogenesis to diverticula of the colon.

FURTHER READING

Van Damme J-P, Bonte J 1990 Vascular anatomy in abdominal surgery. Thieme Medical, New York.

Wright C, Cuschieri A 1987 Jejunal interposition for benign esophageal disease. Ann Surg 205:54–60.

Wong J 1989 Jejunal interposition for oesophageal replacement. In: Jamieson G G (ed) Surgery of the oesophagus. Churchill Livingstone, London.

12 Appendicectomy open and laparoscopic approaches: the anatomy of the vermiform appendix

Glyn Jamieson and Andrew de Beaux

The appendix arises from the posteromedial wall of the caecum, usually 2 cm inferior to and more posterior than the ileocaecal valve. It is often considered a vestigial organ, but the marked lymphocytic aggregation in its wall suggest a specialized function for it although what this may be has never been determined. Its structure, apart from lymphoid masses, is similar to the rest of the large bowel.

It is variable in length but usually of the order of 10 cm long. Its relationship to the caecum can vary and relates to the mode of development from fetal life when the appendix formed the apex of the caecum (Fig. 12.1). Very occasionally, there is duplication of the appendix although in clinical practice this is rarely a source of additional concern. However, if this rare abnormality is not recognized, 'recurrent appendicitis' in the remaining appendix can occur to the embarrassment of the original operating surgeon. The other developmental abnormality which can cause diagnostic difficulty to the surgeon is malrotation of the colon. The caecum, and hence the appendix, may lie in the right upper quadrant or indeed the left upper quadrant.

The literature contains hugely disparate accounts of the normal positions of the appendix relative to the caecum – so much so that it is impossible not to draw the conclusion that the appendix is usually a mobile structure and the findings in any particular site will vary with chance alone as to the frequency with which a particular position occurs. Rather than try and cite figures it is more important for the surgeon to know the various sites where the appendix may be found. These are *perhaps* in order of frequency: retrocaecal, pelvic, subcaecal and paraileal, either behind or in front of the terminal ileum. In spite of its usual mobility the appendix may be fixed, either from previous inflammation and adhesions, or posteriorly if it is sited retrocaecally and the caecum is devoid of peritoneum (Fig. 12.2).

The one certain method of finding the base of the appendix is to follow any of the taeniae of the ascending colon downwards (but in practice the taenia libra, as it is the anterior one and most easily seen), since all the taeniae converge on the base of the appendix. At open appendicectomy, it is possible to deliver the transverse colon, or indeed the sigmoid colon, if it is on a long mesentery and lying on the right side through the wound. The transverse colon is usually easily recognized as it has the fatty omentum attached to it. The sigmoid colon can be more confusing but tracing its mesentery digitally confirms that the mesentery is not attached in the region of the right iliac fossa.

As the appendix is part of the caecum, it has no true mesentery. However, there is usually a peritoneal fold in which the artery runs and this is called the mesoappendix. This attaches on the left side of the appendix and is nearly always shorter than the appendix so that the tip is usually folded on itself to a greater or lesser degree. The appendicular artery is a branch from the ileocolic artery's lower division and it runs behind the ileum to reach the mesoappendix where it usually runs in the free edge. As well as the mesoappendix, there is sometimes a fold of peritoneum in front of the appendix, called the bloodless fold of Treves.

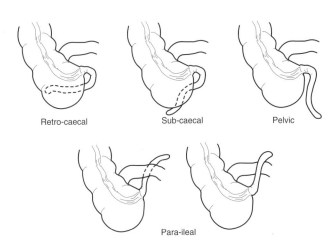

Retro-caecal   Sub-caecal   Pelvic

Para-ileal

FIGURE 12.2   Common sites where the appendix lies.

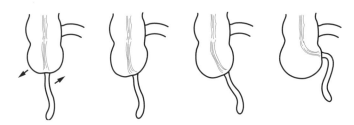

FIGURE 12.1   Development of position of the appendix by differential growth of the caecum in fetal life.

It has been noted previously that McBurney's point (junction of outer and middle thirds of a line joining the umbilicus to the anterior superior iliac spine) bears little relationship to the site of the appendix. Nevertheless, it remains a useful point for two reasons. First, by centering a palpating hand on this point (which clearly palpates an area larger than the point) it often corresponds with the area of maximum tenderness in appendicitis. And second it is a useful surface marking on which to base an incision for appendicitis. (It is often a useful manoeuvre to palpate McBurneys's point again in theatre once the patient is paralysed. Occasionally, the area of maximum fullness can be higher or lower and the incision moved accordingly.)

The incision for open appendicetomy was traditionally an oblique incision, but more commonly is a small transverse incision which heals with better cosmesis. This transverse incision can be extended if alternate pathology is found rather than the traditional method of closing the oblique incision and converting to a midline laparotomy.

Laparoscopy is being increasingly used to aid in the diagnosis of appendicitis in patient's with an atypical history or clinical signs. Laparoscopy can aid placement of the incision over the appendix, but with increasing laparoscopic expertise, removal of the appendix laparoscopically is more likely rather than converting once the diagnosis has been made.

If an inflamed appendix lies retrocaecally, then it may prove necessary to mobilize not only the caecum but the ascending colon in order to remove the appendix. At open surgery, through a small incision, this tends to be carried out in a blunt and somewhat 'blind' manner but it is more easily done under direct vision laparoscopically. Port placement for laparoscopic appendicectomy varies by surgeon but common positions are the laparoscope placed through an umbilical port and two further ports, one in the midline, suprapubically and the other laterally on the right side, somewhere above a horizontal line passing through the umbilicus.

Both at open and laparoscopic surgery, the appendix is never far from the caecum!

13

Colectomy open and laparoscopic approaches; colonic conduits: the anatomy of the colon

Glyn Jamieson, Mehran Anvari and Nicholas Rieger

THE COLONIC WALL

The wall of the colon and caecum is similar to the rest of the gastrointestinal tract with an outer serosa, then longitudinal and circular muscle fibres and a submucosa and mucosa. The colon has several distinctive features however. First, its peritoneal covering varies. The ascending and descending colon are typically retroperitoneal with peritoneum covering only the anterior and to a greater or lesser degree the lateral surfaces. The transverse and sigmoid colons have mesenteries and therefore are completely invested in peritoneum. Second is the presence of small fatty projections from the colonic wall which are peritoneal-covered and are called appendices epiploicae. The reason for their presence is unknown. And third is the fact that the longitudinal muscle layer, although complete, is thickened at three points forming the longitudinally running taeniae coli. The taenia libera lies anteriorly in the caecum and all parts of the colon except the transverse colon where it lies inferiorly. The taenia mesocolica lies posteromedially in the caecum and colon except for the transverse colon where it lies posteriorly in the attachment to the mesocolon (hence its name). The taenia omentalis lies posterolaterally in the caecum and colon; except for the transverse colon where it lies superiorly where the gastrocolic omentum attaches. The taeniae become less obvious as they spread out in the distal sigmoid colon. The sigmoid colon ends at the rectum which has a complete longitudinal layer of muscle and an absence of taeniae. It may not be accurate to say that the sacculations of the colon (haustra), occur because the taeniae are shorter than the rest of the large bowel. However it is an easily remembered concept and division of the musculature does tend to lead to loss of haustration of the bowel wall.

THE CAECUM

In the standing position the caecum often lies in the pelvis but when lying down it usually lies in the right iliac fossa on the iliopsoas muscle. Apart from the fact that it is more distensible than any other part of the large bowel, the caecum's structure is similar to the rest of the colon and its three taeniae

converge on the base of the appendix, as discussed in Chapter 12. It is about 6 cm in depth and 8 cm in breadth in the average individual. In the great majority of subjects the caecum is completely invested in peritoneum. However in a few subjects the caecum is partly or completely retroperitoneal as with the ascending colon. Occasionally the terminal portion of the small bowel mesentery extends across the front of the ileum and attaches to the caecum. The anterior caecal branch of the ileocolic artery runs in this position, either in the extension of the mesentery or usually freely.

The ileum usually enters the caecum posteromedially about 2 cm above the entrance of the appendicular lumen. It gives the impression of pointing into the lumen with superior and inferior lips of mucosa forming an ileocaecal valve. These are joined anteriorly to form the medial frenulum of the valve and laterally to form the lateral frenulum (Fig. 13.1). The valve and its frenulae can often reach quite large proportions and they have been mistaken for a caecal tumour both on barium enema examination and by palpation at operation.

The functional ileocaecal valve may in fact be the circular muscle of the terminal ileum in this area rather than these

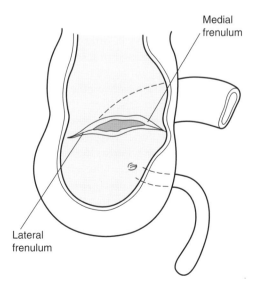

FIGURE 13.1 The ileocaecal valve.

interesting anatomical structures, whose function would then be unknown.

The caecum derives its blood supply from the ileocolic artery. This gives off an ascending branch and then anterior and posterior caecal branches which run across the ileocaecal junction and diagonally across the caecum anterior or posterior to it, as their name suggests. The anterior branch sometimes raises up a fold of peritoneum in front of the ileocaecal junction – the superior ileocolic fold.

The appendicular artery or arteries which may come off the ileocolic itself or either of the anterior or posterior caecal branches almost always pass behind the ileum to reach the appendix. The artery is usually single in western communities but more often may be double in some African communities.

THE ASCENDING COLON

The ascending colon is usually retroperitoneal in position. In a small proportion of cases the colon may be incompletely or even completely invested in peritoneum. In the latter case the ascending colon has a mesentery and is quite mobile. At the other extreme the ascending colon may be bound down by an extension of the peritoneum across the front of it, called Jackson's veil. These variations, i.e. abnormal mobility and abnormal fixation, tend to predispose towards volvulus of the caecum – the former because the mobility allows the caecum to rotate upwards and to the left, the latter because it causes abnormal fixation above the caecum, which is usually mobile.

The ascending colon lies on the quadratus lumborum and psoas muscles and in its upper extent it overlies the lower pole of the right kidney laterally, and medial to this the second and third parts of the duodenum. Its important anterior relation is above where it is overlain by the liver and gall bladder. It turns to the left at the hepatic flexure and becomes the transverse colon.

The ascending colon derives its blood supply from the ascending branch of the ileocolic artery below and the right colic artery above, with a greater or lesser contribution from the middle colic in the region of the hepatic flexure.

The ileocolic artery is the least variable of the colic vessels, and it is the last vessel to arise from the right side of the superior mesenteric artery. It arises about 7 cm from the origin of the superior mesenteric artery and runs in the base of the small bowel mesentery, whereas the superior mesenteric artery runs more anteriorly and to the left within the mesentery. The ileocolic artery gives off superior and inferior colic vessels as well as the caecal arteries and terminal ileal branches.

The right colic artery is the most variable of all the colic vessels (Fig. 13.2). When its origin is from the middle colic artery (30% of cases) it tends to ascend towards the hepatic flexure. When it arises from the superior mesenteric artery (20% of cases) it tends to run more transversely. It is absent

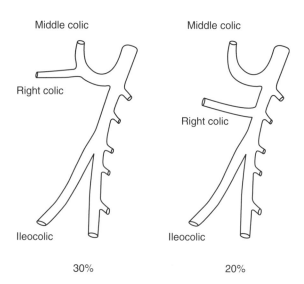

FIGURE 13.2 The right colic artery and its origin. The artery is absent in about 50% of cases.

in about 50% of cases with the ascending colon being supplied by the superior colic branch of the ileocolic below and the middle colic artery from the left. In those cases in which the right colic artery is absent the marginal artery of the colon is sometimes incomplete on the right side.

When the ascending colon is mobilized, its former mesentery is recreated and the blood vessels remain with the mesentery. However, other structures come into view posteriorly with the mobilization – the duodenum and head of pancreas above and the ureter and gonadal vessels below. These latter structures often adhere to the peritoneum (or rather, it is easy for the mobilizing finger to pass behind them) so they must be sought and separated from the peritoneum during the mobilization.

The operation of right hemicolectomy is carried out most often for carcinoma of the caecum or ascending colon. Removal of the regional lymph nodes associated with a cancer is achieved by removing the region of supply of the ileocolic artery and the right colic artery. Few surgeons formally dissect out the origins of the ileocolic and right colic from the superior mesenteric artery (although it is important to be aware of its position) but make their line of dissection a few centimetres to the right of the small bowel mesentery and ligate the respective vessels in this line.

There is little oncological reason to take middle colic territory in tumours of the caecum or proximal ascending colon. But as it is oncologically sound for tumours near the hepatic flexure, and as it is more convenient to carry out an anastomisis centrally in the abdomen, the right side of the transverse colon is usually resected in a right hemicolectomy. Again, most surgeons do not formally dissect out the right branch of the middle colic artery but continue the line of dissection from the right side of the small bowel mesentery out into the mesocolon, keeping well to the right of the midline.

THE TRANSVERSE COLON, MESOCOLON AND GREATER OMENTUM

The transverse colon varies in length from individual to individual, and in position in the same individual depending on whether the supine or upright posture is adopted. It rises higher on the left to the splenic flexure than on the right, where it forms the hepatic flexure. On the left the transverse colon, ascending, often lies partly in front of the left side of the colon, descending.

In the major portion of the transverse colon the mesenteric attachments are straightforward. At either end of the transverse colon the attachments are a little more difficult to comprehend. The straightforward attachments are that the colon retains its mesentery and this hangs down, as shown in Figure 13.3. The former dorsal mesogastrium is redundant and hangs down from the stomach, lying in front of the colon. The posterior layers of this structure pass back over the colon where they are attached to it and they are also attached to the transverse mesocolon which is thus, like the omentum, made up of four layers (Fig. 13.3).

It is because the omentum developmentally has no direct relation to the colon that the blood vessels within it come through the gastrocolic omentum (which is that part of the greater omentum lying between the stomach and the transverse colon). These vessels are from the gastro-omental arcade which runs about 1 cm away from the wall of the greater curvature of the stomach and is formed from the right gastro-omental artery (a terminal branch of the gastro-

duodenal artery) on the right and the left gastro-omental artery (from the splenic artery or one of its branches) on the left. This arcade sends many omental arteries through the gastrocolic omentum to supply the greater omentum, with two branches at either edge being larger and named the right and left omental arteries. Therefore the greater omentum can be dissected off the transverse colon with sharp dissection and relatively little bleeding ensues. In fact if vessels are encountered it usually means the dissection is occurring too deep and the mesocolon has been entered. In practice, it is often easiest to establish the correct plane at one of the flexures of the colon and work towards the centre of the transverse colon. If appendices epiploicae are present, dissection should occur between them behind and the omentum in front, with the dissection breaking through into the lesser sac. In removing the omentum, once the colon has been separated from it, most surgeons do not continue the dissection back to the pancreas but break through the layers just above the colon. However, if the omentum is being taken as part of a D2 gastrectomy the dissection should be continued back to the pancreas and then proceed upwards to take the nodal tissue around the splenic artery.

On the right side as the omentum and mesocolon rapidly shorten they tend to fuse, so that the lesser sac in the region of the antrum of the stomach is often nonexistent and has to be recreated.

The right edge of the greater omentum finishes at the first part of the duodenum and passes upwards over the duodenum to form the free edge of the lesser omentum.

Immediately inferior to the termination of the greater omentum and fused with it is the mesocolon which is here shortening rapidly as the hepatic flexure of the colon becomes retroperitoneal. Thus to mobilize the greater omentum, the pancreatic head is hardly involved in the dissection. But to mobilize completely the mesocolon it is necessary to free the tissue overlying the pancreatic head. As the posterior leaf of the mesocolon tends to fuse with fascia over the pancreas, some care is required in this mobilization, particularly as small pancreatic veins from the head are found here draining to the left into the superior mesenteric vein.

Also in mobilizing the hepatic flexure and first part of the transverse colon off the duodenum and pancreatic head it is necessary to mobilize the root of the mesocolon to the left. Apart from the aforementioned pancreatic veins, as the dissection of the root proceeds to the left, middle colic vessels or their branches may lie in the root of the mesentery. Fortunately by the time such branches are reached the pancreatic head usually is sufficiently cleared to proceed with the transverse colon's removal.

On the left side the gastrocolic omentum is continuous with the gastrosplenic ligament.

The mesocolon shortens here also as the splenic flexure or first part of the descending colon becomes retroperitoneal. This makes dissection of this area one of the difficult points in colonic resection. Although the greater omentum is

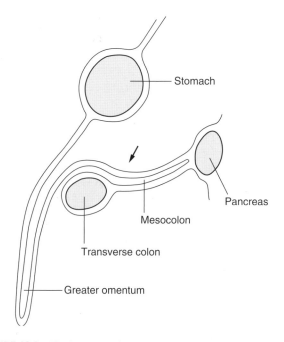

FIGURE 13.3 The formation of the greater omentum and transverse mesocolon. The solid arrow shows the point up to which the greater omentum is often taken in its removal with the stomach.

usually taken in colonic resections for cancer there is often no very good reason why it should be taken unless it is invaded by a tumour. In resections for benign disease the greater omentum should be preserved. If the greater omentum is first dissected off the left transverse colon it makes mobilization of this flexure easier to understand (although the omentum then tends to get in the way of the dissection). The blood supply to the transverse colon is through the middle colic artery. This nearly always arises from the superior mesenteric artery in the region of or just below the pancreatic head. It enters the mesocolon and usually tends to pass towards the right before dividing into right and left divisions which supply the right and left sides of the transverse colon. The point of division is variable but is usually from 5 to 7 cm away from the colon. As mentioned previously, in about 30% of cases the middle colic artery arises as a common trunk with the right colic artery.

Two quite frequent variations are shown in Figure 13.4. It seems that with the tendency of the middle colic artery to be to the right, it is the left side of the transverse colon which needs a helping hand, and it gets it in about 40% of cases with a second left branch being present. In a small percentage of cases the middle colic artery is absent and the transverse colon is then supplied predominantly by the left colic artery.

The operation of transverse colectomy is performed less often now as many surgeons prefer to extend a right hemicolectomy to include the transverse colon. The division of the blood supply to the transverse colon can be done in a relatively blind fashion by dividing the mesocolon from its small bowel mesentery side, or it can be done anatomically and more safely by dissecting the middle colic artery and veins from the lesser sac side. The lesser sac is most easily entered by dividing the phrenocolic ligament near the splenic flexure end of the transverse colon. Then the gastrocolic omentum is divided and the middle colic branches are best seen by transillumination of the mesocolon. The dissection of the trunk of the middle colic in this manner is somewhat timeconsuming but it is the safer and therefore better way to carry out the procedure.

THE DESCENDING COLON

Like the ascending colon, the descending colon has usually lost its mesentery and lies retroperitoneally. Occasionally it retains a mesocolon, although the attachment is usually short and volvulus of the descending colon rarely occurs. The acuteness of the splenic flexure sometimes means that the first part of the descending colon is overlain by the termination of the transverse colon.

The other important relations of the descending colon are posterior as it lies on the lower pole of the right kidney and then the quadratus lumborum and iliopsoas muscles. The greater omentum sweeps up over the splenic flexure and is continuous with the gastrosplenic ligament and the part that 'misses' the spleen passes back to the posterior abdominal wall – this part is called the phrenicocolic ligament and the anteroinferior tip of the spleen lies against it. It may be an important supporting structure for the spleen.

As on the right side, when the left side of the colon is mobilized the ureter and gonadal vessels may be encountered (see below) and they should be sought and safe-guarded.

The blood supply to the descending colon is from the inferior mesenteric artery. This arises from the anterior left side of the aorta about 3 cm above the bifurcation and runs downwards to the left in the retroperitoneal tissues. About 3 cm from its origin, i.e. about 3 cm below the lower border of duodenum, it gives off the left colic branch and the inferior mesenteric continues on into the pelvis as the superior rectal artery (see below).

The left colic artery is the major artery of supply to the descending colon (Fig. 13.5). It usually ascends obliquely and steeply to the left, alongside the vertebral column in the direction of the splenic flexure. It divides into an ascending and descending branch, usually within 2–3 cm of the colon. In a small proportion of cases (10%) an early branch passes

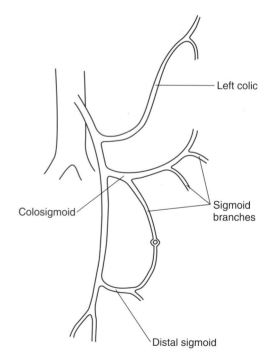

FIGURE 13.5 The left colic artery and blood supply to the sigmoid colon.

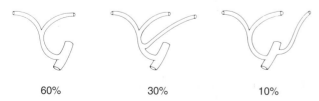

| 60% | 30% | 10% |

FIGURE 13.4 **Left:** The middle colic artery and its two divisions. **Centre, right:** An additional branch to the left side of the transverse colon occurs frequently.

in the base of the mesocolon to join the middle colic – it is called the arc of Riolan. In about 25% of cases a transverse branch to the descending colon is given off (Fig. 13.6). The left colic artery is absent in about 5–10% of cases, in which case an accessory left colic artery usually arises quite proximally on the superior mesenteric artery. This has surgical significance as it may prevent a mobilized splenic flexure having enough length to reach into the pelvis. The surgeon should be aware also that the marginal artery of the colon (see section on colonic blood supply, below) may be deficient in the region of the splenic flexure, so colonic anastomoses in this region should be avoided.

A left hemicolectomy necessitates the removal of the left colic territory and as this encompasses the splenic flexure in about 75% of cases, the left transverse colon should always be removed. The inferior mesenteric artery and its origin from the aorta are readily accessible and it is good practice formally to dissect this to find the left colic origin and divide it (the left colic) at this point. The descending colon is often taken along with the sigmoid colon down to about the sacral promontory, which means some sigmoid vessels are also ligated of necessity. This operation may be deemed a high anterior resection of the upper rectum.

THE SIGMOID COLON

This is that part of the distal colon which possesses a mesentery. The root of the mesentery is often described as an upside-down V. The apex of the V approximately overlies the bifurcation of the left common iliac artery. The left limb passes downwards alongside the left edge of the vertebral column and the right limb passes downwards towards the midline and terminates around the S3 level. Apart from the entry of the inferior mesenteric blood supply, the important relationship of the root of the sigmoid mesentery is the left ureter as it crosses the iliac vessels and lies behind the region of the apex of the mesentery.

It is very common to find the sigmoid colon partially attached to the peritoneum of the left iliac fossa – almost as a *forme fruste* of obliteration of the mesentery. However,

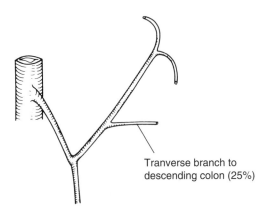

Tranverse branch to descending colon (25%)

FIGURE 13.6 Accessory left colic artery to descending colon.

separation of these congenital adhesions is nearly always a simple matter if they are divided immediately medial to the 'white line' and division allows the sigmoid colon to lie free on its mesentery.

The sigmoid colon receives its blood supply from two to four branches which arise from the inferior mesenteric artery in variable fashion.

The first branch is usually the largest and is called the colosigmoid artery by some authors. In about a third of cases it arises from the left colic and in the remainder it arises from the inferior mesenteric artery at a variable distance below the left colic origin. This vessel may be the origin of most of the sigmoid arteries, but there is usually at least one other sigmoid branch arising from the superior rectal artery (Fig. 13.5) about 2 cm below the level of the sacral promontory.

For the operation of sigmoid colectomy it is usual to divide the inferior mesenteric after it has given off its left colic branch. It is normally necessary to mobilize the left colon in order to carry out an anastomosis, but of course its blood supply is maintained.

ANTERIOR RESECTION

This operation is undertaken for pathology of the sigmoid or left colon (see Ch. 14). Proximal preparation of the bowel is as for left or sigmoid colectomy. The distal line of resection is the upper rectum and in doing so the vessels derived from the inferior mesenteric artery are ligated. If the inferior mesenteric artery is divided at its origin from the area it is called a high ligation. This may be done for two reasons. First to encompass completely the lymphatic drainage of the left colon and second to ensure adequate mobilization of the proximal colon so it reaches easily for a pelvic anastomosis without tension. If there is residual tension (and as a routine with some surgeons), division of the inferior mesenteric vein can be undertaken inferior to the body of the pancreas.

THE PERITONEAL WHITE LINES

At the right and left margins of the ascending and descending colon a white line is sometimes seen and this represents an excellent point of longitudinal division to mobilize the colon. The white line is formed by infolding of the peritoneum at the point where it leaves the colonic wall, i.e. where the peritoneum coming off the colon meets the parietal peritoneum, and there it represents the line of fusion of the former colonic mesentery with parietal peritoneum.

THE LYMPHATIC DRAINAGE OF THE COLON

Lymph nodes have been described in groups such as on the wall of the colon (epicolic), along the marginal artery (paracolic), along the various branches of the superior and inferior mesenteric arteries (intermediate), and at the origins of the main vessels (principal). However these groupings are somewhat arbitrary as in reality the nodes represent a continuum.

Although lymphatic drainage tends to follow the arteries of supply to the colon, blockage of lymphatic channels by tumour can lead to drainage to widely divergent areas, e.g. transverse colon to ileocolic nodes.

Most surgeons believe that it is reasonable to remove the immediately adjacent and perhaps next tier of lymph nodes, but do not carry out a careful dissection of all tissue back to the origin of the main vessel of supply (so-called high ligation). High ligation of the inferior mesenteric artery is at least feasible, i.e. ligation at its point of origin from the aorta, and the procedure has had its proponents over the years for cancers of the left side of the colon. High ligation of the middle colic artery is also technically feasible, although much more difficult as the origin often lies behind or within the pancreas. High ligation for the right side of the colon is only feasible back to the superior mesenteric artery.

THE NERVE SUPPLY TO THE COLON

The colon has a sympathetic and parasympathetic nerve supply. The sympathetic supply to the caecum ascending and transverse colon (proximal two-thirds) is from the coeliac and superior mesenteric ganglia with branches that pass with the arterial supply. The parasympathetic supply is from the vagus nerve. The distal third of the transverse colon and the left side are supplied by the lumbar part of the sympathetic trunk and the parasympathetic supply is from the pelvic splanchnic nerves (nervi erigentes). Although physiologically important these nerves are not surgically relevant. The hypogastric nerves at the pelvic brim are discussed in Chapter 14.

THE URETERS AND THEIR RELATIONSHIP TO THE COLON

The ureters pass from the renal pelvis to the bladder, behind the peritoneum, which in fetal life was the mesocolon to the respective ascending and descending colons. In the abdomen the ureters lie on the psoas muscles in front of the tips of the transverse processes. The gonadal vessels initially lie medially but cross obliquely in front of the ureters to lie laterally. The ureters enter the pelvis in front of the bifurcation of the common iliac artery.

The right ureter lies protected behind the duodenum above and below it is crossed by the right colic and ileocolic vessels where it lies retroperitoneally. Thus in mobilizing the right colon it is easy to mobilize the ureter as well, below the duodenum. If the surgeon makes sure that the gonadal

vessels lie with the retroperitoneal tissues then the ureter should be safe – even if it is not seen.

The left ureter has no such structure as the duodenum protecting it and it is crossed by the left colic and upper sigmoid vessels and at the pelvic brim it lies behind the apex of the sigmoid mesentery.

Thus on both sides the lower courses of the abdominal ureters are easily traced and they should be identified and so should not be at risk. The commonest site where ureteric damage or ligations occur is either near the lower pole of the kidney on the left or in the pelvis if anatomical relationships are distorted by pelvic masses, invasion or scarring.

In the pelvis the ureters lie against the lateral walls initially in front of the internal iliac vessels and then they turn medially across the pelvic floor to enter the bladder.

In the male they cross on the outside of the vasa deferentia to lie in front of them as they pass forwards to the bladder.

In the female the ureters lie immediately posterior to the ovaries then cross in the base of the broad ligaments where they pass behind and then under the uterine arteries. Thereafter the ureters incline more medially away from the cervix.

Thus in operations on the rectum where dissection is occurring within the pelvis, the ureters tend to lie anterior to the field of dissection.

THE COLONIC BLOOD SUPPLY WITH PARTICULAR REFERENCE TO CONSTRUCTION OF COLONIC CONDUITS

In colonic resections for cancer it is important for the surgeon to know in general terms the arterial supply and therefore the field of lymphatic drainage. However, variations are not of great technical importance as the surgeon can resect more colon if the blood supply is in any doubt, as long as adequate mobilization has been done to ensure a tension free anastomosis.

For colonic transposition the blood supply and variations to various areas assumes more critical importance. The pattern of supply to the colon is not dissimilar to that of the small bowel with feeding vessels forming a variable number of arcades which then give off straight arteries (to all intents and purposes end arteries) to the colonic wall. However many arcades are formed, it is the one nearest the bowel which is almost universally known as the marginal artery of Drummond. It is not necessarily of similar size at all sites around the bowel and it is often least well developed in the region of the splenic flexure. For this reason if a length of transverse and left colon is to be developed on the middle colic vessels it is considered wise to ligate the left colic artery well before its bifurcation as it is the bifurcation which most effectively acts as the marginal artery in this area. (It should be pointed out that such a loop would be antiperistaltic and only need to be fashioned in exceptional circumstances.) However the site where the marginal artery is likely to be absent altogether is between the ascending branch of the ileocolic artery and the descending branch of whichever artery is supplying the hepatic flexure and ascending colon.

This deficiency occurs in approximately 5% of individuals and a similar deficiency is occasionally seen, between the ascending branch of the right colic and the right branch of the middle colic artery. The middle colic artery itself is absent in about 5% of cases with the supply to the transverse colon then coming from the left colic artery. In view of the inconstancies of blood supply on the right side, the use of the right colon as a conduit may seem surprising. However dissection of the middle colic vessels and the right side of the colon is somewhat easier than left colonic mobilization, and furthermore the venous drainage of the right colon may be less prone to kinking, so that the use of the right colon continues to have its advocates, although less so today than a few years ago. In all colon preparations the greater omemum should first be separated from the colon. Most often today isoperistaltic loops of colon are used – right colon, transverse colon or left colon.

Right colon preparation

The mesentery of the colon is redeveloped up to the root of the small bowel mesentery to the left and the root of the mesocolon above.

The vessels to be ligated are dissected free. These are from proximal to distal: the arcades of the ileum (and the ileum itself), the terminal ileocolic artery; the right colic artery; the right branch of the middle colic artery (some surgeons would also include the marginal artery at the point of division of the transverse colon (see below)); the colon at the point of division. When these areas have been dissected free, vascular clamps on the arteries (bulldog clamps are used) and non-crushing bowel clamps on the bowel are applied to all areas to be divided. This means the arterial supply is now coming solely from the middle colic artery through its left branch and the marginal artery (Fig. 13.7). It should be possible to feel pulsation in the marginal artery at the level of the caecum and the colour of the small and large bowel should not alter.

Depending on the length of the colon needed and also on the length of the ascending colon, it may not be necessary to divide the right branch of the middle colic artery.

Transverse colon preparation

This is also based on the middle colic artery and is usually used when the length of colon required is not very long (Fig. 13.8). Occasionally and particularly if the transverse colon is long, it is possible to gain enough length to reach up to the neck. The areas which require dissection and ligation are the hepatic flexure of the colon; the ascending branch of the right colic and the marginal artery, if this is not the ascending branch (it usually is); the right branch of the middle colic; the colon proximal to the splenic flexure; possibly

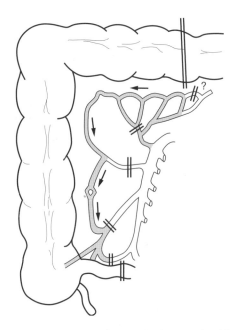

FIGURE 13.7 Construction of a right-sided colonic conduit. The question mark indicates that some surgeons do not think it is necessary to divide the marginal artery. The artery of supply to the conduit is shaded.

the marginal artery at the point of division of the colon distally (see below).

Left colon preparation

This is based on the left colic artery, and as it often uses more of the transverse than the left colon, some surgeons prefer to think of it as an extended transverse colon preparation. Nevertheless it is based on the left colic artery and so it is legitimately called a left colon preparation.

The points to be dissected, preparatory to division, are:

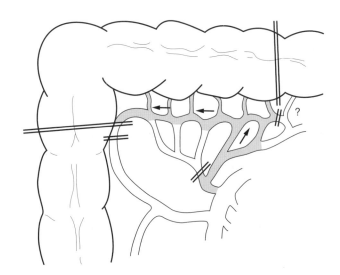

FIGURE 13.8 Construction of a transverse colon conduit based on the middle colic artery (shaded).

❶ The proximal part of the colon, and its marginal artery. It depends entirely on the length required as to where this point of division shall be: it may be in ascending colon, proximal transverse or mid transverse colon.

❷ If the point of division is to be in the right side of the transverse colon then it is preferable to ligate the middle colic, before its division into right and left branches. This is essential if there is only a single arcade, but if – as is more frequent – there are two arcades, it gives a double route for supply of the proximal transverse colon.

❸ The colon at a convenient point in the descending colon.

❹ Possibly the marginal artery at the point of distal colonic division (Fig. 13.9).

If the point of origin of the left colic is unusually distal it may occasionally be necessary to divide the inferior mesenteric vessel distal to the origin of the left colic. This is usually unnecessary but if carried out, the blood supply to the distal colon needs to be carefully checked as it will be receiving its blood supply from the middle and inferior rectal arteries (and possibly also from the marginal artery; see below).

DISTAL DIVISION OF THE MARGINAL ARTERY

The prime aim in the preparation of a piece of colon is to have an adequate length of well vascularized bowel to replace another organ, e.g. the oesophagus or bladder.

With this aim in mind it seems sensible to retain as much blood supply as possible and therefore in the first instance the distal marginal artery of the colonic loop being prepared should not be divided. The intramural anastomoses of arteries within the colonic wall are insufficient to allow removal of much more than 2 or 3 cm of its external blood supply. Thus the straight arteries supplying the colon from the marginal arteries should be treated as end arteries. Nevertheless this is usually sufficient length to allow the colon to be divided and the caudad end to be anastomosed to restore gastrointestinal continuity and the craniad end to be anastomosed to the oesophagus.

Keeping the marginal artery intact distally means that the length of the colonic graft in the abdomen can be tailored to the length required, so that redundancy does not occur. This tailoring is achieved by dividing the colon (but not the marginal artery) level with the point chosen for anastomosis. This technique inevitably means that the cologastric anastomosis and ileocolic or colocolic anastomoses are in close proximity to each other. If for any reason this is thought likely to raise a problem then a length of colon can be removed from the marginal artery, taking great care not to damage the marginal artery (Fig. 13.10).

If it is thought that the distal marginal artery is a major restricting factor in gaining enough colonic length then it can be divided.

VENOUS DRAINAGE OF THE COLON

The venous drainage largely follows the arterial supply, with the caecum and ascending colon draining via the superior mesenteric vein and the descending and sigmoid colon through the inferior mesenteric vein. This latter drains either into the splenic vein or the superior mesenteric vein.

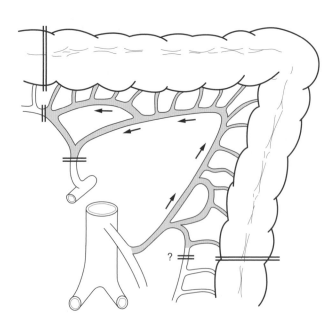

FIGURE 13.9 Construction of a left-sided and transverse colon conduit based on the left colic artery (shaded).

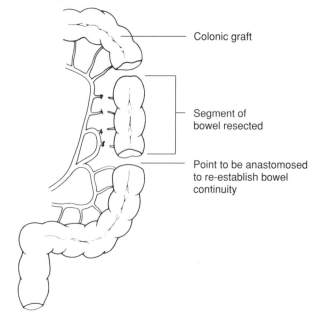

FIGURE 13.10 Tailoring a colonic conduit, and then resecting a portion to separate anastomoses from each other.

Therefore it is important that colonic transplants are not twisted nor kinked, nor have any abnormal pressure placed against their vascular pedicle. Infarction of colonic transplants seems to occur as often because of poor venous drainage as because of insufficient arterial supply.

THE LAPAROSCOPIC APPROACH

Laparoscopic colectomy uses sharp dissection along anatomical planes and requires the sort of detailed knowledge of anatomy of the colon and adjacent structures outlined in this chapter. Blood less dissection of the planes is essential for effective and efficient mobilization of the colon and its mesentery. There is significant discussion in the literature about medial versus lateral or superior mobilization of colon for cancer but to date no studies have demonstrated that any one approach offers a significant oncologic advantage. A number of prospective randomized studies have recently shown that the extent of resection, cancer recurrence and patient survival is comparable between the laparoscopic and the open approach but the former has a number of benefits including early return of bowel function, reduced postoperative pain, early discharge and reduced wound complications.

Use of non-traumatic graspers and minimization of handling the bowel directly during mobilization are important features in the laparoscopic approach which is associated with a reduced rate of postoperative ileus as compared to open surgery. A number of technologies also make the laparoscopic approach easier such as the use of the harmonic scalpel or bipolar cautery dissectors to aid in dissection and division of the mesentery and minimizing blood loss. Infra-red ureteric stents, which are not visible to the naked eye but are brightly visible with a three chip laparoscopic camera are helpful when dealing with difficult pelvic dissections.

Retraction of the small bowel to fully visualize the region of interest is usually aided by patient positioning and tipping side to side and head up or down which is often exaggerated compared to an open approach and requires measures to prevent patient slippage from the table. Also positioning of the surgeon and the assistants is often different from the open approach. Most laparoscopic colectomies can be performed with only one assistant who often stands next to the surgeon rather than on the opposite side.

Intracorporeal ligation and division of the vascular pedicles is performed using endoscopic stapling devices or clips which offer significant time saving. However despite all the technologies and lack of a large incision to close most studies have shown that the laparoscopic approach is associated with longer operating time than open surgery. Also the learning curve with laparoscopic colectomy can be as high as 50 cases. In very experienced hands the laparoscopic approach is associated with conversion rates of less than 5% and operating times no longer than an open approach.

Extraction of the resected specimen is through a 4–6 cm para-umbilical or skin crease lateral/suprapubic incision. Use of wound protectors during extraction minimizes the possibility of wound complications and facilitates specimen extraction and intraperitoneal return of bowel if an extracorporeal bowel anastomosis has been performed.

The laparoscopic approach offers the patient speedier recovery and reduced postoperative pain, enabling some centres to consider same day discharge for an operation (colectomy) which once was associated with a 7–10 day hospital stay.

FURTHER READING

Bourgeon A, Richelme H, Ferrare C, Candau A 1981 The anatomical bases of colon oesophagoplasty. Anat Clin 3:183–193.

De Meester T R, Johansson K E , Franz I et al 1988 Indications, surgical technique and long term functional results of colon interposition or bypass. Ann Surg 208:460–474.

Hong D, Tabet J, Anvari M 2001 Laparoscopic versus open resection for colorectal adenocarcinoma. Dis Colon 44(1):10–19.

Lacy A M, García-Valecasas J C, Delgado S, Castells A, Taurá P, Piqué J M et al 2002 Laparoscopy-assisted colectomy versus open colectomy for treatment of non-metastatic colon cancer: a randomized trial. Lancet 359:2224–2249.

Powers J C Fitzgerald J F, McAlvanah M J 1976 The anatomic basis for the surgical detachment of the greater omentum from the transverse colon. Surg Gynaecol Obstet 143:105–106.

The Clinical Outcomes of Surgical Therapy Study Group 2004 A comparison of laparoscopically assisted and open colectomy for colon cancer. New Engl J Med 350(20):2050–2059.

Van Damme J-P, Bonte J 1990 Vascular anatomy in abdominal surgery. Thieme Medical, New York.

14 | Anterior resection; abdominoperineal resection of the rectum; mesorectal excision: the anatomy of the rectum and associated structures

Glyn Jamieson and Robert Baigrie

THE RECTUM

The rectum commences in direct continuity with the sigmoid colon at the rectosigmoid junction. The precise point at which the sigmoid colon becomes rectum is established anatomically by: cessation of the mesocolon; cessation of the colonic haustra, and by a blending of the lateral and antimesenteric taeniae to form a flat anterior muscular band.

When related to the bony pelvis this junction is situated approximately opposite the body of the S3 vertebra, some 6 cm distal to the sacral promontory.

At operation, a more practical way of determining it, is to stretch the rectum lightly against the promontory of the sacrum. The upper limit of the 'surgical' rectum is measured from the anal verge using a rigid sigmoidoscope and is 15 cm from the verge, of which the distal 3 cm is the anal canal. Therefore the 'anatomical' rectum is approximately 12 cm long, and is divided into thirds for the purpose of planning surgery.

Initially the rectum descends in the midline following the sacral concavity and widens significantly in the lateral diameter. It is covered anteriorly and on both sides by peritoneum. As the rectum descends toward the pelvic floor its peritoneal covering becomes significantly diminished, and the peritoneal covering is reflected forward off the rectum onto the base of the bladder or uterine body. The middle third of the rectum is the widest part and lies on the anterior surface of the sacrum separated from it by the mesocolon. The lower third (4 cm) of the rectum turns forward prior to penetrating the levator ani. It lies on the superior surface of that muscle before abruptly turning backwards to penetrate the pelvic floor, ending at the anal canal. The mesorectum thins out so that it is virtually absent over the last 1 cm (Fig. 14.1). Division of the rectum at this level will result in total mesorectal excision provided the surgeon has not breached the mesorectum during the rectal dissection.

The rectum terminates and becomes the anal canal as it passes through the levator ani. At this point the muscle coat of the rectum becomes continuous with the sphincter mechanism. The anal canal is discussed in Chapter 15.

From an intraluminal viewpoint, the rectum has infoldings of the mucosa and muscle layer (the valves of Houston),

initially left, then right, then left again. These valves are very obvious on sigmoidoscopy. Their purpose is uncertain. As a result of the peritoneal reflection forward onto the bladder in the male and uterus in the female, the immediate anterior relations of the distal rectum are the seminal vesicles and prostate and the vagina respectively.

BLOOD VESSELS OF THE RECTUM

The superior rectal artery

This is the continuation of the inferior mesenteric artery and it runs in the base of the mesocolon. This shortens as the rectum

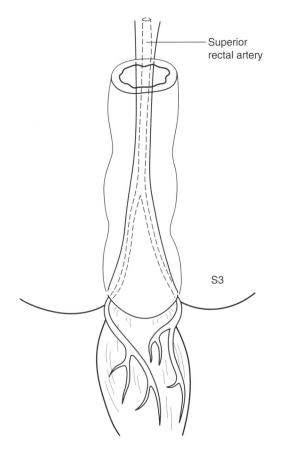

FIGURE 14.1 The peritoneal reflections of the rectum.

is approached, so the artery comes to lie immediately posterior to the rectum and it divides into right and left branches at a variable level, but in the vicinity of the S3 level. These give off branches which are closely applied to the rectal wall and supply the arteries which lie in the anorectal columns. There is an excellent anastomosis between the superior rectal and the lower sigmoid arteries of the inferior mesenteric artery, and also probably with the middle rectal arteries. Thus the superior rectal artery can usually be interrupted at any level without ischaemia of the rectal stump occurring.

The middle rectal arteries

These arteries arise directly from the internal iliac artery or from one of its branches, most often from the internal pudendal branch. One or other side is often absent. They cross to the rectum in the so-called lateral ligaments, and so they are divided during meso-rectal excision. They supply mainly the muscle coat of the rectum but anastomose freely with the superior rectal artery. These facts mean that the rectum can be safely mobilized to the pelvic floor, after division of the superior rectal artery, even though anastomoses between the inferior rectal artery and the other rectal arteries is rather doubtful. The middle rectal artery, when present, runs superior to the S3 nerve root.

The inferior rectal arteries

These arteries are not well named as they supply mainly anal structures. They arise from the internal pudendal artery and cross as one or more branches through the fat of the ischiorectal fossa to reach the anal region where they supply the muscle of the anal sphincter. It is doubtful that any anastomoses of consequence occur between these vessels and the higher rectal arteries.

VENOUS DRAINAGE

In broad terms the venous drainage of the rectum follows the arterial supply. Older texts divide the venous plexuses into an internal plexus, which is the plexus within the anorectal columns which drain into the superior rectal vein (the portal venous system), and an external plexus, which is the plexus of inferior veins which drain into the inferior rectal vein (the systemic venous system). There is no doubt that this anatomical description is correct and very rarely one can see varicosities of these veins in portal hypertension, as it is a watershed area between the portal system and the systemic venous system.

Dilatation of one group or other of these veins was then regarded as leading to internal or external haemorrhoids. However haemorrhoids are not directly related to these veins but are arteriovenous structures (cushions) in the region of the pectinate line. There seems little doubt that the veins and the arteriovenous structures have a complex relationship with each other as occlusion of the veins, in constipation or straining at stool, seems to be a definite aetiological factor in haemorrhoids (see below).

LYMPHATIC DRAINAGE

As with the rest of the large bowel the lymphatic drainage of the rectum follows the arterial supply so that the lymphatic drainage is first to perirectal nodes and thence to nodes along the respective arteries, reaching internal iliac nodes for the middle rectal and periaortic nodes for the superior rectal artery. It is generally regarded that lateral spread of carcinoma only occurs when proximal draining routes are blocked. There may be an exception to this as the rectum passes through the levators and for this reason it is usually recommended in resections for rectal cancer that the levators should be taken as widely as possible.

THE NERVES ASSOCIATED WITH RECTAL SURGERY

The hypogastric plexuses and related nerves

The superior hypogastric plexus is a fenestrated network of sympathetic fibres situated just below the aortic bifurcation. It connects above with sympathetic trunks while caudally fibres exit as the hypogastric nerves. These connect the superior hypogastric plexus with the inferior hypogastric (or pelvic) plexuses. The inferior hypogastric plexus connects with sacral roots from S3 and S4 and sometimes S2.

The hypogastric nerves are 2–3 mm in diameter and lie approximately 1 cm lateral to the midline and 2 cm medial to the ureters. They lie between the leaves of the endopelvic fascia (see below) and are adherent to the posterolateral aspect of the mesorectum. They are connected to the mesorectum by small unimportant rectal branches. Initially they lie superficially under the peritoneum and are at risk at the beginning of rectal mobilization. These nerves eventually migrate away from the mesorectum to the pelvic sidewall and inferior hypogastric plexuses. At surgical dissection, they do not present themselves to the operator. Rather, they need to be deliberately sought, and if not positively identified, they are often divided. This situation is not dissimilar to avoiding damage to the recurrent laryngeal nerve in thyroid surgery.

Nervi erigentes

These are the pelvic parasympathetic (splanchnic) nerves, which arise from S2–4. They pierce the parietal layer of the endopelvic fascia and fuse with the sympathetic hypogastric nerves to form the inferior hypogastric plexus (or pelvic plexus). This lies between the parietal and visceral layers of the endopelvic fascia lateral to the lower third of the rectum. Small rectal branches enter the mesorectum, providing parasympathetic supply to the rectum; however, most splanchnic fibres continue to the anterior visceral compartment, i.e. the genitourinary organs. For this reason the preservation of the inferior hypogastric plexus is very important during mobilization of the rectum, especially the so-called lateral ligaments.

The lateral ligaments

This is a misnomer, as no ligaments, per se, exist. Instead, the middle rectal artery and vein (branches of the pudendal artery and vein) send branches medially to pierce the visceral fascia about 4 cm from the midline, and enter the mesorectum. Outside the fascia, these branches cross the splanchnic nerves which are *en route* to the inferior hypogastric plexus. All these nerves and vessels are embedded in fat and fibrous tissue and resemble a ligament when the dissector pulls the mesorectum medially. This so-called ligament extends between the pelvic side wall and the mesorectum. The middle rectal vessels are usually absent or only small arterioles of less than 0.5 mm. However, in about 10–20% of cadavers they are as large as 1–2 mm in diameter. However, achieving haemostasis during dissection can result in diathermy injury to the splanchnic nerves. Ligation is even more likely to include nerve tissue and is usually very difficult and unnecessary.

Thus the lateral ligament is the complex of middle rectal vessels, splanchnic nerves entering the mesorectum, and their accompanying connective tissue. These form a band like structure extending from the pelvic side wall to the mesorectum. It is worth emphasizing that the splanchnic nerves and inferior hypogastric plexus are particularly prone to injury when this lateral attachment is divided during surgery.

THE FASCIA AND FASCIAL SPACES OF THE RECTUM (Fig. 14.1)

In many ways it is the fascia and its associated spaces which are the key to removal of the rectum, whether by anterior or abdominoperineal resection.

The two important fascial layers are the fascia of Denonvilliers in front and the endo-pelvic fascia behind (Waldeyer's fascia).

The fascia of Denonvilliers is a well developed layer which is adherent to anterior mesorectal fat rather than the wall of the bladder and prostate, or vagina (Fig. 14.1). It is attached to these structures by loose areolar tissue. There is divided opinion in the surgical literature about which side of the fascia the surgeon should dissect, but it does seem oncologically sounder to dissect anterior to it when resecting the rectum. The cavernous nerves run in neurovascular bundles at the lateral border of Denonvilliers fascia, and eventually run anterior to the fascia at the posterolateral border of the apex and base of the prostate. This is probably where most parasympathetic nerve damage occurs, and may explain why erectile dysfunction is more common with very low rectal resections.

Posterior to the rectum the endopelvic fascia of Waldeyer is a two layered structure which separates the rectum and mesorectum from the sacrum and various nerves are within or behind the fascia (Fig. 14.2). The two layers of the endopelvic fascia, visceral and parietal, are connected anterior to the 4th sacral vertebra by a short dense bank known as the rectosacral fascia. This connection to the sacrum probably anchors the rectum to the sacral curvature, preventing rectal prolapse. It is important not to avulse this band from the sacrum since it may be followed by troublesome bleeding from presacral veins. Instead, a bloodless dissection through the retrorectal space which lies between the parietal and visceral layers, will ensure an intact mesorectum. This plane is often referred to as the 'holy plane', a term coined by Heald (Fig. 14.2).

In the distal midline posteriorly, the visceral fascia becomes continuous with the parietal fascia and the endopelvic fascia passes off the sacrum and coccyx to line the pelvic floor so that it must be broached in this region during an abdominoperineal resection. It should be pointed out that dissecting the rectum from the perineal approach very easily takes the surgeon into the plane *posterior* to the endopelvic fascia with consequent damage to the splanchnic nerves. For this reason many surgeons no longer recommend a synchronous abdominoperineal resection. Instead full mobilization of the rectum is carried out by the abdom-

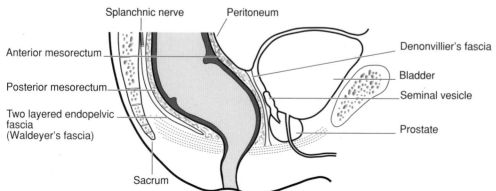

FIGURE 14.2 The fascia and fascial planes associated with the rectum.

inal operator before the perineal operator commences the resection from below.

THE PERINEAL MUSCULATURE AND RECTAL SURGERY

The perineal musculature is almost universally approached from below by surgeons and so it will be considered from this aspect.

The levator ani muscle

This is really a group of muscles with a similar nerve supply. The most posterior muscle is the iliococcygeus. This is a flat muscle which arises from the ischial spine and from the fascia over obturator internus – the arcus tendineus of levator ani. Its fibres pass transversely and backwards to insert into the coccyx and the anococcygeal ligament in front of the coccyx (Fig. 14.3).

The more anterior part of the muscle is the pubococcygeus which arises from the back of the pubic body and obturator fascia. Its fibres sweep backwards and are inserted into the pelvic viscera which pass through the pelvic floor. Behind the anus the fibres are inserted into the anococcygeal ligament. From the perineal aspect the most medial and most superficial fibres of pubococcygeus are the thickest part of the levator and they sling around the anorectal junction and are called the puborectalis muscle. The puborectalis can be quite clearly felt on digital rectal examination and furthermore these are quite clearly the thickest fibres which are encountered during the perineal part of abdominoperineal resection of the rectum.

The rectum and anus are intimately attached to the levator ani. The longitudinal muscle of the rectum gives off muscle as the rectourethralis (vaginalis) in front and the rectococcygeus behind. These blend with the subjacent levator ani. The puborectalis is blended with the deepest portion of external anal sphincter and sends fibres into the longitudinal muscle of the anus.

The levator ani is supplied by branches from the fourth sacral spinal nerve and the inferior rectal nerve from the pudendal nerve.

There seems little doubt that the puborectalis/external anal sphincter complex is the most important factor in rectal continence.

The anterior perineal muscles

These are insubstantial muscles but it is useful to know of them because they are landmarks in surgery of the area.

Many of them insert into the perineal body, which is a fibromuscular junction lying between the anus and the urogenital structures.

The transverse perineal muscles, superficial and deep, arise from the ischium and cross to insert into the perineal body. The bulbospongiosus arises from the perineal body and a midline raphe extending anteriorly. Its fibres surround the penile bulb and corpus spongosium or the vaginal orifice. The ischiocavernosus lies along the ischial tuberosity covering the penile or the clitoral crura.

They are all supplied by the perineal branch of the pudendal nerve (S2-4).

The perineal approach in abdominoperineal resection

It is usual to commence the dissection posteriorly as there are no important structures which might be damaged. An incision behind the anus is deepened until the tip of the

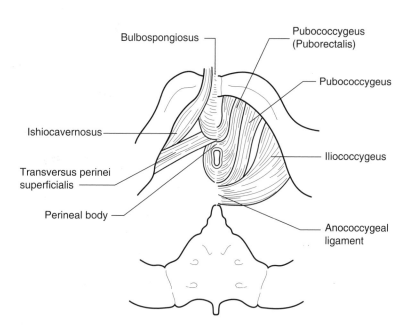

FIGURE 14.3 Perineal muscles involved in rectal operations.

coccyx is reached. Division of the anococcygeal ligament provides access to the pelvis on the superior surface of the levator complex. Provided the mesorectal dissection has been completed by the abdominal surgeon, the perineal surgeon's fingers can then be swept on the pelvic side of the levator lateral to the rectum, allowing division of the muscle with impunity.

Of course in order to reach the muscle the areolar and adipose tissue of the ischiorectal fossa must first be divided. This is relatively avascular except for the branches of the inferior rectal artery which cross to the anus. These are often small and usually cause inconsequential bleeding when divided. If a patient has had radiotherapy, bleeding here may be more noticeable.

In front the incision is deepened through the perineal body. The transversus perinei muscles are useful landmarks as the surgeon should stay behind the line of these muscles when deepening the excision. Certainly if the diverging muscle fibres of bulbospongiosus are seen the surgeon is too far anteriorly. The situation in the female is simpler because the dissection is between the anus and the vagina rather than between the anus and the urethra, as in the male. With anteriorly based tumours in females, the posterior vaginal wall is excised in continuity if there is thought to be any risk of involvement.

The most important points for the perineal surgeon to grasp is the necessity to stay in *front* of the presacral fascia posteriorly and to aim toward the sacral promontory after dividing the transverse perinei muscle. It is much safer for the abdominal operator to guide the perineal surgeon rather than allowing blind upwards anterior dissection.

FURTHER READING

Heald R J, Moran B J, Brown G, Daniels I R 2004 Optimal total mesorectal excision for rectal cancer is by dissection in front of Denonvilliers fascia. Br J Surg 91:121–123.

Havenga K, DeRuiter M C, Enker W E, Welvaart K 1996 Anatomical basis of autonomic nerve preserving total mesorectal excision for rectal cancer. Br J Surg 83:384–388.

Jones O M, Smeulders E M, Wiseman O, Miller R 1999 Lateral ligaments of the rectum: an anatomical study. Br J Surg 86:487–489.

Lindsey I, Guy R J, Warren B F, Mortensen N J 2000 Anatomy of Denonvilliers 'fascia' and pelvic nerves, impotence and implications for the colorectal surgeon. Br J Surg 87:1288–1299.

Van Damme J-P, Bonie J 1990 Vascular anatomy in abdominal surgery. Thieme Medical, New York.

15 Surgical procedures of the anus: the anatomy of the anal canal and associated structures

Glyn Jamieson and Nicholas Rieger

THE ANAL CANAL

The anal canal and anus are perhaps more bedevilled by confusing nomenclature than any other area in the body. Fortunately most of the anatomical controversies do not have a great deal of practical relevance and this account will use only generally accepted nomenclature.

At the outset it should be stated that the anal canal is that part of the bowel that commences at the termination of the rectum at the pelvic floor. Here it is angulated by the muscles of the pelvic floor, and passes backwards down to the cutaneous anal margin. It is 3–5 cm long and is divided into an upper part above the line of the anal valve cusps and a lower part below the anal cusps. The six to 10 columns of mucosa should be called anal columns and the valves at their lower limit constitute the pectinate or dentate line (Fig. 15.1). This pectinate line is situated opposite the middle of the internal sphincter.

It used to be taught that the pectinate line marked the junction of the embryonic gut and the dimple growing in to meet it, the proctodeum, the valves themselves representing remnants of the membrane separating these two portions – the proctodeal membrane. As a result, the anal canal was divided into a proximal portion which was endodermal in origin and a distal portion which was ectodermal in origin. Unfortunately this is unlikely to be completely true. It has recently been suggested that the attachment of the anal membrane undergoes differentially rapid growth and enlarges in area to become the whole of the 15 mm of the anal transitional zone; that is, the whole of the anal transitional zone represents the endoderm–ectoderm boundary.

In the newborn the pectinate line does delineate the mucosal junction between the stratified squamous epithelium below and the columnar epithelium above. With advancing age this border becomes less defined and stratified squamous epithelium often occurs proximal to the pectinate line. The epithelium of the anal canal can thus be divided into four regions. The proximal limit of the anal canal is at the level of the anorectal ring or levator ani. The angle between rectum and anal canal is maintained by the active contraction of the puborectalis loop. This proximal point is not marked by any apparent epithelial or developmental boundary. The epithelium consists of rectal type mucosa with mucus-secreting or goblet cells and columnar epithelium and this region is approximately 10 mm long.

This variably changes to the anal transitional zone (mentioned above) where the mucosa consists of stratified columnar or stratified squamous epithelium with islands of columnar epithelium within it. This lasts for about 5–10 mm and then changes at, or just below, the anal valves to the third region which is 10–15 mm long and is lined by thicker stratified squamous cell epithelium. It is essentially modified skin but is devoid of hair and sebaceous and sweat glands and it is closely adherent to underlying tissues. It is thin, smooth, pale and stretched and is known as the pecten.

This then gives way to the distal anal canal which is lined with hairy skin containing sebaceous and sweat glands and large apocrine glands, with this area extending to the distal limit of the anal margin. As a point of interest, squamous cell cancer of the anus should be subdivided into those tumours arising below the pectinate line and those arising above it. The tumours above the pectinate line arise from the anal transitional zone and, although they are all squamous in nature, they have been labelled by various names, such as basaloid, squamous, mucoepidermoid, cloacogenic or transitional according to the predominant cell type present in the tumour. These tumours are usually treated with chemoradiotherapy.

The pecten band is a term that was used to describe a so-called circumferential band of fibrous tissue situated between the skin of the lower part of the anal canal in the region of the pecten and the sphincter musculature, and was said to be associated with anal fissure and haemorrhoids. It is this band that is stretched deliberately or torn during an anal dilatation. However, no such fibrous tissue is apparent on histological examination of the area and the band probably represents no more than the rounded inferior border of the internal sphincter.

At approximately the distal limit of the pecten there is often a groove, which is readily palpable, known as the intermuscular or intersphincteric groove. It is produced by the space which lies between the end of the internal sphincter proximally and the subcutaneous portion of the external sphincter distally (Fig. 15.2).

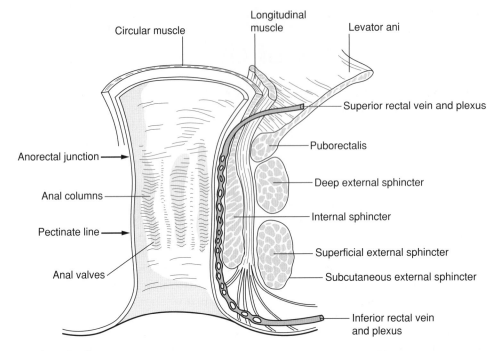

FIGURE 15.1 The anus and associated structures.

Hilton's white line is a term which should be avoided. It was said to be a line which marked the intersphincteric groove. However most evidence suggests that this line does not exist in reality.

THE ANAL GLANDS AND DUCTS

Some anal glands are confined to the submucosa but two-thirds have one or more branches which enter the internal sphincter and 50% of these pass across the internal sphincter completely to reach the intersphincteric longitudinal muscle layer. There are usually five or six glands per individual. Each gland drains via a duct into the base of the sinus created by an anal valve. They are not evenly located but tend to drain mainly into the posteriorly situated sinuses.

It is doubtful whether the anal glands have any very important secretory function.

Although not universally accepted, most surgeons believe that blockage of a duct from an anal gland is a major cause of perianal sepsis, including abscess and fistula formation.

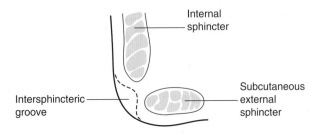

FIGURE 15.2 The intersphincteric groove.

THE ANAL SPHINCTERS AND SPHINCTEROTOMY

The internal anal sphincter

The internal anal sphincter is approximately 3 cm long and is an extension of the circular muscle of the rectum. This muscle tends to thicken as it passes distally. It finishes about 1 cm below the pectinate line and its distal margin is easily palpable digitally. Its smooth muscle fibres are grouped into discrete elliptical bundles. It is separated from the external sphincter by the longitudinal muscle and its ramifications. The resting anal pressure recorded manometrically is largely produced by tonic contraction of the internal sphincter. This is innervated by sympathetic nerves via the hypogastric (presacral) nerves derived from the fifth lumbar segment. Its parasympathetic innervation is derived from the sacral outflow via the pelvic splanchnic nerves. Older texts reported that sympathetic stimulation caused contraction of the internal sphincter. However, recent observations show that stimulation of the presacral sympathetic nerves causes relaxation of the internal sphincter. The rectoanal inhibitory reflex consists of internal sphincter relaxation in response to rectal distension. This was previously thought to be under parasympathetic control via sacral nerves. However, recent evidence suggests that the reflex is predominantly intramural, although subject to some sacral nervous control.

The longitudinal muscle

The taeniae of the colon widen and descend as the longitudinal muscle of the rectum. As this passes through the levator ani it gives off slips of muscle posteriorly (rectococcygeus muscle) and anteriorly (rectourethralis muscle – this runs to the back of the urogenital diaphragm at the membranous urethra and lies between the medial borders of the two puborectalis muscles; it has to be divided at the same time as the puborectalis in order to open up the plane between rectum and prostate). However, more importantly, the longitudinal muscle receives striated muscle fibres from the pubococcygeus part of the levator ani, so that some voluntary muscle passes downwards with the basically smooth muscle of the longitudinal muscle, which splits to pass on either side of the external sphincter.

The more substantial division descends between the internal and external sphincter in the intersphincteric plane. The longitudinal muscle here loses its voluntary muscle elements and many elastic fibres and some fibrous tissue fibres appear. The muscle ends with these fibres radiating as septa through the lowermost part of external sphincter to the pecten region and perianal skin. The fibres to the perianal skin are responsible for the puckering which occurs there and are known as the corrugator cutis ani. Some of these fibroelastic fibres pass directly through the internal sphincter and attach to the mucosa below the pectinate line and are called the musculus submucosae ani. One rather stronger band of longitudinal fibres passing directly from the inner aspect of the lower part of the internal sphincter to the lining of the anal canal just below the anal valves has been called the mucosal suspensory ligament.

Pulling down the mucosa as in a haemorrhoidectomy may thus pull the internal sphincter down as well. In addition, an anaesthetic causes relaxation of the external sphincter and so the lower end moves laterally. This may be the reason why it is the internal sphincter which is the muscle seen deep to a haemorrhoid in haemorrhoidectomy, when in fact in health it is the subcutaneous part of the external sphincter which is usually the most superficial muscle in the region. The musculus submucosae ani fibres also mean that the voluntary muscle of puborectalis is attached, not only to the longitudinal muscle of the anal canal, but also to the internal sphincter. Elevation of the levators thus elevates all the musculature of the anal canal and this no doubt aids in the expulsion of faeces.

The external anal sphincter

This muscle is derived from the posterior part of the cloacal sphincter and extends further downward than the internal sphincter. The lowermost portion curves medially to occupy a position below and slightly lateral to the lower rounded edge of the internal sphincter. Although traditionally divided into subcutaneous, superficial and deep parts, the terminology is not particularly helpful as there are no separate parts to the muscle, which is one continuous sheet. It is a somewhat cone-shaped muscle with the most distal part (subcutaneous portion) lying distal to the internal sphincter, and this portion has no ventral or dorsal attachments. The

middle portion (superficial) lies around the longitudinal muscle and the internal sphincter and is elliptical in shape and attaches posteriorly to the coccyx. The most proximal portion (deep) blends intimately with the puborectalis muscle and is itself encased by longitudinal muscle fibres running down on both sides of it. Its fibres decussate anteriorly to blend with the perineal muscles.

The external sphincter receives its nerve supply from the inferior rectal branch of the pudendal nerve (S2, 3) and from the perineal branch of the fourth sacral nerve. There is crossover of fibres so that unilateral transection of the motor fibres does not abolish tonic discharge. Stimulation of these nerves causes contraction of the external sphincter which thus, along with puborectalis, produces the anal squeeze pressure. Childbirth or chronic straining at stool may stretch these nerves, causing a pudendal neuropathy and this may result in faecal incontinence.

An anal fissure is a split in the anal mucosa. It is a painful condition which is thought to lead to spasm of the sphincters. Why overcoming the spasm by either stretching or division of muscle should lead to healing of the mucosa is something of a mystery – perhaps tight spasm of the area interferes with the blood supply and thus prevents normal healing.

Sphincterotomy may be performed closed (percutaneous), or open. A closed sphincterotomy away from the fissure deliberately seeks the intersphincteric groove to insert the knife, and then cut towards the mucosa, dividing the lower fibres of the internal sphincter.

The intersphincteric groove (and the lower border of the internal sphincter) is usually readily identifiable, but can be made more prominent if the patient is not given muscle relaxation and if a gentle anal retractor is used to put the sphincters on the stretch. An open sphincterotomy is performed via a perianal incision. The internal sphincter is visualized, grasped with an Allis forcep, and then divided under direct vision. Either procedure can be done equally well in the lithotomy position, prone jack-knife, or in the left lateral position. Classically, a sphincterotomy divides the internal anal sphincter to the level of the pectinate line. This may cause incontinence and hence a shorter `tailored' sphincterotomy to the upper level of the fissure may be performed, reducing the risk of incontinence, but increasing the likelihood of recurrence.

ANAL BLOOD SUPPLY, VENOUS DRAINAGE AND HAEMORRHOIDS

The inferior rectal artery supplies blood to the muscle of the anal sphincters and lower anal mucosa, whilst the superior rectal artery supplies the mucosa in the region of the anal columns. The middle rectal artery also supplies the wall of this part of the bowel, but the extent and significance of its contribution have been a matter of debate. The superior rectal artery is the direct continuation of the inferior mesenteric artery and travels in the root of the sigmoid mesocolon, giving off numerous branches before it divides into several branches which descend on either side of the distal part of the rectum. The paucity of the vessels on the anterior *and* posterior walls of the rectum has been advanced as a reason for the high leakage rate of low anterior resections. Mucosal branches of the superior rectal arteries are said to run in the columns of Morgagni, with those vessels in the left lateral and the right posterior and right anterior quadrants being particularly well developed. Reports about the extent of anastomoses between the arterial supply to the rectum and the anal canal vary in their conclusions. However, there is abundant clinical evidence that much of the rectum and the anal canal can survive the division of both the superior and middle rectal arteries.

The venous drainage follows the arteries. Older texts regarded dilatation of the submucous veins of the anal columns as responsible for internal haemorrhoids and dilatation of the veins below the pectinate line as responsible for external haemorrhoids. However, it now seems that haemorrhoids are not simple varices of these veins at all but dilated cushions of arteriovenous tissue which lie in this area and which are normally found at an early stage in development.

This would explain the bleeding of bright red blood which is seen in patients with haemorrhoids. The cushions are submucosal and comprise dilated blood vessels, smooth muscle and connective tissue. They are concentrated in the 4, 7 and 11 o'clock positions in the anal canal at or above the level of the anal valves. Thus the current hypothesis is that haemorrhoids are due to a breakdown in the connective tissue and smooth muscle which provided support for these cushions. This results in their prolapsing into the lumen of the distal canal.

There are also now good clinical data to confirm that there is no association between haemorrhoids and portal hypertension (although some patients with this condition do develop true varices within the anorectal mucosa).

If haemorrhoids are injected it is usual to insert the needle above the pectinate line as cutaneous-type nerve fibres are less likely to be found there. From 10 to 15 mm above the anal valves down to the boundary with hairy skin, the epithelium has a rich sensory nerve supply made up of both free and organized nerve endings. Touch, pinprick and heat and cold stimuli are readily perceived in the anal canal up to 15 mm above the anal valves. The sensitivity of this region of the canal has been postulated as a mechanism to aid continence by discriminating between fluid and faeces. Patients with neuropathic incontinence have been shown to have a decreased sensitivity of the upper anal canal. Furthermore, it has been suggested that this region of the upper anal canal should be preserved in the operation of proctocolectomy and ileoanal pouch in order to obtain better functional results.

THE LYMPHATIC DRAINAGE OF THE ANUS

The lymphatic drainage of the anus exhibits a curiosity. The upper anal canal and sphincters follow the normal rule of drainage following the arterial supply, thus draining to inferior mesenteric and internal iliac nodes respectively. However, the pecten of the anus does not drain to internal iliac nodes but follows the drainage of perianal skin to superficial inguinal nodes.

The pectinate line is a watershed area between lymphatic drainage to intra-abdominal and extra-abdominal nodes. There is some communication across the area and it is possible (although unusual) for squamous cell cancers of the anus to metastasize to internal iliac or inferior mesenteric nodes, and on rare occasions for carcinoma of the lower rectum to metastasize to superficial inguinal nodes.

16 Inguinal and femoral hernia operations, open and laparoscopic approaches: the anatomy of the inguinal and femoral regions

Glyn Jamieson and Guy Maddern

The anatomy of the inguinal region has received a lot of attention from surgeons with an interest in the area. However while it has been shown that some of the anatomy in standard texts is wrong, the corrections have often been couched in terms of a particular repair being advocated. This has led to a certain amount of confusion about nomenclature in the area. Perhaps the best example of this confusion is what actually constitutes the transversalis fascia.

The basic anatomy of this area is not difficult and many of the named fascial bands, e.g. reflected inguinal ligament, interfoveolar ligament, have no surgical relevance and will receive scant attention in this account.

Definition of the regions

The inguinal ligament is the inrolled lower edge of the external oblique aponeurosis and it is attached to the anterior superior iliac spine laterally and the pubic tubercle medially. Some of its medial terminating fibres tend to fan out posteriorly to insert along the pecten into other strong ligamentous fibres which lie along the pecten – the pectineal ligament.

The space deep to the inguinal ligament is divided into two by the strong fascia which lies over the iliopsoas muscle and which is called the iliopectineal arch (Fig. 16.1).

This fascia blends with the inguinal ligament in front and the pectineal ligament and pectineus fascia behind so that the only way under the inguinal ligament here is beneath the iliopsoas fascia, e.g. iliopsoas abscess. Medial to the iliopectineal arch is a space through which the iliac vessels pass into the thigh. It is here that the various types of femoral hernia occur. Inguinal hernias all occur above the inguinal ligament.

The external iliac artery and vein pass forwards and inferiorly from the retroperitoneal area to pass under the inguinal ligament. At this point the inferior epigastric artery arises and passes anteriorly towards the midline. It lies on the peritoneum in the extraperitoneal tissue which in this area some surgeons call the preperitoneal space. All of the fascial, aponeurotic and muscular structures lie in front of this plane. They will be described, building up the picture from within outwards.

THE TRANSVERSALIS FASCIA

This is the fascia which lines all of the inner side of the abdominal muscles. It is perhaps better characterized (and certainly more notorious) here than in other regions because it fills in the gap left by the transversus muscle below and also has some thickenings within the region. The distinction between the lower border of the flat tendon or aponeurosis of transversus and the transversalis fascia, which lines the posterior surface of the muscle, is not clear-cut and as aponeurotic fibres pass with the transversalis fascia to a greater or lesser degree, the stage is set for surgical and anatomical argument as to what constitutes the transversalis fascia in this region.

There are two thickenings often found in the transversalis fascia. The first is the iliopubic tract. This arises from the iliopectineal arch and tends to run parallel with but deeper than the inguinal ligament. It curves around the femoral vessels and femoral canal to blend with the pectineal ligament (Fig. 16.2).

It can be regarded as the inguinal ligament of the transversus/transversalis fascia, being the lower limit of the structure in this area. Below this point the iliopubic tract gives rise to the anterior and medial walls of the femoral

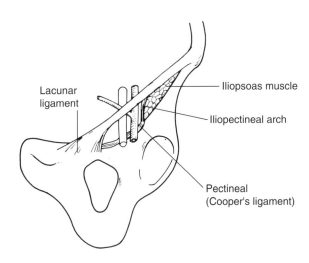

FIGURE 16.1   The left inguinal ligament and associated structures.

Lacunar ligament

Iliopsoas muscle

Iliopectineal arch

Pectineal (Cooper's ligament)

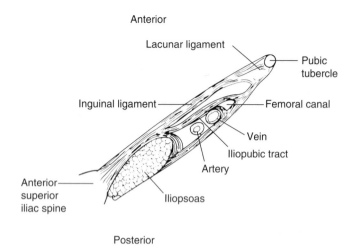

FIGURE 16.2 The left inguinal ligament and iliopubic tract seen from above.

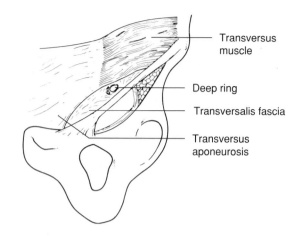

FIGURE 16.4 The transversus muscle and transversalis fascia in the region of the inguinal ligament.

sheath. The other thickening of the transversalis fascia is a sling around which the spermatic cord structures turn to enter the inguinal canal. This forms the superior and inferior pillars or crura of the deep ring (Fig. 16.3).

The transversalis fascia in the absence of any aponeurotic fibres from transversus is a definite but not very substantial layer. As one gets closer to the transversus tendon the transversalis fascia becomes a more substantial structure and, as mentioned, where the actual tendon begins is not definite. As we are talking of a distance of between 1 and 2 cm, i.e. pubic bone to transversus arch, arguments about nomenclature seem somewhat trivial. The point is that all surgeons who use transversalis fascia as a repair use a structure which is substantial and clearly holds sutures. They are not using tenuous endoabdominal fascia and whether they are actually using the aponeurosis of the transversus muscle (which we think seems likely) can remain an open question.

THE TRANSVERSUS MUSCLE

The lower part of transversus muscle arises from the iliac crest and outer third of the inguinal ligament (Fig. 16.4).

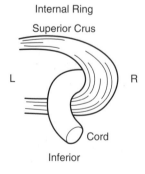

FIGURE 16.3 The crura of the deep inguinal ring seen from within. L = Left or lateral; R = right or medial.

Some authors suggest it is the iliopsoas fascia from which the muscle arises but as the inguinal ligament is fused with iliopsoas fascia in this region the distinction is not important.

The muscle fibres pass medially and give way to an aponeurosis about halfway across the abdomen. In the lower abdomen they join with the aponeurosis of internal oblique to pass in front of the rectus muscle as the anterior layer of the rectus sheath.

The lowermost part of the muscle arches downwards as well as medially and the aponeurosis is inserted into the pubic crest and ramus to a somewhat variable extent. Older anatomy texts suggested that the transversus aponeurosis usually fused with the internal oblique aponeurosis in this region to form a conjoint tendon. However fusion other than the aponeurosis forming the rectus sheath is rare, and the term should be dropped. Whether there is any need to use the term falx inguinalis for the fibres of transversus aponeurosis which sometimes insert into the pubic ramus is a moot point. Once again aponeurotic fibres blending with the transversalis fascia tend to blur the lower limit of transversus. It is probably best to regard the transversalis fascia as a direct extension of the transversus muscle and aponeurosis, thinking of it as the transversus musculoaponeurotic layer. This layer is then strong where muscle and aponeurosis are well formed but progressively weaker as muscle and aponeurosis give way to fascia. The testis in its descent never manages to penetrate this layer which it pushes in front of itself. However the testis traverses beneath the arching muscle fibres of transversus so that the layer it takes with it is fascia! and surrounds the cord and testis; it is called the internal spermatic fascia.

THE INTERNAL OBLIQUE MUSCLE

The lower fibres of the internal oblique muscle also arise from the iliac crest and the lateral half of the inguinal ligament or, perhaps more correctly, the iliopsoas fascia. Like transversus they arch medially and downwards and form an aponeurosis more medially than transversus (so that in the inguinal region this layer is mainly muscular). It blends with the transversus aponeurosis forming the anterior sheath of the rectus muscle. The lowermost fibres also may insert into the pubic crest and ramus, but here they are nearly always more medial and separate from the aponeurosis of transversus.

Because of the more medial origin of the muscle the testis has to push through the muscle and its fascia in its descent. Therefore once again it merely pushes muscle and fascia in front of it as the cremasteric muscle and fascia (Fig. 16.5). Usually the testis pushes through the lowermost fibres of internal oblique so that the cremaster muscle predominates on the anterior surface of the cord, but sometimes it pushes through slightly higher, leaving internal oblique muscle below the cord. These fibres travel parallel with the inguinal ligament and give way to aponeurotic fibres at a variable point. They can make the lowermost margin of the inguinal ligament difficult to define – the fibres can be confused with the inguinal ligament.

THE EXTERNAL OBLIQUE MUSCLE

In its inguinal part the external oblique muscle is entirely aponeurotic. As the fibres pass downwards and medially they split to form a triangular opening – the superficial inguinal ring. The upper of the margins is called the medial crus and the lower the lateral crus. The lower limit of the lateral crus is really the inguinal ligament at the point where it inserts into the pubic tubercle. The triangle is not as distinct as it might be for two reasons. First transverse fibres, called intercrural fibres, tend to truncate it by binding the apical portion of the crura together. Second there is a fascial layer which covers the external oblique muscle, including this ring. Therefore the testis in its descent through the external ring has to push this layer as well; this is the final covering of the cord – the external spermatic fascia.

The lower edge of the external oblique aponeurosis forms the inguinal ligament which runs from the anterior superior

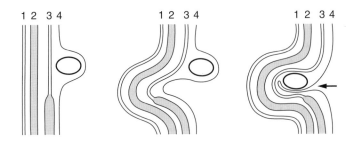

FIGURE 16.5 This shows how the testis pushes the abdominal wall layers in front of itself, thus producing the coverings of the spermatic cord. (**1**) External oblique aponeurosis (giving rise to external spermatic fascia); (**2**) internal oblique muscle (giving rise to cremaster muscle); (**3**) transversalis fascia (giving rise to internal spermatic fascia); (**4**) peritoneum (giving rise to the processus vaginalis).

iliac spine to the pubic tubercle. It is folded inwards with the concavity directed upwards. It is not a cord-like structure, as is often depicted, but a rather flat band. It is not free-lying but intimately attached to the fascia over iliopsoas laterally and the fascia lata of the thigh medially. Although its main insertion is into the pubic tubercle some fibres pass backwards to insert into the pecten. These fibres constitute the lacunar ligament – so named because it forms the most medial boundary of the vascular lacuna or opening through which the iliac vessels pass. The more direct boundary is the iliopubic tract as it curves posteriorly (Fig. 16.2).

The extension of tissue laterally from the lacunar ligament along the pecten of the pubis is known as the pectineal ligament. This is a very thick, tough fibrous band and consequently holds stitches well. The pectineus muscle and its fascia arise from it.

THE DEEP INGUINAL RING

This is the point of entry of the spermatic cord structures into the inguinal canal. As already pointed out, the testis and its cord in one sense do not leave the abdominal cavity at all – they just push the structures in front and so make the scrotum an extension of the abdomen.

The deep ring lies below the arching transversus muscle but behind the internal oblique. Because the spermatic cord structures hook medially (Fig. 16.3), the fascia tends to be heaped up as superior and inferior crura as already mentioned. The inferior epigastric artery rises vertically directly medial to the deep ring and also occasionally inconsequential tissue – dignified unnecessarily with the name the interfoveolar ligament – lies medially.

The condensation of the transversalis fascia called the iliopubic tract runs below the ring. It is clear that there is not really a ring at all but an area where the cord enters the canal. This area has quite well developed upper and lower boundaries, a less well developed medial and no lateral boundary at all to speak of.

The surface marking for the deep ring is the so-called mid inguinal point, which is the midpoint of a straight line between the anterior superior spine and the upper end of the symphysis pubis. This point is slightly medial to and above the midpoint of the inguinal ligament.

THE INGUINAL CANAL

This is the area between the deep and superficial inguinal rings which contains the spermatic cord or round ligament and the ilioinguinal nerve.

Its anterior wall is formed by the aponeurosis of the external oblique muscle. As the cord usually passes through the lowermost fibres of internal oblique (acquiring the cremaster muscle), this muscle cannot also be in front of the cord.

The inferior wall of the canal is the incurved edge of external oblique and the iliopubic tract and lacunar ligament further medially.

Its posterior wall is transversalis fascia and medially the aponeurosis of transversus (if it inserts into the pubic ramus) and the rectus muscle.

The area between the inguinal ligament below and the rectus muscle medially and the inferior epigastric artery rising to meet the rectus laterally is often called the inguinal triangle (Hesselbach's triangle). The lower part of this triangle is the posterior wall of the inguinal canal and, as it is formed of transversalis fascia only, it is a point of weakness in the lower abdominal wall. It is through this weakness that direct hernias develop.

The superior wall of the canal is formed of the arching fibres of the internal oblique and transversus muscles.

THE NERVES ASSOCIATED WITH THE INGUINAL CANAL

The iliohypogastric and ilioinguinal nerves arise primarily from the LI nerve root and descend, piercing the various muscle layers as they do so. About 3 and 2 cm respectively medial and superior to the anterior iliac spine the nerves pierce the internal oblique muscle to lie between it and the external oblique muscle. The iliohypogastric nerve lies in the same plane as and runs parallel with the spermatic cord but about 1–2 cm superior to it, eventually supplying skin of the suprapubic area. The ilioinguinal nerve in a sense continues its same relationship by running on the cord lying on cremaster muscle between it and the external oblique muscle. Initially it is anterior to the cord and then inferior to it and it exits with the cord through or adjacent to the superficial ring to supply scrotal or labial skin and skin in the pubic region.

The genital branch of the genitofemoral nerve (S2, 3) enters the inguinal canal with the cremasteric vessels and lies posterior to the cord. It also emerges from the superficial ring to supply scrotal/labial skin and skin of the inner side of the thigh. It also supplies the cremaster muscle.

With their relatively superficial locations the ilioinguinal and iliohypogastric nerves are usually seen without difficulty, although if the cord layers are incised (or removed) then the ilioinguinal nerve is at risk and must be dissected free in order to protect it. It is also at risk when the superficial ring is being repaired at the end of the procedure, when a suture closing the external oblique can easily but inadvertently pick up the nerve.

The iliohypogastric nerve may only be seen if the upper external oblique flap is mobilized for 2 cm more. If a darn or mesh is used the nerve is at risk of being picked up by the superiorly placed sutures, or if a relaxing incision is made in the rectus sheath the nerve may be divided.

The genital branch is at risk unless it is identified running with the cremasteric vessels. When cleaning the region of the deep ring, the nerve is at risk of damage. Its division can lead lo some loss of labial/scrotal skin sensation and in the male can lead to a low-lying testicle.

BLOOD VESSELS OF THE INGUINAL CANAL

In the female these are all very small and of no importance and will not be considered further.

In the male the testicular artery arises from the aorta and traverses the cord to be the main artery of supply to the testis.

The cremasteric artery arises from the inferior epigastric artery and it supplies the cremasteric muscle and the cord surroundings.

The artery which accompanies the ductus deferens, the deferential artery, arises from the superior vesical branch of the internal iliac artery.

There is also a small artery which arises from the inferior epigastric artery called the pubic branch. It runs along the iliopubic tract and follows it around the medial margin of the femoral ring to anastomose with the obturator vessels. Occasionally this can be greatly enlarged, when it is called an accessory obturator artery. If it replaces the obturator artery it is called an abnormal obturator artery. While it can be damaged by operations in the area it should be noted that accompanying veins are often moderately large and they are also a source of haemorrhage on occasions.

The testicular veins make up a plexus called the pampiniform plexus which usually narrows down to a single vein by the time the deep inguinal ring is reached. The left testicular vein drains into the left renal vein and the right testicular vein drains into the inferior vena cava.

The cremasteric vein usually drains into the inferior epigastric vein and the deferential vein into the internal iliac system.

THE FEMORAL SHEATH

The femoral sheath is formed from the fascia which is adjacent to the iliac vessels as they exit under the inguinal ligament and become the femoral vessels.

Posteriorly is the pectineal ligament and below it the pectineus fascia. Because of the obliquity of the iliopsoas muscle mass the fascia covering this muscle forms part of the posterior wall also but it is mainly a lateral relation (Fig. 16.4). The anterior part of the sheath arises from the iliopubic tract part of the transversalis fascia. As this curves medially to the pecten it also bounds the medial part of the opening into the femoral sheath.

The sheath descends with the vessels becoming progressively narrower and eventually ending about 4 cm below the inguinal ligament by fusing with the adventitia of the vessels. Anteroposteriorly running septa divide the femoral sheath into three compartments. The lateral compartment contains the femoral artery, the middle the femoral vein and the medial compartment is the femoral canal.

THE FEMORAL CANAL AND THE FEMORAL RING

The femoral canal is empty of structures apart from some fat, lymphatics and a lymph node (Cloquet's or Rosenmuller's node) and the canal's function is said to be to allow expansion of the femoral vein, which seems highly unlikely as vein walls are not very elastic.

The femoral ring is the entrance to the femoral canal (Fig. 16.2) and it is bounded by the tissue of the femoral sheath which in turn derives from, or is intimately related to structures as follows. Anteriorly is the iliopubic tract of transversalis fascia and in front of it the inguinal ligament; medially the iliopubic tract as it turns medially and beyond it the lacunar ligament, while posteriorly is the pectineal ligament and laterally the femoral vein. The femoral ring is closed by a tenuous fascial layer and as the transversalis fascia actually forms the anterior boundary and wall there is only extraperitoneal fat between the ring and the peritoneum.

Note that when the femoral ring is expanded, as in femoral hernia, the more unyielding structures form its boundaries, i.e. the inguinal ligament in front and lacunar ligament medially.

The femoral canal is only about 1–2 cm long before its walls fuse.

When a femoral hernia occurs it is initially deep to fascia lata and so may be difficult to feel. As it enlarges it tends to protrude through the weakest area in the region, which is the region of the saphenous vein penetrating to the deep vein – the fossa ovalis. However the deep layer of the superficial fascia descending from the abdomen inserts into the distal margin of this fossa. Thus as a sac enlarges this fascial attachment tends to prevent the downwards extension of the sac so it bulges upwards. Therefore large femoral hernias can give the appearance of being above the inguinal ligament.

TESTICULAR DESCENT AND INGUINAL HERNIA

After the sixth month of fetal life the testis pushes its way through the abdominal wall, pushing the various structures ahead of it, as already mentioned. A peritoneal evagination precedes this descent and the peritoneum comes to cover most of the testis (Fig. 16.5).

This peritoneal evagination is called the processus vaginalis and it usually becomes obliterated during the first year of extra uterine life – except around the testis where it persists as the tunica vaginalis. If it persists either in totality or

in part, the potential exists for an indirect hernia to occur, as shown in Figure 16.6.

ANATOMICAL FEATURES OF LAPAROSCOPIC HERNIA REPAIR

While the anatomy is unchanged whether an open or laparoscopic approach is chosen, the perception and relevance of the anatomical features is different. The laparoscopic features are similar whether viewed pre-peritoneally or trans-peritoneally.

Umbilical ligaments – inferior epigastric artery

A pneumoperitoneum distorts normal anatomy as it stretches and inflates hernias and some ligaments and tenses parietal peritoneum. When viewed laparoscopically, the midline fold that arises from the dome of the bladder reaching towards the direction of the umbilicus is the median umbilical ligament. This is inconsistently present. More frequent, however, are the folds from the lateral pelvic wall proceeding towards the umbilicus. These are known as the lateral and medial umbilical folds or ligaments. Each medial ligament is formed by the obliterated umbilical artery which is the terminal branch of the anterior division of the internal iliac artery. The lateral umbilical folds are formed by the inferior epigastric vessels. Inguinal and femoral hernias usually lie lateral to these folds.

The inferior epigastric vessels

The inferior epigastric vessels usually lie lateral to the medial folds and are readily seen as they course along the lateral edge of the rectus abdominus muscle below the level of the arcuate line. The inferior epigastric artery can occasionally form a prominent peritoneal ridge (the lateral fold) but it is never as evident as the medial umbilical fold. The inferior epigastric artery along with the edge of the

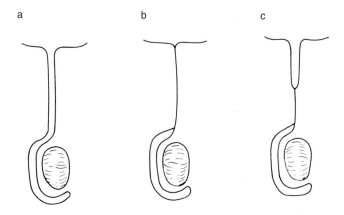

FIGURE 16.6 The processus vaginalis and inguinal hernia. (a) Congenital hernia; (b) normal; (c) indirect hernia.

rectus muscle and the unseen inguinal ligament complete Hasselbach's triangle, the boundaries of direct inguinal herniation. The inferior epigastric artery arises in the male immediately medial to the point of convergence of the vas deferens and spermatic vessels at the internal inguinal ring. At this point in the male are the external iliac artery and vein. The artery lies anterolateral to the vein; both disappear distally from view and have been described as the triangle of doom to warn against laparoscopic dissection in this region.

Nerves

Although not easily seen, nerves can be readily traumatized by dissection, staple, screw or suture. The lateral cutaneous nerve of the thigh lies on the iliacus muscle and is found midway between the anterior-superior iliac spine and the epigastric vessels then passes deep to the fascia iliacus and below the iliopubic tract. Fixation of mesh should be avoided in this region to avoid inadvertent injury.

The genitofemoral nerve trunk is located beneath the fascia iliacus between the spermatic vessels and the iliac artery and bordering the psoas. The nerve is smaller than the lateral cutaneous nerve of the thigh and bifurcates close to the deep inguinal ring, the femoral branch proceeding first laterally and then anteriorly to the artery beneath the iliopubic tract and entering the femoral sheath which it then perforates to supply sensation to a small area beneath the inguinal ligament. The genital branch passes from the anterior surface of the external iliac artery to pierce the fascia iliacus and into the inguinal canal where it lies on the posterio-inferior aspect of the spermatic cord. It supplies sensation to the lateral scrotal skin or labium magus.

The femoral nerve lies in a groove between psoas and iliacus muscles and is not seen during normal dissection in this region. It lies approximately midway between the genitofemoral and lateral cutaneous nerves. It is at risk from deep stapling or suturing in this area.

The ilio-inguinal nerve, although rarely seen in laparoscopic groin surgery, bears mentioning because it can also be injured by mesh fixation in this region.

FURTHER READING

Condon R E 1964 The anatomy of the inguinal region and its relationship to groin hernias. In: Nyhus L M, Harkins H N (eds) Hernia. JB Lippincott, Philadelphia.

Hughes D F R 1997 Anatomy, laparoscopic. In: Maddern G J, Hiatt J R, Phillips E H (eds) Hernia repair. Open vs laparoscopic approaches. Churchill Livingstone, London.

17 Operations on the scrotum and testis: the anatomy of the scrotum and testis

Glyn Jamieson and Colm O'Boyle

THE TESTIS AND ITS COVERINGS

In fetal life the testis develops on the posterior abdominal wall and it moves downwards into the scrotum taking the various layers of the abdominal wall with it (see Ch. 16). The testis is therefore surrounded by the coverings derived from the anterior abdominal wall, which are the same as the coverings of the spermatic cord, i.e. internal spermatic fascia, cremasteric fascia (there is usually no muscle around the testis) and external spermatic fascia. These various layers have little clinical importance other than the blood supply to the cremaster which anastomoses with the other vessels that supply the testis. The testis is preceded in its descent by an outpouching of peritoneum, the processus vaginalis, which it comes to invaginate posteriorly. Thus the testis and its coverings are in turn covered by the remnant of the processus vaginalis, the tunica vaginalis on its anterior and lateral borders. Posteriorly the epididymis sits above and behind the testis.

If the space between the layers of the tunica vaginalis becomes fluid-filled this forms a vaginal hydrocele which, if tense, makes the testis difficult to palpate, although the hard epididymis can usually be felt posteriorly. Other types of hydrocele result from differing degrees of obliteration of the processus vaginalis (Fig. 17.1). If the processus vaginalis remains completely open and there is free communication with a peritoneal cavity containing ascites, it is called a congenital hydrocele. If only a part of the processus remains patent it can form an encysted hydrocele of the cord. If the processus retains a communication with the peritoneal cavity but is obliterated at varying points above the scrotum, it is called a funicular hydrocele. And if the opposite – proximal fusion of the processus but open distally – it is called an infantile hydrocele.

The testis is covered by a dense whitish-blue coat called the tunica albuginea and beneath this is a filmy coat in which run many blood vessels – the tunica vasculosa. The tunica albuginea is thickest posteriorly where it penetrates into the testis as the mediastinum testis and gives off incomplete septa which radiate forwards. For this reason if the testis is to be decompressed it is best to divide the tunica albuginea on the anterior convexity of the testis.

Blood supply and collateral circulation of the testis

The blood supply of the testis is predominantly from the testicular artery, which arises from the aorta. The artery to the vas deferens from the superior vesical artery also contributes to the testicular blood supply and anastomoses with the branches of the testicular artery. The cremasteric artery (a branch of the inferior epigastric artery) and branches to the scrotal skin from the internal pudendal and external pudendal vessels also anastomose with the testicular artery.

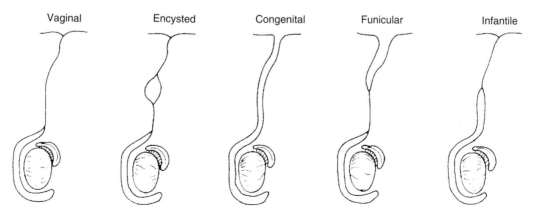

Vaginal   Encysted   Congenital   Funicular   Infantile

FIGURE 17.1   The processus vaginalis and different types of hydrocele.

If the testicular artery is divided within the peritoneal cavity it is uncommon for significant ischaemia of the testis to occur. Even after severance of the spermatic cord, and hence division of the major blood supply to the testis, it is unusual to get overt necrosis of the testis, although testicular atrophy will usually occur.

Venous drainage and varicocele

The testis and epididymis drain into a plexus of veins, which lie mainly anterior to the vas deferens, although a smaller plexus often lies posteriorly. These veins unite to form three or four vessels and then unite again and usually ascend in the cord as two veins where the veins usually join and continue into the abdomen where the left testicular vein drains into the left renal vein and the right testicular vein drains into the inferior vena cava. Within the abdomen the testicular veins may be single or double.

The veins in the spermatic cord (particularly the left side) sometimes become varicose, when they are known as a varicocele. Although it has been argued that cremasteric veins can cause a varicocele, this must be so unusual as to be discounted. The condition can be cured or greatly ameliorated by ligation of the testicular vein or veins at the level of the internal inguinal ring, although the need for surgery is uncommon.

Lymphatic drainage

The testis drains with the testicular vessels to para-aortic nodes. As the scrotal coverings drain to a completely different set of lymph nodes, it is surgical lore that testicular neoplasms should not be biopsied through scrotal skin. Rather the testis should be delivered into the inguinal region for direct-access biopsy, with a soft clamp applied to the spermatic cord.

The scrotum

The scrotum is divided into two compartments, each having a distinct blood supply and lymphatic drainage. The main distinctive feature of the scrotum is the presence of smooth muscle fibres in the superficial fascia – this muscle is named the dartos muscle. When it contracts, as it does under cold conditions or through stimulation of its nerve supply (the genital branch of the genitofemoral nerve), the skin is thrown into rugose folds and the testis is brought close to the perineal area.

The superficial fascia of the scrotum is continuous with the superficial fascia of the anterior abdominal wall so that any bleeding deep to that fascia in the abdominal wall can, and often does, track down into the scrotum.

The lymphatic drainage of the scrotum is to superficial inguinal nodes, and its nerve supply is the ilioinguinal nerve (LI) to the anterior third of scrotal skin and the poste-rior scrotal branches of the perineal nerves (S2–4) and the perineal branch of the posterior cutaneous nerve of the thigh to the posterior two-thirds of the scrotal skin.

THE SPERMATIC CORD

Torsion of the testis and vestigial elements

The spermatic cord is covered by the layers it acquires in its passage through the anterior abdominal wall. It contains the blood vessels and lymphatics already mentioned, the ductus deferens and a variable amount of fat. This latter can be quite marked and is sometimes described as a lipoma of the cord.

The ductus deferens tends to travel medially or posteriorly in the cord behind the obliterated processus vaginalis and the blood vessels. If a hernia occurs, the ductus and the blood vessels tend to lie behind an indirect sac.

There is often a high termination of the tunica vaginalis in patients susceptible to the condition of torsion of the testis, so that the testis is said to hang in the tunica vaginalis like a clapper in a bell.

When torsion occurs the testis turns but it is the twist in the structures of the spermatic cord which causes the vascular obstruction and consequent ischaemic necrosis of the testis.

The twist in the cord may be caused by excessive contraction of the cremaster muscle. The direction of twisting is said to be towards the midline anteriorly, so that viewed from below the right testis turns clockwise and the left anticlockwise. The significance of this is that if seen very early, within an hour of onset, untwisting of the cord has been recommended. This should not be regarded as definitive treatment but, if successful, allows testicular fixation to be performed with slightly less urgency. Although untwisting should proceed as outlined above, it is the alleviation of worsening of pain which should be the ultimate guide as to whether untwisting is proceeding in the correct orientation. The conditions leading to torsion are nearly always bilateral although an episode of torsion is usually unilateral. Therefore fixation of the uninvolved testis should be undertaken at the same time as detorsion and fixation of an affected testis.

Vestigial elements which can undergo torsion

There are three structures which are thought to be vestiges of the mesonephros and paramesonephros which have been described as undergoing torsion and causing testicular pain (Fig. 17.2). First is the appendix of the testis which is situated superiorly on the testis near the head of the epididymis. Second is the appendix of the epididymis which is found superiorly on the head of the epididymis, and third are some inferior aberrant ductules which are attached to the tail of

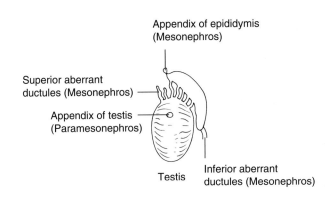

FIGURE 17.2 Vestigial elements in the testis.

the epididymis. There are also some superior aberrant ductules associated with the superior part of the testis in the region of the head of the epididymis. It is possible that these latter ductules can give rise to a collection of sperm-rich fluid in this region, called a spermatocele.

18

Adrenalectomy: the anatomy of the adrenal gland and open and laparoscopic approaches to the retroperitoneum

Glyn Jamieson and Lee Swanstrom

The adrenal glands sit on the upper medial poles of the kidneys and are contained within a compartment of the fascia investing the kidney – Gerota's capsule. However their position is not determined by the kidneys in that if the kidneys are ptosed or abnormal in position, e.g. horseshoe kidney, then the adrenals tend to be found in their normal position. In other words, their relationship to the inferior vena cava (right adrenal) and aorta (left adrenal) are the constants in their position. Apart from the blood supply, anatomic variations are unusual for the adrenals. Although the adrenals have a rich sympathetic nerve supply it is of little direct surgical or physiologic significance.

THE RIGHT ADRENAL GLAND

Perhaps emphasizing that the adrenals are independent structures from the kidneys is the fact that the right adrenal tends to be a little higher than the left adrenal gland, whereas the right kidney is normally lower than the left kidney.

The right adrenal gland is pyramidal in shape with its base lying against the upper pole of the kidney and usually well superior to the renal vasculature (Fig. 18.1). The plane of the gland is well posterior to the inferior vena cava, as a CT scan view indicates (Fig. 18.2). The gland lies on the diaphragm behind, and in front medially is the inferior vena cava and laterally the liver. The inferior leaf of the coronary ligament crosses it so that the lower surface is covered by peritoneum and the upper surface lies in the bare area of the liver (Fig. 18.1).

The right adrenal vein is usually short (less than 1 cm in length); it leaves the anteromedial area of the gland at the hilus and enters the posterolateral surface of the inferior vena cava. It may enter in a transverse direction or descend somewhat in direction. Occasionally it is longer and enters the inferior vena cava closer to the right renal vein. It is preferable to gently mobilize as much of the adrenal gland as possible before mobilizing the vein for ligature in adrenalectomy. This is particularly true in laparoscopic adrenalectomy when it is often the last substantial structure taken.

THE LEFT ADRENAL GLAND

The left adrenal is lower than the right. It is more crescenteric in shape and lies to a greater degree along the medial surface of the left kidney rather than superiorly. It is not uncommon for the inferior aspect of the gland to be close to or in contact with the left renal vessels. It is the opposite of the right gland in that its upper part is directly related to peritoneum (the floor of the lesser sac) whilst its lower half lies behind the pancreas (Fig. 18.1). It lies on the diaphragm which separates it from the aorta.

The left adrenal vein leaves the hilus near the middle of the anteromedial border. It runs downwards medial to the lower pole (but applied to it) and enters the left renal vein.

The blood supply and lymphatic drainage of the adrenal glands

There are multiple small arteries which supply the adrenal glands arising from above, below and medial to the gland. They all enter the gland peripherally rather than at the hilus.

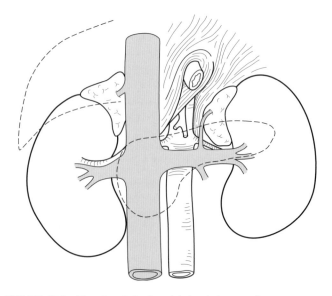

FIGURE 18.1 The adrenal glands and their relations to other structures.

The arteries are derived from the inferior phrenic artery above, the aorta medially and the renal artery below. The vessels are usually so small (less than 2 mm) that individual ligation is not necessary, and cautery or ultrasonic coagulation is sufficient in removing the gland. Occasionally one of the groups is replaced by a slightly larger vessel, particularly those arising from a renal artery. This can cause troublesome bleeding if divided without ligation and so should always be looked for in either adrenalectomy or mobilization of a renal artery.

The lymphatic drainage of the adrenal glands is to para-aortic nodes.

OPERATIVE APPROACHES TO THE ADRENAL GLANDS

The glands can be approached anteriorly, posteriorly or laterally by an open approach. Most surgeons use an anterior or lateral approach for laparoscopic removal of the glands.

The open anterior approach

This approach has the advantage of allowing both glands to be exposed through the one incision (either midline or bilateral subcostal) and allows exploration of the remainder of the abdominal cavity. It has the disadvantage of being the least direct approach to the glands (they are further away from the surgeon) and there is the attendant morbidity from the necessarily large laparotomy incision.

The right gland is approached by mobilizing the colon (hepatic flexure) and duodenum off the right kidney and

inferior vena cava and then incising the peritoneum in front of the inferior vena cava where it lies behind the foramen of the lesser sac. Although the adrenal glands are contained within a part of Gerota's capsule they are easily separated from the kidney. The glands are recognized by the brightness of their yellow colour which distinguishes them from the adipose tissue, which is in abundance in the region. The vascularity of the retroperitoneum and Gerota's fat make careful haemostasis important, as bleeding will stain the tissues and make identification more difficult.

As mentioned, the short course of the right adrenal gland's vein makes it the more difficult gland to resect, particularly as the superior aspect of the gland lies high behind the liver and inferior vena cava and within the bare area of the right lobe.

The left gland can be approached in a similar fashion by mobilizing the left side of the colon (splenic flexure) off the left kidney. However a more direct approach is through the lesser sac which is entered through the gastrocolic omentum. The peritoneum along the lower border of the pancreas is then divided. This takes the operator down to the left renal vein and the left adrenal vein. The adrenal gland is next sought by dissecting the adrenal vein proximally in the area between the aorta and the medial border of the kidney.

The anterior (antero-lateral) laparoscopic approach

Patients are positioned either supine with the left side propped about 45° off the horizontal, or in the left complete lateral position. The peritoneal 'white line' at the splenic flexure is divided to take the surgeon retroperitoneally and then the suspensory ligament of the spleen is divided and occasionally a little of the splenorenal ligament. This allows the spleen to fall medially and opens a space which contains the kidney laterally, the tail of the pancreas below and the left adrenal gland medially. It is worth emphasizing at least two points about this procedure. The first, as in other laparoscopic procedures, veins do not look blue as in open surgery, but white. Second, if a vein is divided without sealing, it may not bleed much, or at all, until the gas pressure is released.

The posterior approach

This is the most direct approach to the adrenal glands and is associated with the least morbidity. It has the further advantage that both adrenal glands can be exposed, either seriatim without moving the patient, or synchronously with two operating teams. Its disadvantage is that the exposure is limited by the ribs and the paraspinous muscles medially.

Because the approach is also a useful one to the retroperitoneum generally and can be used to approach some abdominal structures, e.g. spleen, tail of pancreas, it will be described in some detail.

The approach can either be through the bed of the 11th or 12th ribs (or occasionally through the bed of the 10th rib) or

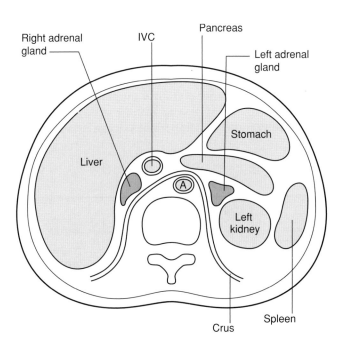

FIGURE 18.2 CT scan-type coronal section through the adrenal glands. IVC = Inferior vena cava; A = aorta.

just above the appropriate rib. In practice it does not matter very much, although removal of the rib tends to provide slightly better exposure.

Because the right adrenal gland lies higher than the left it is best to approach it with an incision over the 11th rib, while for the left adrenal gland an 11th or 12th rib approach can be used (Fig. 18.3).

Most surgeons find the anatomy difficult to visualize as they are more used to approaching structures from the front.

The latissimus dorsi muscle is divided in the line of the rib (Fig. 18.4). Depending on the degree of exposure required this incision can be extended into the flank muscles – external oblique, internal oblique and transversus. These muscles take attachment from the rib or its costal cartilage and have to be divided if a rib is removed.

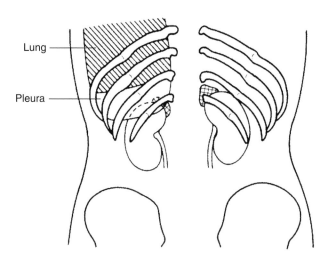

FIGURE 18.3 Relation of the adrenal glands and the kidneys to the ribs – posterior view.

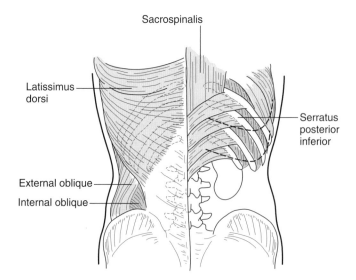

FIGURE 18.4 The muscles related to incisions approaching the adrenal glands or the retroperitoneum. On the right side the latissimus has been left out to show the deeper muscles.

Under latissimus dorsi, some fibres of serratus posterior inferior muscle are divided and the incision is extended medially until the vertical fibres of sacrospinalis are seen.

As shown in Figure 18.5, the pleura is related to the medial half of the 12th rib and to the medial three-quarters of the 11th rib. Therefore care must be taken if pleural damage is to be avoided. Because blunt dissection or pushing of the pleura away from the rib and the diaphragm often leads to a hole in the pleura, some surgeons prefer deliberately to incise it and then incise the diaphragm. Such a mini-intrathoracic approach adds very little to the morbidity of the procedure. Whichever approach is used, the next step is to divide the diaphragm which lies directly beneath the incision. While it is possible to remove the adrenal glands without division of the diaphragm, such division facilitates exposure, particularly on the right side, and is best regarded as an essential step.

During the procedure the neurovascular bundle should be sought as it lies below the 12th rib and the bundle is protected. The superior pole of the kidney is the only structure easily found by this incision and the adrenal is then sought in the usual way.

Laparoscopic posterior approach

A laparoscopic posterior approach is possible as well. It is particularly useful for bilateral adrenalectomy as performed for patients with Cushing's syndrome as sequential adrenalectomy can be accomplished without repositioning the patient. Because of the limited space with this approach, larger adrenal masses are considered a relative contraindication. Three ports per side are usually adequate, with the ports placed in a line 2 cm below the 12th rib. It is often helpful to use transcutaneous ultrasound to map out the adrenals at the beginning of the procedure to help with port placement and to help localize the glands once inside. Dissecting balloons help to create an adequate retroperitoneal space to manoeuvre in. Once the posterior portion of the gland is identified, it can be dissected out in the same manner as described above. Meticulous haemostasis is important as it can be very difficult

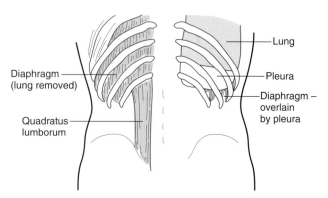

FIGURE 18.5 Relations of the lung, the pleura and the diaphragm to the ribs.

to identify the gland in the midst of the retroperitoneal fat if it becomes stained by blood.

Other approaches

The lateral approach is an extension of the posterior approach but while providing good access to retroperitoneal structures on the side undergoing operation, it produces more morbidity and precludes a bilateral approach without repositioning of the patient.

A thoraco-abdominal approach is sometimes advocated for large adrenal tumours but with adequate subcostal retraction such operations can usually be as well accomplished by an abdominal approach alone.

PART 2

GENERAL SURGICAL OPERATIONS IN THE THORAX

19 | Thoracic and thoracoabdominal incisions: the anatomy of the thoracic wall and diaphragm

Glyn Jamieson and Michael Griffin

Access to the left or right side of the chest is usually through an intercostal space or bed of a rib. Such access involves division of all or some of the flat muscles associated with the chest wall. These are the rhomboids, the trapezius and the latissimus dorsi posteriorly, laterally the serratus anterior and anteriorly pectoralis major and minor. The external oblique and rectus muscles also overlie part of the lower rib cage.

THORACIC WALL MUSCULATURE

The rhomboids

The rhomboid minor and major extend from the spine downwards to the medial border of the scapula. Rhomboid minor extends from the spines of C7 and Tl to the base of the scapular spine and rhomboid major runs parallel to and in the same plane as rhomboid minor from the spines of T2–5 to the medial border of the scapula down to the inferior angle (Fig. 19.1). These muscles are divided to a varying degree in the posterior part of the posterolateral approach, depending on how high the incision is taken between the medial border of the scapula and the vertebral column.

Trapezius

The trapezius is one of the flat muscles covering the thorax posteriorly and it is encountered in posterior or posterolateral thoracic incisions. It arises from the occiput and the spinous processes and associated ligamentous structures of all the cervical and thoracic vertebrae. Its fibres then sweep laterally downwards or upwards to insert into the clavicle, the acromion and the spine of the scapula (Fig. 19.1). Its nerve supply is the accessory nerve (the spinal portion), which enters it from the posterior triangle of the neck, and this supply is therefore not at risk in thoracic incisions.

Latissimus dorsi

The latissimus dorsi is the other major flat muscle of the back. It arises from the lowermost three or four ribs, the spinous processes of the lower six thoracic vertebrae, the lumbosacral vertebrae and the iliac crest. The fibres sweep upwards across the inferior tip of the scapula (where more muscle fibres may arise) and then pass in a spiral fashion around the lower border of teres major to insert into the intertubercular (bicipital) groove of the humerus (Figs 19.1 and 19.2). The nerve supply is from the thoracodorsal nerve arising from the posterior cord of the brachial plexus and this nerve supply is not at risk except during transaxillary approaches to the thorax.

Serratus anterior

The serratus anterior is a large muscle covering the lateral aspect of the thorax (Fig. 19.2). It arises by slips from the first eight or nine ribs and inserts into the superior angle, medial border and inferior angle of the scapula. The upper part of the muscle anteriorly is covered by pectoralis major. The nerve supply is from the fifth, sixth and seventh anterior rami of the cervical nerves which join to form the long thoracic nerve. This courses behind the brachial plexus and in the lower part of its course it lies behind the mid axillary line where it is relatively exposed on the surface of the muscle. It is therefore in danger during many thoracotomy incisions and is no doubt damaged or divided more often than is usually recognized. This probably produces little morbidity because only the distal two or three slips of the muscle are denervated. Damage to the serratus anterior can be minimized by keeping the incision as low as possible.

Pectoralis major

The pectoralis major is a large flat muscle covering most of the anterior part of the chest (Fig. 19.2). It arises from the clavicle, manubrium and sternum, the upper six costal cartilages and aponeurosis of the external oblique muscle. It inserts into the intertubercular (bicipital) groove of the humerus. Its nerve supply arises from the brachial plexus as the medial and lateral pectoral nerves and these nerves are not at risk during thoracotomy incisions.

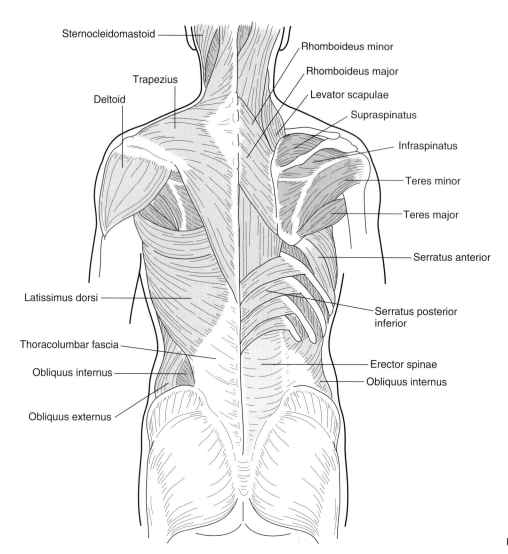

Sternocleidomastoid
Trapezius
Deltoid
Rhomboideus minor
Rhomboideus major
Levator scapulae
Supraspinatus
Infraspinatus
Teres minor
Teres major
Serratus anterior
Latissimus dorsi
Serratus posterior inferior
Thoracolumbar fascia
Obliquus internus
Erector spinae
Obliquus internus
Obliquus externus

FIGURE 19.1 Muscles of the back.

Pectoralis minor

The pectoralis minor lies deep to pectoralis major and arises from the third to the fifth ribs anteriorly and inserts it into the coracoid process. The nerve supply is from the medial pectoral nerve.

External oblique

The external oblique muscle has its origin from the lowermost six or seven ribs interdigitating with the serratus anterior where the two have a common origin (Fig. 19.2). It therefore covers the lowest part of the anterolateral thorax. Its nerve supply from the intercostal nerves is not in jeopardy from thoracic incisions.

The rectus muscle

The rectus muscle arises from the fifth, sixth and seventh costal cartilages and the xiphoid process and so it is not usually encountered in thoracic incisions.

THE THORACIC WALL

The ribs

There are typically 12 ribs although occasionally a cervical rib can occur (see Ch. 39) and even more rarely a 13th lumbar rib, somewhat picturesquely known as a gorilla rib – presumably because a gorilla has 13 ribs. Its only importance is that it can direct the surgeon too low in approaching, for example, the adrenal gland through an 11th or 12th rib incision.

The first seven ribs usually attach to the sternum via their costal cartilages while the remainder attach to each other through the cartilage which makes up the lateral half of the costal margin (the medial half of the costal margin is usually made up of the costal cartilage of the seventh rib).

When a posterolateral approach is to be made the surgeon's hand can be placed under the scapula to find the first rib for counting downwards. In other incisions the sternal

ing the intercostal space – the external anteriorly where in the region of the costal cartilages it is replaced by the anterior intercostal membrane and the internal posteriorly where it is replaced by the posterior intercostal membrane.

The transversus muscle may be represented by muscle fibres which lie deep to the intercostal neuromuscular bundle, the innermost intercostal muscle, and also the transversus thoracis muscle which arises from the deep surface of the lower half of the sternum and fans outwards and upwards to join the costal cartilages of the upper six or so ribs.

These muscles are usually either incised under direct vision or separated from their attachments by blunt dissection. These muscles assume their greatest importance in the raising of a muscle flap for bolstering various anastomoses within the thorax. A flap is fashioned by detaching the muscles from the rib above and the rib below from anterior to posterior. The feeding posterior intercostal vessel is maintained by entering the periosteum of the ribs to detach the muscles. This provides a long viable muscle flap for use intrathoracically.

The intercostal neurovascular bundle

The upper nine intercostal arteries arise from the supreme intercostal artery and the thoracic aorta. They anastomose anteriorly with anterior intercostals from the internal thoracic and the musculophrenic arteries.

The intercostal nerves terminate either as anterior cutaneous branches near the sternum (the upper six) or as nerves of supply to abdominal structures (the lower five and the subcostal nerve). The neurovascular bundle posteriorly lies about midway in the intercostal space, but from the costal angle on comes to lie in the subcostal groove of the rib above, where it is partly protected by the downward projection of the lower border of the rib. Like the nerves and vessels of the abdominal wall, it lies in the plane deep to the outer two muscles, i.e. the external and internal intercostals, between them and the vestiges of the transversus muscle. The intercostal artery lies between the vein above and the nerve below.

Thus in making an incision in an intercostal space, anteriorly it can be made in the middle of the intercostal space, but as one passes posteriorly the incision should be closer to the rib below, in order to avoid cutting the artery or damaging the nerve. If a rib is being mobilized, to enter the pleural cavity through its bed then, for similar reasons, the intercostal muscles are stripped off the rib's upper border. If the neck of a rib is excised the length of the accompanying intercostal nerve can be excised from the neck region and anteriorly. This may reduce postoperative thoracotomy pain.

The internal thoracic artery

This artery arises from the subclavian artery and passes downwards with its accompanying veins, about 1–2 cm lat-

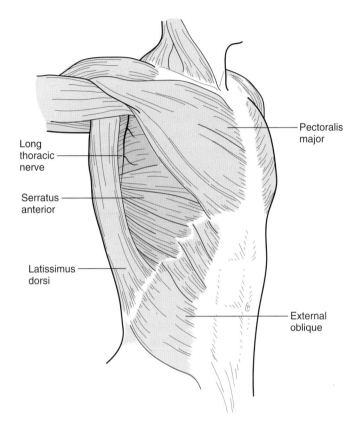

FIGURE 19.2 Anterolateral view of thoracic wall muscles.

Long thoracic nerve

Serratus anterior

Latissimus dorsi

Pectoralis major

External oblique

angle is sought and this lies opposite the second rib. The position of the sternal angle varies only very occasionally.

The ribs articulate posteriorly with the vertebrae and anteriorly with the sternum. The head of a typical rib articulates with the lower part of one vertebra, the intervertebral disc and the upper part of the vertebra below. It also articulates further laterally with the transverse process of the same numbered vertebra and the costotransverse ligaments are the limiting factor posteriorly in dividing the tissue between the ribs. In fact the lateral border of the costotransverse ligament is thick and strong and can be felt as a landmark for the posterior extent of the division of the intercostal muscles in any thoracotomy. Resection of the neck of the rib in a posterolateral thoracotomy can give wider exposure in the chest.

As the ribs are arched (a rib has been likened to a bucket handle), if all but their anterior and posterior attachments are divided, they can he spread to a considerable degree without breaking.

The intercostal spaces

The external intercostal muscle runs obliquely from the rib above to the rib below with its fibres running in the same direction as the fibres of the external oblique muscle. The internal intercostal runs obliquely from the rib below to the rib above with its fibres similar in direction to the internal oblique muscle. Both of these muscles are incomplete in fill-

eral to the sternal edge. At the sixth intercostal space it divides into the superior epigastric artery and the musculophrenic artery. It gives off mediastinal branches, perforating branches (of importance in mastectomy) and two anterior intercostal branches for each intercostal space. These travel along the upper and lower borders of the ribs bounding the intercostal space.

The artery is separated from the pleura through most of its course by the transversus thoracis muscle, except in the upper one or two intercostal spaces above the insertion of the transversus thoracis. Occasionally there is an aberrant branch which runs parallel but lateral to the internal thoracic, which may also require securing in opening an intercostal space anteriorly.

THE ANATOMY OF THORACIC INCISIONS

Posterolateral thoracotomy

The posterolateral thoracotomy incision is a standard approach for operations on the mid and upper thorax. Because the aortic arch curves across the oesophagus in the left chest the right-sided approach is preferable for approaching mid and upper oesophageal lesions. Some surgeons prefer the left approach because of its better exposure of the distal oesophagus and the proximal stomach. The patient is placed in the lateral position with the side to be entered uppermost. The upper arm is lifted towards the head and placed on a rest. A standard incision links three points: the first, three fingers' breadth below the nipple, the second two fingers' breadth below the inferior angle of the scapula and the third the midpoint between the medial border of the scapula and the vertebral column. The posterior end of the incision may be extended upwards as far as is considered necessary (Fig. 19.3).

The muscles divided by this incision are, from behind forwards, the trapezius and rhomboids, latissimus dorsi and serratus anterior. The division of pectoralis major depends on how far anteriorly the incision is taken. Care is taken to divide the serratus anterior as close as possible to its origin from the rib cage in order to minimize functional loss. The object of a lateral thoracotomy is to detach sufficient of the scapula from the chest wall to allow adequate exposure of the target rib or intercostal space. A scapula retractor can be used to improve exposure of the chest wall.

Once the chest wall is exposed four modes of entry to the chest are available:

❶ through an intercostal space;
❷ through a rib bed with excision of the rib;
❸ through a rib bed without excision of the rib;
❹ through a rib bed with excision of the neck of the rib only.

Personal choice on the part of the surgeon usually dictates which route is chosen. The ribs are kept open by some form of self retaining retractor such as an Omnitract or Finochietto.

Anterior thoracotomy

The patient is placed in a supine position with the side of the table elevated on the side of the operation. The arm is placed on an arm board in the mid abducted position.

In females a submammary incision is used. In males an incision is made over the interspace to be entered. For oesophageal operations this is usually the fourth or fifth interspace. The incision extends from the edge of the sternum medially to the axilla laterally. The obliquity of the ribs laterally is quite marked so that the incision needs to be directed superiorly as well as laterally.

The incision is taken through the pectoralis major muscle which is then reflected upwards with the skin. Coagulating diathermy (on a high setting) or cutting diathermy can be used to divide the muscles.

Division through the intercostal space is begun anteriorly at a point midway between the ribs and lateral to the inter-

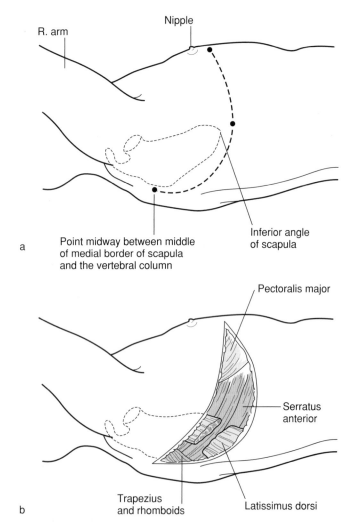

FIGURE 19.3 (a) Posterolateral skin incision; (b) muscles divided by this incision.

nal thoracic artery. The pleura is punctured with a blunt instrument. The incision is then taken posteriorly, keeping towards the rib below in order to avoid damaging the main neurovascular bundle.

The division of the intercostal musculature should be taken back much further posteriorly than the skin incision. In fact it is best to take it back to the unyielding costotransverse ligament arising from the tubercle of the rib posteriorly. The posterior reaches of the intercostal muscles can be divided by blunt dissection using a swab on a holder or can be done under vision from within the chest once the anterior portion of the incision has allowed entry to the chest.

One, two or three costal cartilages can be divided just lateral to the internal thoracic artery if it is necessary to improve access to the chest. Nevertheless, if rib separation is undertaken gradually over several minutes it is unusual for this to be necessary.

Thoracoabdominal incisions

The use of sternal retraction in abdominal surgery provides excellent exposure to the upper abdominal contents so it is not as common to perform a thoracoabdominal incision now as it was in the past. Nevertheless, the exposure of the upper abdomen obtained with a thoracoabdominal incision, is excellent and in difficult cases it is still an appropriate approach.

The skin incision begins anteriorly approximately halfway between the xiphisternum and the umbilicus and passes transversely to intersect the costal margin at the level of the seventh or eighth left interspace. The skin incision then follows the interspace obliquely upwards to about the mid axillary line (Fig. 19.4).

The rectus muscle and abdominal flat muscles are divided and the peritoneum entered. A 1 cm piece of the costal margin may be resected and the incision is continued back in the seventh or eighth interspace, keeping towards the lower rib. Depending on the degree of thoracic exposure required the intercostal incision can be taken further posteriorly than the skin incision, as for the anterior thoracotomy approach.

THE DIAPHRAGM

The diaphragm arises from the posterior surface of the xiphoid process, the inner sides of the lowest six ribs, from the fascial arches known as the medial and lateral arcuate ligaments and from the upper lumbar vertebrae via the crura. The muscle fibres pass centrally to insert into the central tendon.

The aortic hiatus lies between the two crura of the diaphragm and transmits the aorta and the thoracic duct and sometimes the azygos and hemiazygos veins.

The oesophageal hiatus lies in muscle usually of the right crus adjacent to the posterior border of the central tendon, a little to the left of the midline.

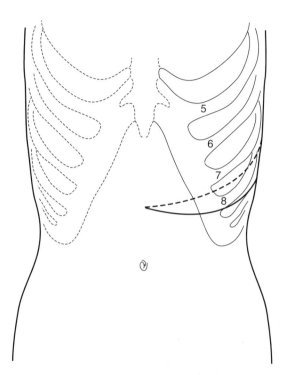

FIGURE 19.4 Thoracoabdominal incision through either the seventh interspace (interrupted line) or eighth interspace (solid line).

The foramen for the inferior vena cava is slightly to the right of the midline, somewhat anterior and superior to the oesophageal hiatus.

The motor nerve supply to the diaphragm is through the phrenic nerves (C3–5) which enter the diaphragm near the midline and supply the muscle in a radial fashion. The lower intercostal nerves supply some sensory fibres to the periphery of the diaphragm.

The major blood supply is from the inferior phrenic arteries which arise from the aorta just beneath the diaphragm and enter the diaphragm from its abdominal surface. The superior phrenic arteries are smaller vessels arising from the aorta in the thorax. Thus most of the blood supply comes from posteriorly.

An anterior blood supply comes from the musculophrenic arteries which are terminal branches of the internal thoracic arteries.

Incisions in the diaphragm

Major incisions in the diaphragm are usually made via the transthoracic route and it is important to remember that innervation arises centrally and passes peripherally. Therefore radial incisions may divide a part of a phrenic nerve and denervate a portion of the diaphragm, while circumferential incisions close to the rib cage are unlikely to cause any area of the diaphragmatic muscle to lose its nerve supply.

Usually the incision is from the left chest and the position of the patient is the same as for a left posterolateral thoracotomy. The incision is through the bed of the left seventh or eighth rib and the costal margin is divided in the same line. The pleura and diaphragm are now incised parallel to the costal margin and about 1.5 cm from it. The incision is taken from where it can be comfortably made anteriorly (about 5 cm from the sternum) to the region of the kidney posteriorly. Some surgeons advocate division of the peritoneum in a slightly different line from the incision to make separate closure of the layer easier at the end of the procedure, but the usefulness of this point has not been established.

Smaller incisions are often made in order to enlarge the oesophageal hiatus. This can be done by dividing the right and left pillars of the hiatus laterally. The division of the pillars should be made well posteriorly as the left hepatic vein is close to the right crus anteriorly and is in some danger if the division is made in a blind fashion anteriorly. The only structure of note on the left is the pleura and this should be swept off the pillar prior to division.

The hiatus can also be enlarged by anterior division. The muscle fibres prior to their insertion into the central tendon are divided. Once the tendon is reached care must be taken as it blends with the pericardium and it is preferable to avoid opening the pericardial sac.

20 | Oesophagectomy, open and thoracoscopic approaches; oesophagomyotomy, open and laparoscopic approaches; oesophageal bypass: the anatomy of the thoracic oesophagus and mediastinum

Glyn Jamieson and David Gotley

THE OESOPHAGUS

General anatomy

The oesophagus begins at the lower border of the cricoid cartilage at the level of the sixth cervical vertebra and it passes through the hiatus in the diaphragm at about the T10 level and terminates at about the T11 level.

It begins in the midline, curves to the left in the neck and superior mediastinum and then curves to the right below the bifurcation of the trachea. It then passes back to the left side as it enters the hiatus (Fig. 20.1). Three points of narrowing occur in the oesophagus: first, the upper oesophageal sphincter at the beginning of the oesophagus; second, where the aortic arch crosses the oesophagus and third, where the oesophagus passes through the diaphragm. These points lie very approximately at 15, 22 and 40 cm respectively from the incisor teeth and are the levels at which foreign bodies tend to lodge in the oesophagus.

Cervical oesophagus

This is considered in detail in Chapter 22.

The thoracic oesophagus

The thoracic oesophagus lies behind the trachea and its bifurcation. The left main bronchus lies in front of it. Below this level the oesophagus passes to the left, with the pericardium and left atrium in front, the thoracic aorta to the left, and the anterolateral part of the vertebral bodies to the right. More distally the aorta crosses obliquely to lie in the midline. The aorta is posterior to the oesophagus above the diaphragm and posterior and to the right of the oesophagus in the abdomen.

The right intercostal arteries cross behind the oesophagus and various accompanying veins, and occasionally the right subclavian artery crosses behind rather than lying in its usual distant anterior position. The thoracic duct also lies behind the oesophagus. The duct crosses obliquely, passing from the right of the posterior surface of the oesophagus to lie on its left. It is most usually directly posterior to the oesophagus at about the level of the arch of the azygos vein (as seen from the right) or the arch of the aorta (as seen from the left), at which point it is most at risk from damage during oesophageal mobilization. Distally the duct lies medial to the azygos vein, to the right of the oesophagus, and after it has crossed behind the oesophagus it lies medial to the left subclavian artery and to the left of the oesophagus.

The entire length of the right side of the oesophagus is related to the pleura, except where the azygos vein arching forwards separates it. Hence, division of the azygos vein and visceral pleura exposes the entire length of the thoracic oesophagus in the right thorax. On the left side the aortic arch and its branches lie between the oesophagus and the pleura above, but below the arch the pleura is in direct relation to the lower oesophagus. In fact posterior to the lower thoracic oesophagus the two pleural cavities almost touch so that if care is not exercised it is easy to enter the left pleural cavity when dissecting the oesophagus from the right side and vice versa.

The vagus nerves cross the oesophagus laterally on their course to lie posterior to the root of the lungs, and after forming a plexus around the mid oesophagus they usually emerge as two or more trunks which come to lie anterior (mainly left vagus) and posterior (mainly right vagus) to the body of the oesophagus. The left recurrent laryngeal nerve is also a lateral relation above the arch of the aorta. It can be damaged during dissection from the right chest where the nerve lies medial to the aortic arch and then between trachea and oesophagus more proximally.

OESOPHAGEAL WALL AND MUSCULATURE

The oesophageal mucosa consists of stratified squamous non-keratinizing mucosa overlying a lamina propria and muscularis mucosa, whose fibres are mainly running longitudinally. Deeper is the submucosa which contains

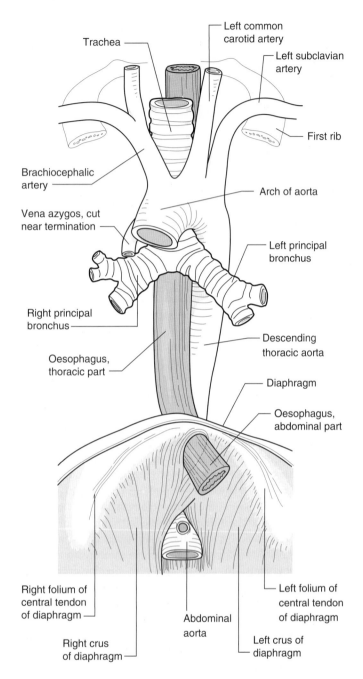

FIGURE 20.1 The oesophagus and its major relations.

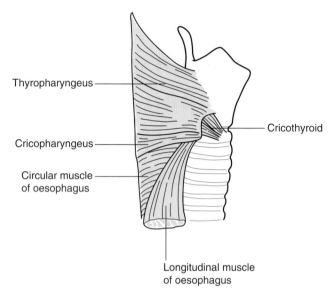

FIGURE 20.2 Cricopharyngeus and related muscles.

elastic and fibrous tissue. It is this layer which is usually regarded as the strongest layer of the oesophagus for holding sutures.

As in the rest of the alimentary tract, the oesophagus has an outer longitudinal and inner circular muscle coat. The longitudinal muscle arises from the back of the cricoid cartilage by a tendon which gives rise to two fasciculi which spread out to constitute the longitudinal muscle (Fig. 20.2). The circular muscle is a continuation of the cricopharyngeus muscle.

The oesophageal muscle is most uniform in its type in its lowermost portion where it is typical smooth muscle. As one ascends, more and more voluntary muscle is found so that the proximal portion of the oesophagus is predominantly skeletal muscle. As a generalization one can state that the lower third of the oesophagus is composed of smooth muscle, the middle third is a mixture of smooth and skeletal muscle and the proximal third is predominantly skeletal muscle. But note the word predominantly. The fact that a variable amount of smooth muscle is found in the proximal oesophagus has been the reason why some surgeons have advocated myotomy of the total oesophagus when surgery is used in the treatment of diffuse spasm – an affliction of the smooth muscle of the oesophagus.

There is little doubt that contraction of the longitudinal muscle plays a role in the development of a sliding hiatus hernia, and it is also responsible for the shortening of the oesophagus of 5 cm or more after division of the organ. After division of the oesophagus the muscle contracts so that the edge separates from the mucosa, which means that the mucosa protrudes beyond the muscle for 1 cm or so.

The loose connection between the mucosa and the oesophageal muscle facilitates the operation of myotomy in any region of the oesophagus. Sharp dissection can be carried down to the mucosa and a blunt instrument such as artery forceps or scissors can then be insinuated between the mucosa and the muscle and gently opened out. The plane is relatively easy to develop and the muscle can then be split longitudinally. The separation of the mucosa from muscle leads to the mucosa tending to balloon out through the myotomy.

At the distal end of the oesophagus in the region where it becomes difficult to be certain whether one is dealing with lowermost oesophagus or uppermost stomach (particularly on the lesser curve side), there is a slight muscular thickening which may correspond with the manometrically determined lower oesophageal sphincter. This thickening has been noted in anatomical studies but is not evident at operation.

NEUROVASCULAR SUPPLY TO THE OESOPHAGUS

Nerve supply

The skeletal muscle of the oesophagus is supplied by the recurrent laryngeal nerves and the smooth muscle receives parasympathetic supply from the vagus nerve and its plexuses and sympathetic supply from the sympathetic trunk and its ganglia and the greater and lesser splanchnic nerves. Within the oesophageal wall there are both myenteric and submucosal plexuses.

At the present time local myogenic and vagal influences seem to be the most important factors associated with oesophageal function and the role of the sympathetic nervous system remains to be determined.

Blood supply

Generally speaking the oesophagus can be divided into four regions in terms of its blood supply. The cervical oesophagus is supplied by branches from the inferior thyroid arteries; the thoracic oesophagus above the tracheal bifurcation is supplied by branches from right and left bronchial arteries; the infratracheal oesophagus is supplied by one, two or three branches from the thoracic aorta and the abdominal oesophagus is supplied by the left gastric artery.

However none of the arteries of supply are large and just about any artery in proximity to the oesophagus can give small branches of supply to the organ. While the arterial supply tends to anastomose freely, at least externally the weakest area of anastomotic linkage is between the aortic and bronchial regions of supply.

The fact that the inferior thyroid arteries anastomose freely with the superior thyroid arteries may be the reason why ligation of an inferior thyroid does not appear to jeopardize the blood supply to a cervical stump for oesophago-enteric anastomoses.

There is also a rich intramural network of anastomoses within the wall of the oesophagus which communicate with anastomoses in the wall of the upper stomach, which is responsible for the adequate vascularization of an oesophageal anastomosis even though as much as 4 or 5 cm of oesophagus has been mobilized from its bed.

There are at least two reasons why procedures such as non-thoracotomy, oesophagectomy and oesophageal eversion extraction can be carried out without encountering major bleeding. The first is, as already emphasized, oesophageal arteries tend to be small and many, and second they tend to arborize into even smaller branches outside the oesophageal wall, so that providing dissection is made close to the wall it is only these extremely small vessels which are divided or avulsed.

Venous drainage

The gross venous drainage is similar to the arterial supply above and below with the cervical oesophagus draining into the inferior thyroid veins and the abdominal oesophagus draining into the left gastric vein (the coronary vein) and thence into the portal venous system. The thoracic oesophagus drains into the azygos and its system of veins.

The venous drainage of the lower oesophagus has received a lot of attention because it is a watershed area between the systemic and portal venous system and therefore is an area where varices develop in portal hypertension.

There is a plexus of veins in the submucosa and also external to the oesophagus and these are in communication via perforating veins. However, there is also a plexus of veins in the region of the lamina propria, i.e. a subepithelial plexus which is more or less limited to the distal 5 cm of the oesophagus. It is these veins which enlarge and bleed as oesophageal varices. The limitation of these veins to the distal oesophagus probably explains why injection sclerotherapy of veins in the distal oesophagus is not always followed by the development of further varices more proximally in the oesophagus.

The lymphatic drainage

The oesophagus contains plexuses of lymphatic channels in its wall which communicate along its length and also with external channels which lie on the outside of the oesophagus and tend to run longitudinally, often for long distances. This explains the clinicopathological findings of satellite metastases and submucosal tumour deposits some distance from the primary tumour in some patients with carcinoma of the oesophagus. There are nodes associated with the oesophagus at all levels and although functionally continuous, they are loosely classified into anatomical groupings for descriptive purposes, e.g. paratracheal, hilar, subcarinal, para-aortic, paraoesophageal, etc. The free communication between the various lymphatic channels means that in a small proportion of cases with cervical oesophageal cancer coeliac nodes will be involved and similarly in a small proportion of cases with lower third oesophageal cancers, cervical lymph nodes will be involved.

Some surgeons set great store in resecting all of the lymphatic tissue associated with the oesophagus, but as the procedure is time-consuming and the benefit is yet to be established, the radicality of the approach has not gained general acceptance in the western world.

OTHER POSTERIOR MEDIASTINAL STRUCTURES WITH A RELATIONSHIP TO THE OESOPHAGUS

The azygos veins

These are a paired system of veins which are named the azygos vein on the right side and the hemiazygos vein on the left side. There are many variations in their anatomy, none of which are of much surgical importance. The most usual arrangement is that each vein is formed by the union of the subcostal vein and the ascending lumbar vein just below the diaphragm. The azygos vein lies posterolateral to the oesophagus on the vertebral bodies with the thoracic duct medial to it. It receives the terminations of the right intercostal veins on its right side, and some connecting channels from the hemiazygos and the hemiazygos itself on its left side. As it arches forwards over the root of the lung it receives the superior intercostal venous drainage, the tributaries of which usually unite to form a single trunk before joining the azygos vein.

On the left side the situation is similar with the hemiazygos vein draining the lower thoracic wall and the accessory hemiazygos draining the upper thoracic wall, both usually draining into the azygos vein in the vicinity of T7 and T8 respectively.

The azygos veins lie in front of the posterior intercostal arteries from the aorta.

The thoracic duct

The thoracic duct arises variably from the union of the paired lumbar lymphatic trunks and the single intestinal lymph trunk – these form the cysterna chyli. This and the thoracic duct arising from it lie just to the right of the aorta, and the duct passes into the chest through the aortic hiatus. At this level the thoracic duct lies behind and to the right of the oesophagus, between the aorta and the azygos vein, and as it ascends the duct crosses obliquely behind the oesophagus at about the level of the aortic arch and passes up on the left of the oesophagus into the neck and then arches away from the oesophagus at about the level of the inferior thyroid artery, passing behind the vascular structures and then downwards to end in the angle between the union of the internal jugular vein and the subclavian vein. There are many variations, but none of surgical importance.

If the duct is damaged at oesophagectomy the presence of damage may not become obvious until enteral nutrition is resumed, when lymphatic flow from the duct greatly increases and a chylothorax ensues or drainage from a chest drain increases. A leak from the thoracic duct will be more apparent intraoperatively if 100 mL of cream is instilled enterally during the early stages of oesophagectomy.

If damage is identified at the time of operation, usually the best form of treatment is direct repair or ligation of the duct above and below the damage. Because of numerous alternative lymphatic pathways ligation either at the time of operation, or at a later time, can be carried out with impunity.

The thoracic sympathetic trunk

The thoracic sympathetic trunk and its connections and branches have had a somewhat chequered career in surgical terms. Most ablative operations of the sympathetic nervous system have now passed into history, although with the advent of endoscopic surgery it is possible that nerve resections will again be used, particularly in controlling abdominal pain.

The thoracic sympathetic trunk begins at the T1 ganglion which is usually (80% of cases) fused with the inferior cervical ganglion to form the stellate ganglion which lies in front of and below the neck of the first rib. The trunk then passes down in front of the heads of the ribs and it usually lies in front of all the intercostal structures in the thorax and lateral to its corresponding azygos vein. The one more or less constant exception is the first (supreme) intercostal vein which usually lies anterior to it and, more variably, other intercostal veins may cross in front of it. It usually exits from the thorax beneath the medial arcuate ligament. There are usually ganglia corresponding to each intercostal nerve, although at the distal end the arrangement is less constant. Each ganglion gives off one grey and one white ramus to each intercostal nerve. The sympathetic chain and its section are considered in detail in Chapter 38.

The splanchnic nerves

The sympathetic trunk gives off three splanchnic nerves on each side as well as branches to the aortic, pulmonary and cardiac plexuses. All of these nerves show great variability but the most common pattern for the splanchnics is outlined below.

The greater splanchnic nerves arise from the fifth to the ninth thoracic ganglia and slope obliquely across the vertebral bodies to exit through the crura of the diaphragm. Most of their fibres pass to the coeliac ganglia while a few pass to the aorticorenal ganglia.

The lesser splanchnic nerves arise from ganglia 10 and 11 and the least splanchnics from the 12th thoracic ganglia. These nerves also exit through the crura of the diaphragm and their fibres are destined for the aorticorenal ganglia and associated renal plexuses.

It is reckoned that of the order of half of the nerves travelling in the splanchnic nerves are not sympathetic nerves but pain fibres from abdominal viscera. In order to be sure of dividing the splanchnic nerves completely it is necessary to remove thoracic ganglia 4–12 bilaterally. In the past, even in patients with intractable pain from cancer, a bilateral thoracotomy in order to achieve this was regarded as too formidable a procedure. However, with the advent of endoscopic surgery it is likely that such denervation procedures are due for a reassessment in the management of patients with intractable pain.

THE SUPERIOR AND ANTERIOR MEDIASTINUM AND RETROSTERNAL OESOPHAGEAL BYPASS

These spaces are of interest to the general surgeon mainly because of the occasional need to split the sternum or to create a space for oesophageal bypass.

The anterior portion of the superior mediastinum contains the thymus gland which atrophies to a variable degree after puberty. It is contained in a capsule which remains quite strong and which lies in front of the brachiocephalic vein and the great vessels in the root of the neck. It lies behind the upper sternum and the attachment of the sternohyoid and sternothyroid strap muscles. These muscles are invested by the deep cervical fascia which attaches retrosternally down to the manubriosternal junction.

The surface anatomy of the brachiocephalic veins is that of broad bands 1.5 cm wide which begin behind the respective sternal ends of the clavicle. The right is short, 2–3 cm long, and descends to finish behind the right first costal cartilage. The left brachiocephalic vein crosses obliquely behind the upper portion of the manubrium to end behind the right first costal cartilage where it joins the right vein to form the superior vena cava.

The left vein is separated from the left sternoclavicular joint and the manubrium by the sternohyoid and sternothyroid muscles, the remains of the thymus and loose areolar tissue.

The anterior mediastinum contains adipose tissue in front of the pericardium. The pleural reflections pass downwards behind the sternoclavicular joints, tending towards the midline and they come close together at about the level of the manubriosternal joint. Behind mid sternum the reflections usually diverge again – mainly because of the heart tending to push the left pleural reflection laterally.

When this space is to be used for the stomach, as in bypass of the oesophagus, it is entered below by dividing the slips of the diaphragm arising from the xiphisternum and developing the space by blunt dissection, staying close to the back of the sternum. The pleura is gently separated from the sternum also by blunt dissection. The plane so developed is anterior to the thymus (and therefore the brachiocephalic vein) but will pass behind the strap muscles and deep cervical fascia.

When the space is being entered above, the surgeon mobilizes behind the manubrium and this is anterior to the plane which is developed from below with the strap muscles and deep cervical fascia separating the two areas. This separating layer must be divided in order to have the two areas freely communicate.

The surface area of the thoracic inlet can be diminished substantially by the posterior aspect of the sternoclavicular joints, which therefore sometimes are excised.

The sternoclavicular joint and its excision

The sternal end of the clavicle, the manubrium and the first costal cartilage all take part in the formation of the sternoclavicular joint. The head of the clavicle has a significant posterior portion which juts out into the retromanubrial space, and can therefore compress the organ – usually stomach or colon – which is being brought up to bypass the oesophagus.

The joint has anterior and posterior sternoclavicular ligaments and also a strong costoclavicular ligament binding it to the first rib.

It is usually the left joint which is removed in oesophageal bypass. Providing the surgeon stays close to the bone there is no real danger to any vital structure in removing the joint. The left brachiocephalic vein is a direct posterior relation but it is separated from the joint by the sternohyoid and thyrohyoid muscles and the thymic capsule.

The fibres of origin of pectoralis major muscle in front, sternocleidomastoid muscle above and the sternohyoid muscle behind require division from the medial end of the clavicle. However it is the joint ligaments which provide the strongest attachment and in particular the costoclavicular ligament below and the anterior sternocostal ligament in front.

The corresponding half of the manubrium sterni and part of the first rib are usually removed as well as the joint.

MOBILIZATION OF THE OESOPHAGUS

The cervical oesophagus

The cervical and superior mediastinal oesophagus curves slightly to the left, making a surgical approach from the left side to the cervical oesophagus most appropriate. The omohyoid muscle and middle thyroid veins are usually divided. A plane is readily apparent between the carotid sheath and strap muscles and thyroid to the prevertebral fascia posteriorly. The oesophagus is found behind the trachea, and may be encircled at the thoracic inlet. The close proximity of the left recurrent laryngeal nerve to the oesophagus, ascending in the tracheo-oesophageal groove, demands meticulous care in this dissection.

The thoracic oesophagus

From the right side the only structure preventing the full mobilization of the oesophagus is the azygos vein and this can be divided without causing untoward effects. The root of the lung can be pushed away by dividing the pleural fibrous tissue envelope, called the inferior pulmonary ligament, which extends down from the root of the lung.

On the left side the oesophagus is slightly less accessible, but there are two areas above and below where the oesophagus is beneath pleura only. The superior area is a triangle formed by the vertebral column as a base, with the converging limbs the arch of the aorta and the left subclavian artery (Fig. 20.3). The inferior triangle is bounded by the aorta as the base and the diaphragm and heart as the converging limbs of the triangle.

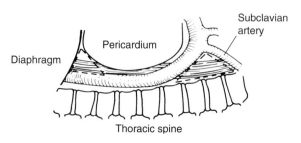

FIGURE 20.3 Diagrammatic representation of the surgeon's view of Zenker's diverticulum, showing the indenting of the lumen by cricopharyngeus.

The abdominal oesophagus

The abdominal oesophagus is covered by peritoneum on its anterior and anterolateral faces only. However, on dividing the peritoneum, the oesophagus is attached to the endo-abdominal and endothoracic fascias by the phreno-oesophageal ligament (see Chapter 10). If the oesophageal hiatus is difficult to delineate either in a re-operative situation or because of a bulky tumour, then division of the diaphragm immediately anterior to the hiatus will take the operator into the mediastinum, and this can allow for a safer mobilization of the distal oesophagus. It should always be remembered that the left hepatic vein is an important structure close by – particularly in situations where the anatomy is distorted.

THORACOSCOPIC PROCEDURES

Positioning a patient for thoracoscopic procedures such as oesophagectomy is similar in most respects to positioning a patient for a thoracotomy, with the exception of the prone position. Some surgeons like the prone position for operations on posterior mediastinal structures, as gravity causes the lung to fall away from the field. It is worth noting that the first time one sees the mediastinum with the patient in the prone position, it can cause the surgeon some cognitive dissonance, and it is worth constantly reminding oneself that the aorta is above (towards the ceiling!) and the hilum of the lung is below (towards the floor) the oesophagus.

As noted in Chapter 19, the neurovascular bundle lies about midway between the ribs posteriorly, and the further anteriorly it passes, the higher it lies in the intercostal space. Thus when placing trochars they should be placed as close as possible to the top of the rib below.

The space between the pectoral muscles in front and the latissimus dorsi behind is the part of the chest wall which has the least thickness of muscle, and chest entry with trochars proves easiest through this area.

For thoracotomies the approach to the mediastinum via the right or left chest is more a matter of the surgeon's choice than anything else. For thoracoscopic procedures the lower oesophagus is best accessed through the left chest and the mid and upper oesophagus through the right chest.

HEAD AND NECK OPERATIONS

21 | Head and neck incisions: the anatomy of cervical skin, musculature and cutaneous nerves

Glyn Jamieson and R Gwyn Morgan

HEAD AND NECK SKIN AND INCISIONS
(Fig. 21.1)

Langer determined the lines bearing his name in supine cadavers and these lines generally are not appropriate for head and face incisions. The correct placement of incisions should be parallel to the lines of skin creases or lines of expression. These are best seen in the animated face, i.e. prior to induction of anaesthesia.

In the neck these lines correspond to Langers lines with a gentle downward slope posterior to anterior.

When considering incisions for ablative surgery on the face, which may require local flap reconstruction, one should look for the areas of skin availability where there is always 'spare' skin. These areas are the glabellar area of the forehead, the upper lateral forehead, the temple, the pre-auricular skin and the nasolabial folds. In the older patient the upper eyelids may also be a potential donor site.

CERVICAL CUTANEOUS NERVES

The cervical cutaneous nerves arise from C2–4 spinal nerves. They emerge from the posterior surface of the sternomastoid muscle, as shown in Figure 21.2. The lesser occipital nerve (C2) passes upwards and backwards along the posterior border of the sternomastoid muscle and supplies skin from the auricle back to the occipital region. The great auricular (C2, 3) passes upwards immediately behind the external jugular vein to supply skin of the auricle and preauricular region. The transverse cervical nerve (C2, 3) passes horizontally across sternomastoid to supply the skin of the anterior neck region. The supraclavicular nerve (C3, 4) passes downwards and divides into branches which pass over the clavicle supplying the more lateral reaches of the neck.

CERVICAL FASCIA

Hollinshead states that there is no generally accepted definition as to how dense connective tissue must be before it can be regarded as forming a fascia and perhaps this statement

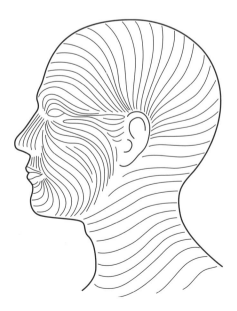

FIGURE 21.1   Relaxed skin tension lines in the head and neck.

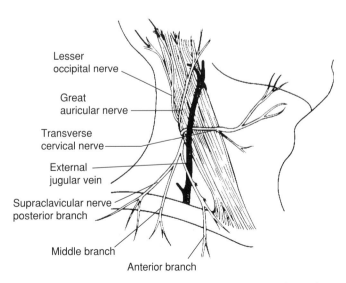

Lesser occipital nerve

Great auricular nerve

Transverse cervical nerve

External jugular vein

Supraclavicular nerve posterior branch

Middle branch

Anterior branch

FIGURE 21.2   The cervical cutaneous nerves and their relationship to the external jugular vein.

is particularly appropriate with regard to the fascia of the head and neck. It is overstating the case to say that the fascial layers are figments of various anatomists' imagination, because in some areas the fascial layers have surgical relevance. But anyone who spends time in the living looking for something justifying the name 'sheath' around the carotid artery, internal jugular vein and vagus nerve will be sorely disappointed.

Even in the preantibiotic era some surgeons doubted the usefulness of classifying various fascial spaces in the neck and no attempt will be made to perpetuate outmoded and useless anatomical concepts.

The superficial fascia refers only to the subcutaneous tissue, but in the head and neck it contains the platysma and facial muscles. The anterior and external jugular veins and the cervical cutaneous nerves all lie deep to the platysma in the neck.

The deep fascia is often divided into various layers but the divisions are arbitrary and it is only in certain areas where the fibroareolar tissue becomes thicker or has an important anatomical relationship that it assumes any clinical importance. Thus a superficial condensation around the omohyoid muscle tends to hold that muscle tendon in its position (by attaching it to the clavicle). And a fascial condensation overlies the phrenic nerve as it lies on the scalenus anterior muscle while the emerging nerves of the brachial plexus tend to take some fascia with them as the axillary sheath. On the other hand, the accessory nerve lies deep to the trapezius muscle on levator scapulae but superficial to the condensation on that muscle.

At risk of overemphasizing their surgical importance, a diagrammatic representation of the deep fascia is shown in Figure 21.3 and a description of some of the more important layers follows.

The investing layer of the deep cervical fascia

This fascial layer surrounds the neck like a collar. It splits to enclose the sternomastoid and trapezius muscles and the parotid and submandibular glands.

The investing layer is attached behind to the ligamentum nuchae and in front to the hyoid bone. Above it attaches to the skull base at the origins of the sternomastoid and trapezius muscles and to the lower border of the mandible.

Between the angle of the mandible and the tip of the mastoid process it splits into two layers which contain the parotid salivary gland. The deep layer attaches to the lower border of the tympanic plate and blends with the carotid sheath at the carotid foramen. Part of the deep layer of the parotid fascia, between the styloid process and the angle of the mandible is thicker than the rest and is called the stylomandibular ligament. The space between this ligament and the ascending ramus of the mandible anteriorly is the stylomandibular tunnel. Deep lobe parotid tumours extend medially through this tunnel, often expanding on either side of the ligament to create the so-called dumb-bell tumour, the medial extent causing distortion of the soft palate near the upper pole of the palatine tonsil.

The lower attachment of the investing fascia is to the pectoral girdle. Between the insertions of trapezius and sternomastoid to the clavicle the investing fascia splits, the deeper layer forming a fascial sling which binds the omohyoid muscle to the clavicle.

The prevertebral fascia

This firm membrane lies in front of the prevertebral muscles that form the floor of the posterior triangle and it thus forms the floor of a radical neck dissection. It is important not to breach it in a neck dissection as the cervical plexus and trunks of the brachial plexus lie deep to it. Large cutaneous branches of these cervical plexus pierce the prevertebral fascia and must be divided as a neck dissection proceeds.

CERVICAL MUSCLES

In descriptive terms the division of the neck region into anterior and posterior triangles is quite useful.

The posterior triangle consists of the trapezius behind and the sternomastoid in front, with the clavicle forming the base (Fig. 21.4).

STERNOCLEIDOMASTOID MUSCLE

This muscle arises from the front of the manubrium sterni and the superior surface of the medial part of the clavicle and ascends obliquely backwards to insert into the outer surface of the mastoid process and the anterior part of the superior nuchal line. Because of its course across the neck it is related to many structures of the neck and is one of the keys to the surgical anatomy of the area.

The external jugular vein courses across it from below the ear lobe to about the midpoint of the clavicle where the vein plunges deeply to join the subclavian vein.

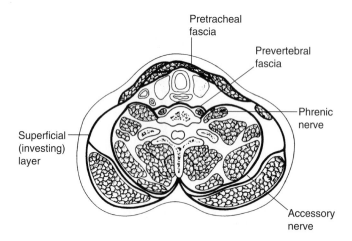

Pretracheal fascia

Prevertebral fascia

Phrenic nerve

Superficial (investing) layer

Accessory nerve

FIGURE 21.3 Some named layers of the deep fascia in the neck.

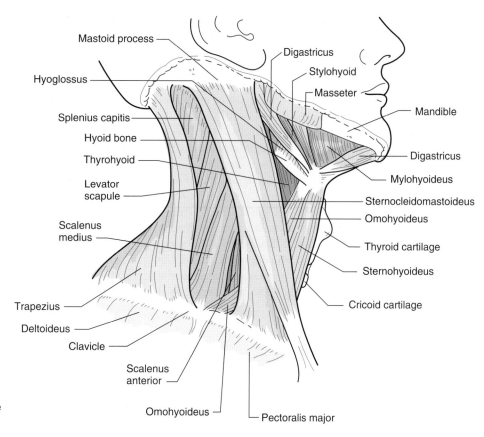

FIGURE 21.4 The muscular triangles of the neck.

Emerging from the posterior border and ascending across sternomastoid, behind and parallel to the external jugular vein, is the great auricular nerve, and emerging from the same point but passing transversely across the muscle is the transverse cervical nerve (Fig. 21.2).

The lower part of the parotid gland lies over the uppermost portion of the muscle.

Its nerve supply is from the accessory nerve, which supplies it from the muscle's deep surface about 5 cm below the mastoid process.

As the muscle lies over the carotid vessels, the internal jugular vein and the deep cervical lymph nodes, it is easy to see why it is such a key muscle in operations of this area, and several neck operations commence with an incision along the line of the anterior border of sternocleidomastoid muscle.

The movement of pushing the chin to one side against resistance tenses the muscle on the opposite side. But acting together, level rotation of the head is probably the main function of the muscles.

The infrahyoid strap muscles

There are four muscles – superficially the sternohyoid and omohyoid and deeply the sternothyroid and thyrohyoid muscles (Fig. 21.5).

The sternohyoid muscle originates from the back of the manubrium sterni and ascends, inclining medially to lie alongside its fellow, superficial to the thyroid gland, to insert into the body of the hyoid bone.

The superior belly of omohyoid muscle inserts immediately lateral to the sternohyoid muscle on the hyoid and passes downwards, lying lateral to sternohyoid but inclining away from it until it reaches its intermediate tendon behind the sternocleidomastoid. This tendon is held in position by a condensation of cervical fascia which attaches it to the clavicle and the inferior belly then passes obliquely to join the upper border of the scapula near the scapula notch.

The sternothyroid muscle arises from the back of the manubrium, inferior to the origin of sternohyoid, and passes

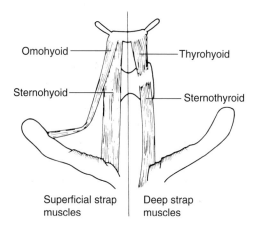

FIGURE 21.5 The strap muscles of the neck.

upwards deep to that muscle in front of the thyroid to insert into the oblique line on the front of the thyroid cartilage. The thyrohyoid muscle arises from this line and is a direct extension of the sternothyroid muscle. It inserts into the body and greater cornu of the hyoid bone.

These muscles are important in swallowing, acting as depressors of the larynx and hyoid bone.

Their nerve supply is derived from spinal nerve roots C1–3 (Fig. 21.6) via the ansa cervicalis. The innervation of the sternohyoid and sternothyroid muscles is usually double and the innervation pattern can be variable. In spite of this, the innervation of the muscles proximally usually occurs above the level of the lower border of the thyroid cartilage and the innervation of the muscles distally is usually close to the level of the suprasternal notch. Therefore if the strap muscles and/or the descending limb of the ansa cervicalis are to be divided it is best to do it midway between the lower border of the thyroid cartilage and the suprasternal notch (Fig. 21.6).

Other cervical muscles

Most of the other muscle groups in the neck need not concern us in any detail, although certain individual muscles will be described in reference to other structures, e.g. the mylohyoid muscle in reference to the submandibular gland.

The scalene muscles descend from the transverse processes of the first six or seven cervical vertebrae to insert in the first two ribs. The posterior scalene muscle arises from the fifth and sixth cervical vertebrae and is not easily separated from the middle scalene muscle, except that it passes beyond the first rib to insert into the second rib. The middle scalene is the largest of the three, arising from the sixth or seventh cervical vertebra and passing down to insert into the first rib behind the subclavian artery and brachial plexus. These latter structures separate the middle scalene from the scalenus anterior muscle, which arises from the cervical transverse processes of C3–6 and inserts into the first rib in front of the subclavian artery but behind the subclavian vein.

The lateral border of the sternomastoid muscle approximates the lateral border of the scalenus anterior muscle, which is also where the brachial plexus and subclavian artery emerge from behind the anterior scalene muscle. This muscle is considered again in the section on resection of the first rib (Ch. 39).

The scalene muscles are supplied by branches of the cervical nerve roots.

A pad of fibroareolar and lymphatic tissue lies behind the sternomastoid muscle on the anterior scalene muscle. Aspiration cytology in diagnosis has almost made the procedure of scalene node biopsy obsolete. However occasionally it may still be undertaken. After division of the clavicular fibres of the sternomastoid muscle the tissue can be removed by sweeping them towards the medially lying internal jugular vein.

The thyrocervical trunk of the subclavian artery typically arises alongside the medial border of the scalenus anterior muscle and two of its branches run transversely in front of the scalene muscle (Fig. 21.7).

Deep to all is a fascial condensation beneath which the phrenic nerve crosses the muscle from lateral to medial. On the left side the thoracic duct lies in the lower part of the field as it curves to its termination at the junction of the subclavian and internal jugular veins.

THE ANSA CERVICALIS

This is the nerve loop which supplies the strap muscles of the neck. Its upper root comes from fibres from the C1 nerve root which travel with the hypoglossal nerve and exit from it as the hypoglossal curves forwards around the occipital artery. The upper root then runs down on the anterior aspect of the internal carotid artery to join the lower root at a level just above the crossing omohyoid muscle.

The lower root usually comes from the C2, 3 nerve roots and it passes down on the lateral surface of the internal jugular vein before inclining forward to join the upper root. The distribution of its fibres to the strap muscles is shown in Figure 21.6.

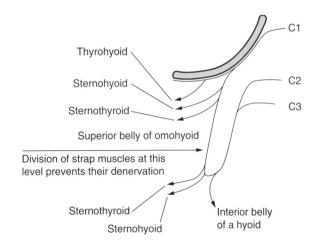

FIGURE 21.6 The ansa cervicalis and the innervation of the strap muscles.

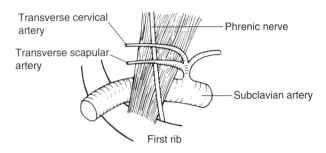

FIGURE 21.7 Some important relations of scalenus anterior muscle.

BRANCHIAL CYSTS AND SINUSES

Older texts of anatomy and surgery often ascribed probable congenital remnants of various branchial clefts with a degree of certainty which was unwarranted. Nevertheless a branchial fistula probably arises from the second branchial pouch. Most commonly it is blind internally but occasionally it can be blind externally or complete, in which case it is a branchial fistula.

A branchial fistula is most likely to open on the skin anterior to the lower third of the sternomastoid muscle, while a cyst is more likely to lie deep to the middle third of the sternomastoid muscle. However, the most important point to know is their relationship to the carotid vessels. A fistula always passes between the internal and external carotid arteries and a cyst tends to lie in this vicinity. The internal opening of a fistula is also relatively constant, into the tonsillar fossa of the pharynx.

FURTHER READING

Last R J 1959 Anatomy, regional and applied, 2nd edn. J A Churchill, London.

22 | Exposure of the cervical oesophagus for oesophageal anastomoses or excision of Zenker's diverticulum: the anatomy of the cervical oesophagus

Glyn Jamieson and André Duranceau

THE CERVICAL OESOPHAGUS

The cervical oesophagus lies behind the lower part of the larynx and trachea. It is important to realize that the first 1–2 cm of the oesophagus lies behind the larynx and is not easily separable from it, so that a 'total' oesophagectomy nearly always leaves behind about 2 cm or more of the proximal oesophagus. Laterally the cervical oesophagus is separated from the lobes of the thyroid gland by the deep cervical fascia, under which also lie the inferior thyroid arteries emerging from behind the carotid sheaths. The recurrent laryngeal nerves lie in the tracheo-oesophageal groove in about 50% of cases. In about 10% of cases the nerves are more posterior and in a direct lateral relation to the oesophagus. In the remainder of cases they lie more anteriorly as a direct lateral relation of the trachea.

Posteriorly the oesophagus lies on the vertebral bodies and the longus colli muscles which lie along the lateral sides of the anterior part of the vertebral bodies. The oesophagus is separated from these structures by the prevertebral fascia.

The thoracic duct lies to the left of the oesophagus in the region of the thoracic inlet. More proximally it passes laterally behind the carotid sheath and out of the field.

The cervical oesophagus is composed predominantly of skeletal muscle and receives its nerve supply from the recurrent laryngeal nerves, and its blood supply from small branches of the inferior thyroid arteries.

INFERIOR CONSTRICTOR OF THE PHARYNX AND THE UPPER OESOPHAGEAL SPHINCTER (CRICOPHARYNGEUS)

The inferior constrictor muscle arises from the cricoid cartilage and the thyroid cartilage and sweeps upwards and backwards to insert in the midline raphe with its fellow of the opposite side (Fig. 22.1). Morphologically there is no distinction to be found between any of the muscle fibres of the inferior constrictor or indeed between the lower fibres of inferior constrictor and the circular oesophageal muscle, except for a small area anteriorly where the inferior

constrictor arises from the cricoid cartilage (known in some texts as the Killian–Jamieson area). Nevertheless the lowermost fibres of the inferior constrictor differ physiologically from the contiguous fibres on either side of it in being maintained in tonic contraction. Physiologically this is the upper oesophageal sphincter and morphologically it seems to correspond best with the part of the inferior constrictor arising from the cricoid cartilage and thus called cricopharyngeus. This part may have a different nerve supply from the rest of the muscle, via the recurrent laryngeal nerve. The remainder of the inferior constrictor muscle arises from a tendinous arch over the cricothyroid muscle and the oblique line on the thyroid cartilage and so it is sometimes called thyropharyngeus to distinguish it from the cricopharyngeus. The thyropharyngeus obtains its nerve supply through the pharyngeal plexus.

Incision of the inferior constrictor

The digestive tube cannot be removed proximal to the cricoid cartilage without entering the pharynx. On occasions it may be necessary to make an anastomosis between the pharynx and the stomach or colon. It is best to make an incision as posterior as possible in order to avoid damaging or constricting the arytenoid muscles and other muscles of the laryngeal inlet. Posteriorly the incision (theoretically) can be taken as high as the base of the skull.

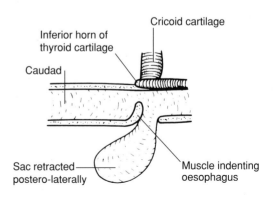

FIGURE 22.1 Cricopharyngeus and related muscles.

PHARYNGEAL DIVERTICULUM AND CRICOPHARYNGEAL MYOTOMY

The primary defect in patients with a pharyngeal diverticulum is an inability of the cricopharyngeus to open adequately. This is related to fibrosis affecting the muscular fibres. In order to squeeze food through the narrowing, high pressures are generated in the pharynx and the mucosa bulges immediately proximal to the fibrotic zone. Why this mucosa tends to bulge posteriorly and to the left is unknown but obviously this is the weakest point of the general area.

In removing a symptomatic diverticulum it obviously makes sense to divide the narrowed zone of muscle and this is known as a cricopharyngeal myotomy. Division of this muscle is also sometimes undertaken for other conditions.

As already mentioned, there is no dividing line between the muscle fibres above and below cricopharyngeus. Therefore it is usual to mobilize the upper oesophagus and divide from the proximal 2 or 3 cm of the oesophagus upwards for 4–5 cm. The pharynx above usually tends to balloon more in its wall than the oesophagus. Other approximate landmarks for the level of cricopharyngeus are the point where the inferior belly of omohyoid crosses the viscera, the cricoid cartilage itself, or the inferior horn of the thyroid cartilage which is about level with the distal most fibres of origin of cricopharyngeus. When a pouch is present the cricopharyngeus indents its neck considerably and it is important to be sure that all muscle and fibrous tissue fibres are divided. This inevitably means that the myotomy should include the lowermost fibres of the thyropharyngeus. The mucosa will bulge without restriction from the oesophagus or the neck of the sac when complete division is achieved. The cervical oesophagus part of the myotomy does not alter the resting pressure in the upper sphincter. When cutting the muscle in relation to the cricoid cartilage, this decreases the upper sphincter resting pressure by approximately 50%. When thyropharyngeal fibres are divided, the resting pressure of the upper sphincters falls even further.

As the pouch tends to arise posteriorly it is usual to undertake the myotomy towards the midline posteriorly, or as close to it as practicable. A more lateral myotomy may well achieve the same effect.

Exposure of the cervical oesophagus

The cervical oesophagus can be approached through an incision in the right or left side of the neck. Because the oesophagus tends to lie to the left of the midline, the left side is often chosen, although in practical terms there is little to choose between the two sides.

An incision along the anterior border of sternomastoid (or a transverse incision) is made from the sternal notch below to a few centimetres below the ear lobe above and deepened through the subcutaneous tissues and platysma.

A branch of a cervical cutaneous nerve is usually seen in the upper part of the incision and should be preserved if possible. The omohyoid muscle is divided. It usually contains a blood vessel within its substance which requires ligature or cautery. The prethyroid muscles and their investing fascia may need to be divided to expose the carotid sheath. This is retracted laterally and the middle thyroid veins are divided. The ansa cervicalis lying on the carotid artery and internal jugular vein is always exposed, and branches from it to the prethyroid strap muscles usually need to be divided. (They receive a dual nerve supply, so this does not cause problems for the patient – see Chapter 21.) The inferior thyroid artery is then sought. Although it can be divided with apparent impunity, it is one of the major arteries of supply to the cervical oesophagus and it is probably sensible practice to preserve it, if practicable, during oesophagectomy only.

Whether the recurrent laryngeal nerve should be sought and dissected free is a moot point. Such an approach is often followed by nerve dysfunction and although usually only temporary it may deprive the patient of an ability to cough normally over a vital postoperative time. The nerve can usually be seen or palpated along its course and it is our practice to keep the dissection very close to the oesophageal wall without identifying the nerve and separate the oesophagus from its investing fibroalveolar attachments by a mixture of sharp and blunt dissection.

Anteriorly and proximally it is not easy to be sure where the oesophagus commences. The inferior cornu of the thyroid cartilage can usually be palpated and is a useful landmark for the commencement of the oesophagus. One encounters difficulty in mobilizing the anterior 1–2 cm from the trachea in front, and as the blood supply enters here it is better to leave this part of the cervical oesophagus undissected.

Using a dissecting swab it is not difficult to mobilize the oesophagus by blunt dissection well down into the superior mediastinum.

The right side of the oesophagus is not always easy to determine, but using judicious retraction and a curved clamp it can usually be dissected free under direct vision. The pharyngo-oesophageal junction can usually be lifted and pushed toward the operating surgeon, rendering the right lateral limits of the cervical oesophagus available for direct dissection. Once again it is important to stay close to the oesophageal wall in order to avoid the right recurrent laryngeal nerve.

The sternoclavicular joint and its excision

The sternal end of the clavicle, the manubrium and the first costal cartilage all take part in the formation of the sternoclavicular joint. The head of the clavicle has a significant posterior portion which juts out into the retromanubrial space, and can therefore compress the organ – usually stomach or colon – which is being brought up, for instance, to bypass the oesophagus.

The joint has anterior and posterior sternoclavicular ligaments and also a strong costoclavicular ligament binding it to the first rib.

It is usually the left joint which is removed in oesophageal bypass. Providing the surgeon stays close to the bone there is no real danger to any vital structure in removing the joint. The left brachiocephalic vein is a direct posterior relation but it is separated from the joint by the sternohyoid and thyrohyoid muscles and the thymic capsule.

The fibres of origin of pectoralis major muscle in front, sternocleidomastoid muscle above and the sternohyoid muscle behind require division from the medial end of the clavicle. However it is the joint ligaments which provide the strongest attachment and in particular the costoclavicular ligament below and the anterior sternocostal ligament in front.

Using some form of bone cutters, or performing a proximal sternotomy with subsequent use of a Gigli saw, the corresponding half of the manubrium sterni and part of the first rib are usually removed, as well as the joint. If the lateral portion of the head of the clavicle is left attached to the corresponding anterior portion of the first rib, this leaves a 'stable' clavicle while still providing a more capacious proximal chest inlet.

23 | Thyroidectomy; tracheostomy: the anatomy of the thyroid gland and related structures

Glyn Jamieson and Leigh Delbridge

THE THYROID GLAND

The thyroid gland develops as an outpouching from the floor of the embryonic pharynx, this point becoming the foramen caecum of later life. It descends in the midline and the track of its development forms the thyroglossal duct which may persist or differentiate into thyroid tissue at any level – thus explaining the origin of a lingual thyroid. The distal portion of the duct, just superior to the thyroid isthmus, becomes the pyramidal lobe of the thyroid. This lobe is important in thyrotoxicosis as, if it is not resected along with the rest of the gland, it may be responsible for recurrent thyrotoxicosis. Embryological descent of the thyroid sometimes continues into the anterior mediastinum. This descent can result in isolated thyrothymic thyroid rests, which may be the origin of retrosternal goiters. During embryological development the thyroid also receives a contribution from the 4th branchial pouch and ultimobranchial body. This contribution is the origin of the C-cells of the thyroid, and frequently persists as the Tubercle of Zuckerkandl, a small visible projection from the posterolateral border of the thyroid. The importance of the Tubercle of Zuckerkandl is its constant relation to the recurrent laryngeal nerve.

Occasionally cystic differentiation occurs in the thyroglossal duct with the development of a thyroglossal cyst. Such cysts are usually located close to the hyoid bone, either above or below it.

The isthmus of the thyroid gland usually lies over the second and third tracheal rings and the lobes lie behind the strap muscles on either side of the trachea. The carotid sheath structures lie posterolaterally. The upper lobes are limited by the insertion of the sternothyroid muscles into the thyroid cartilage.

The thyroid gland has a capsule which surrounds the thyroid follicles and beneath which lie the plexus of tertiary vessels. The gland is surrounded by fibroareolar tissue which is most noticeable on the medial aspect of the upper lobes where bands of fibrovascular condensation attach the gland to the trachea. These are called the lateral ligaments of the thyroid gland (Ligaments of Berry).

The parathyroid glands may lie within the thyroid capsule, immediately outside the capsule, or completely separate from the thyroid gland.

The fibroareolar tissue which surrounds the thyroid allows the gland to be dissected away from the overlying strap muscles by gentle blunt dissection. On the anterolateral and inferior aspects of the lobes the only structures interfering with this mobilization are the middle and inferior thyroid veins. In thyrotoxicosis, or in patients with Hashimoto's thyroiditis, the fibroareolar tissue is often thicker and less easy to dissect.

With the gland fully exposed it is important on each side to routinely identify:

❶ the middle thyroid vein or veins;
❷ superior and inferior thyroid arteries;
❸ the external branch of the superior laryngeal nerve;
❹ the recurrent laryngeal nerve;
❺ two parathyroids during the procedure of thyroid resection.

The parathyroid glands can be identified by their tan colour, their wheat-grain size, their soft, consistency (which is very different from the firm feel of a small lymph node), and their mobility within their capsule.

The inferior gland, derived from the endoderm of the 3rd branchial pouch is found in an anterior–inferior location, specifically anterior to the line of the recurrent laryngeal nerve, either on the surface of the inferior pole of the thyroid gland, in the region of the thyrothymic ligament, or within the thymus.

The superior gland, derived paradoxically from the 4th branchial pouch, is found in a postero–superior location, usually posterior to the recurrent laryngeal nerve on the posterolateral aspect of the upper half of the thyroid, frequently in close relation to the upper border of the Tubercle of Zuckerkandl.

Minor trauma to the glands causes them to become plum-coloured from subcapsular haemorrhagic discoloration.

In an operation on the thyroid gland, early identification of the trachea medially, and the pre-vertebral fascia adjacent to the carotid vessels laterally, provides clear orientation for all subsequent dissection.

Arterial supply

The thyroid gland is richly supplied with blood from the two thyroid arteries on each side.

The superior thyroid artery arises from the external carotid artery near its origin and descends on the inferior constrictor muscle to reach the upper pole of the thyroid where it gives off a branch to the posterior surface and continues on the anterior and medial border of the upper pole of the lobe. The artery is relatively constant and lies in close proximity to the external branch of the superior laryngeal nerve, usually inferior and lateral (superficial) to it (Fig. 23.1), although the nerve may occasionally pass around the artery and be found anterior to the upper pole of the thyroid, a situation commonly seen in large multinodular goitres. Division of the strap muscles during thyroidectomy enables the surgeon to obtain a better view of the external branch of the superior laryngeal nerve and the superior thyroid artery by retracting the upper pole lateral to open up the avascular space between the cricothyroid muscle and medial surface of the thyroid. This division however is by no means universally practised, nor always required, although if any technical difficulty is encountered it is usually wise to divide the strap muscles.

Opening of the avascular space allows ready identification of the external branch of the superior laryngeal nerve in almost all cases, except where it lies within the substance of the cricothyroid muscle. This nerve supplies the cricothyroid muscle, i.e. the tensor of the vocal cords, and damage causes a loss of high-pitched phonation and projection.

The inferior thyroid artery is not quite as constant and is absent in about 5% of cases. It arises from the thyrocervical trunk of the subclavian artery, loops up on scalenus anterior and turns medially behind the carotid artery. As it emerges here it runs down on longus colli and in front of the cervical sympathetic chain to enter the thyroid gland. Before entering the gland it usually divides into two to three primary branches – one branch providing the blood supply to the inferior parathyroid gland. Ligature of the trunk of the inferior thyroid artery should be avoided as it may threaten the viability of the parathyroid glands whose blood supply should be protected by capsular dissection, dividing only the tertiary branches of the artery on the thyroid capsule. Its relationship to the recurrent laryngeal nerve is discussed subsequently.

As well as the four main arteries the relatively inconstant thyroidea ima artery rises from the brachiocephalic or other artery in the area in about 5% of patients. It can occasionally replace the inferior thyroid arteries in which case it is larger. Its main surgical importance is that it usually ascends in front of the trachea and may be encountered at tracheostomy.

All of the arteries anastomose with each other and with oesophageal and tracheal branches, such that brisk back-bleeding from the thyroid surface will still be seen despite almost complete surgical separation of the gland from its major blood supply.

Venous drainage

The venous drainage from the thyroid gland is variable with the superior thyroid veins, like their companion arteries being the most constant. The veins form from a plexus on the surface of the gland and run parallel but inferior and lateral to the superior thyroid arteries, and drain into the internal jugular vein or the facial vein.

The middle thyroid veins are variable in size and number and presence. On each side there is usually one emerging posterolaterally from the lower part of the lobe and draining into the internal jugular vein. Occasionally there are two veins and quite often the veins are absent.

There are usually two inferior thyroid veins, also of differing sizes, which exit from the lower border of the gland and drain into the brachiocephalic veins of their respective sides. These veins commonly communicate in front of the trachea and can therefore cause troublesome bleeding if they are damaged during tracheostomy, and they may also be encountered when displaying the pretracheal region during thyroidectomy. In patients with venous obstruction secondary to a large retrosternal goitre the veins are greatly engorged and may be a source of brisk bleeding until the retrosternal component is delivered.

Lymphatic drainage

In most cases, the lymphatic drainage of the thyroid gland initially goes to the 'central nodes' comprising the paratracheal nodes in the tracheo-oesophageal groove (level 6 nodes), the delphic node superior to the isthmus, as well as to perithyroidal nodes. It is these nodes that are primarily involved with metastases from papillary or medually thyroid cancer. Subsequently drainage to the jugular nodes (levels 2, 3 and 4), and later to the lateral nodes (level 5) or anterior mediastinal nodes (level 7) occurs.

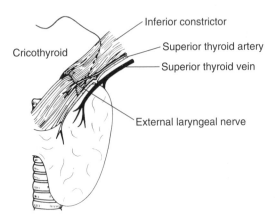

FIGURE 23.1 The superior thyroid artery and its relationship to the external laryngeal nerve.

So-called lateral aberrant thyroid was initially regarded as embryonic tissue which had developed separately from the rest of the gland. When it was realized that, occasionally, follicular carcinoma of the thyroid produced extremely well differentiated metastases in lymph nodes, the diagnosis of lateral aberrant thyroid fell into disrepute. However some pathologists are now suggesting that such a condition can, in fact, exist.

THE RECURRENT LARYNGEAL NERVES AND THE THYROID GLAND

The right recurrent laryngeal nerve arises from the right vagus nerve and passes around the right subclavian artery to pass upwards approximately in the tracheo-oesophageal groove and it disappears from view beneath the inferior-most fibres of the inferior constrictor muscle (the cricopharyngeus) behind the inferior cornu of the thyroid cartilage.

The left recurrent nerve passes from lateral to medial under the arch of the aorta just lateral to the obliterated ductus arteriosus but thereafter its course is similar to the right nerve. The right nerve may be non-recurrent in 0.5% of cases, associated with a 4th branchial arch anomaly involving the right subclavian which takes off from the distal aortic arch.

Direct communicating branches between the sympathetic chain and the recurrent laryngeal nerves are common, with the branches being as large as the recurrent laryngeal nerve in up to 2% of cases (and thus potentially being mistaken for a non-recurrent nerve).

There are several important facts to know in regard to the relationship of the nerve to the inferior thyroid artery.

Although the nerve lies in the tracheo-oesophageal groove in about 50% of cases, in the remainder it lies either further laterally or more anteriorly alongside the trachea and occasionally more posteriorly alongside the oesophagus. In the past the nerve has been described as traversing the substance of the thyroid gland but it is now recognized that, in these cases, the nerve is actually passing into a groove medial to an enlarged Tubercle of Zuckerkandl (Fig. 23.2).

There is perhaps only one essential fact to know in regard to the relationship of the recurrent laryngeal nerve to the inferior thyroid artery and that is that the two always have a very close relationship. The most usual relationship is for the nerve to pass between the two branches of the inferior thyroid artery (Fig. 23.2), but it may pass in front of or behind the artery, and as often as not the relationship differs on the two sides. Careful capsular dissection on the thyroid surface allows the recurrent laryngeal nerve to be 'encountered' most commonly at the site where it is in a close relationship to the artery. Dividing only the tertiary branches of the artery protects both the recurrent laryngeal nerve as well as the blood supply of the parathyroids.

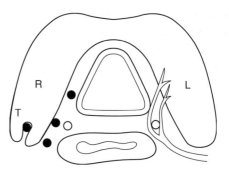

FIGURE 23.2 The relationship of the recurrent laryngeal nerves to the thyroid gland and related structures. Viewed from below, on the right (R) are five different positions of the nerve (the commonest position is the open circle). One position is shown medial to the tubercle (T). On the left (L) is the commonest position between branches of the inferior thyroid artery.

In spite of the fact that much surgical attention is focused on the close relationship of the recurrent laryngeal nerve and the inferior thyroid artery this is now so well known that injury to the nerve at this site is unlikely. In total removal of a lobe the nerve is perhaps in more danger adjacent to the medial surface of the upper pole of the thyroid gland. The thyroid is attached to the trachea by quite dense fascia here and depending on the relationship to the thyroid the nerve can be bound up in this fascia (see Fig. 24.1). Therefore it is important to observe the course of the nerve from the artery up to its point of disappearance behind the inferior cornu of the thyroid cartilage, in order to be certain that it is not damaged during removal of a lobe.

Attention is also drawn to the fact that when the thyroid lobe is forcefully retracted anteriorly, the nerve tends to travel at an angle of 45° to the line of the tracheo-oesophageal groove and can thus be mistaken for a blood vessel.

One further point worth mentioning is that the nerve not uncommonly divides before disappearing from view. This generally (but not always) occurs cephalad to the inferior thyroid artery. When branching does occur, the anterior branch contains the principal motor supply to the intrinsic laryngeal muscles, with the posterior branches primarily supplying sensory fibres to the oesophagus and trachea. There is however some crossover. An internal constant communication between the external branch of the superior laryngeal nerve and the recurrent laryngeal nerve (the Nerve of Galen) may also have some motor function).

NERVE INJURY DURING THYROIDECTOMY

Damage to the external branch of the superior laryngeal nerve leads to loss of function of the cricothyroid muscle, and therefore loss of ability to tighten the cord on the side of the nerve. This makes it difficult for the patient to make high-pitched sounds, or to project the voice.

Damage to one recurrent laryngeal nerve may produce some weakening of the voice but as the cricothyroid muscle is unaffected (assuming the external branch of the superior laryngeal nerve has not also been damaged) the cord lies close to the midline and the opposite cord can cross the midline to compensate for the injury. Damage to both the recurrent and external nerves on the same side leads to the cord assuming the cadaveric position of mid adduction, so that there is hoarseness of the voice and an inability to cough.

Bilateral recurrent laryngeal nerve paralysis leads to both cords initially being in the semi-adducted position, so that there is not usually early respiratory difficulty. However with time the cords tend to move towards the midline so that the voice improves but respiratory difficulty develops and a tracheostomy is usually required.

It is worth noting that idiopathic unilateral cord paralysis (which is often asymptomatic) is said to occur in about 1% of normal individuals and so it makes both clinical and medicolegal sense to ascertain the state of the vocal cords by laryngoscopic examination before embarking on a thyroidectomy.

THYROGLOSSAL DUCT CYSTS

Cysts sometimes develop along the thyroglossal tract, usually just below the hyoid bone, although they have been described at all sites along the tract.

The tract usually passes deep to the hyoid but in some cases it passes in front of or occasionally through the hyoid. It is for this reason, and because it is difficult to be certain at operation where the tract passes, that it is recommended that the body of the hyoid should be excised when removing a thyroglossal duct cyst and associated track.

THE TRACHEA

The trachea begins at the lower border of the cricoid cartilage and descends in the neck in front of the oesophagus. Its important anterior relations beneath the skin and platysma are the cervical strap muscles which have the anterior jugular veins lying on them. (These veins often communicate but it is usually low in the neck.) Beneath the strap muscles is the thyroid gland and in particular the isthmus of the thyroid. This usually overlies tracheal rings 2–4. Below the isthmus are the inferior thyroid veins which are variable and often form something of a plexus lying on the front of the trachea. If a thyroidea ima artery is present it also lies in front of the trachea.

A tracheostomy tube can be inserted through the area of tracheal rings 2–6 or 7 but it is better to avoid going too high because it can cause dysphagia when the tube is in position and may cause stenosis later.

Therefore tracheal rings 3–5 or 4–6 seem to be ideal as they are either below the isthmus of the thyroid or it can be displaced easily to expose these rings.

The main blood supply to the trachea is through the inferior thyroid arteries and its nerve supply is from the vagus and recurrent laryngeal nerves. The important relationship of these latter nerves to the trachea has already been discussed above.

FURTHER READING

Delbridge L 2003 Total thyroidectomy: the evolution of surgical technique. ANZ J Surg 73:761–768.
Randolph G W 2003 Surgical anatomy of the recurrent laryngeal nerve. Chapter 25. In: Randolph G W (ed) Surgery of the thyroid and parathyroid glands. Saunders, Philadelphia.

24 | Parathyroidectomy, open and minimal access approaches: the anatomy of the parathyroid glands

Glyn Jamieson and Peter Malycha

The upper parathyroid arises from the endodermal lining of the 4th branchial arch and is associated with the developing thyroid which descends to reach the trachea by 11 weeks. This embryological mesenchymal tissue also differentiates into the vessels, nerves, muscle and cartilage of the pharynx. It separates from the pharynx and travels a relatively short distance to its final position near the thyroid. It is more constant in position than the lower gland. Thus an undescended superior gland may be found in the pharyngeal and neurovascular derivatives of the 4th arch from the angle of mandible and carotid bifurcation to the thyroid gland. Ninety-four per cent are found above and lateral to the intersection of the recurrent laryngeal nerve and inferior thyroid artery.

The lower parathyroid arises from the endodermal lining of the 3rd branchial arch and is therefore closely related to the embryological parathymus. At the 6th week of gestation the developing thymus begins to pull the lower glands down towards the lower thyroid pole. At the 18 mm embryo stage the lower glands usually separate from the thymus and take up their position near the lower end of the respective thyroid lobes.

The lower gland's position is less anatomically constant and may be found associated with the 3rd arch mesenchymal derivatives including the thyroid, carotid sheath, thyrothymic ligament and, within the anterior mediastinum, may reach the aorto-pulmonary window.

The average combined weight of the four glands is around 120 mg with individual glands weighing from 30 mg to 70 mg. An adult gland measures $6 \times 5 \times 2$ mm and may be multilobular. Autopsy studies suggested that 3% of the population will have only three glands, and 13% will have supernumerary glands. Superior glands are bilaterally symmetrical in about 80% of cases and inferior glands in 70%. Parathyroid glands increase in size until the 4th decade. They have an increasing fat content with age which provides up to 60% of glandular volume in old age.

LOCATION (Fig. 24.1, Table 24.1)

The superior gland is usually easier to find. It normally lies behind the thyroid capsule adjacent to the terminal divisions

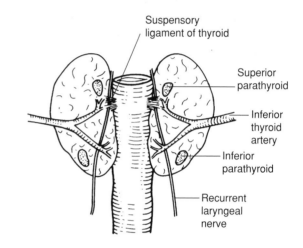

FIGURE 24.1 The thyroid gland and the parathyroid glands viewed from behind.

of the recurrent laryngeal nerve where it passes behind the cricothyroid muscle. The superior gland may not always be obvious until the thyroid capsule is opened. It may also be found at the distal end of a tear-shaped fatty lobule that travels (plombages) down alongside the inferior thyroid

Table 24.1   The percentage of parathyroid glands found in various locations

Location of superior parathyroid glands	
80%	just above and lateral to intersection of the RLN and ITA
14%	behind the superior pole thyroid gland
4%	adjacent to ITA, behind tubercle of Zuckerkandl
1%	retropharyngeal or retro-oesophageal
0.8%	above superior pole of thyroid
0.2%	intrathyroid
Location of inferior parathyroid glands	
46%	behind inferior thyroid pole
26%	thyrothymic ligament
17%	anterolateral to inferior thyroid pole
6%	just below intersection of RLN and ITA
2.8%	above intersection of RLN and ITA
2%	intrathymic
2%	anterior mediastinum
0.2%	intrathyroid

ITA = inferior thyroid artery, RLN = recurrent laryngeal nerve

artery and then into the retro-oesophageal space. When not found in the commonest position it is most likely to be found within the subcapsular tissues of the posterior aspect of the upper thyroid pole at the level of the cricoid cartilage. It may also be partially or completely within the thyroid. When found in the pedicle containing the superior thyroid vessels, most will have an obvious vascular pedicle arising from the upper thyroid pole vessels.

A truly undescended superior gland may be found anywhere within the 4th arch derivatives including the pharyngeal wall, parapharyngeal space and neurovascular structures in the common carotid sheath.

The inferior parathyroid gland is found in more varying positions. It is found most commonly within the thyroid capsule on the posterolateral surface of the lower pole, inferior to the intersection of the inferior thyroid artery and the recurrent laryngeal nerve. Twenty-six per cent of glands are found inferior to the thyroid in association with the thyrothymic ligament and thymus gland. The incidence of an inferior intrathyroid gland is comparable with that of the superior gland even though the thyroid and inferior parathyroid gland share a common origin from the 3rd branchial arch. The inferior gland can also be found in the carotid sheath structures. The embryological 3rd branchial arch vessels fuse with the dorsal aorta to become the first part of the internal carotid artery and thus an undescended lower gland can be found as superiorly as the skull base.

Blood supply

The glands have a rich blood supply from the anastomoses between superior and inferior thyroid arteries and division of all four thyroid arteries does not devascularize them. However, their direct blood supply is mainly from the inferior thyroid artery (Fig. 24.2). The small end-vessel entering the broader end of the gland is easily seen and will often enable the surgeon to identify the parathyroid gland. When rubbed too vigorously the gland changes from a London tan to brown or purple due to venous bruising beneath the capsule. A deeply discoloured or devascularized parathyroid gland should be sliced into 1–2 mm pieces and placed in a sternomastoid muscle pocket as a free graft. Function can be expected to return in 6 weeks.

ANATOMICAL POINTS DURING OPEN PARATHYROIDECTOMY

Successful parathyroid surgery needs a bloodless field. Meticulous care, gentle dissection and appropriate retraction is needed for absolute haemostasis as connective tissue discoloration makes identification of normal parathyroid glands difficult or impossible. Normal parathyroid glands are slightly different in colour from the fat. They are described as being a London tan colour.

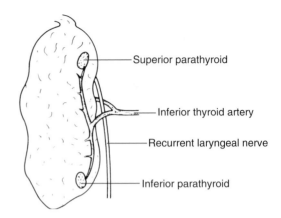

FIGURE 24.2 This shows the parathyroid glands receiving their blood supply from the inferior thyroid artery.

While colour can differentiate a parathyroid gland from fat, it is often movement (wobble) within the capsule which draws the surgeon's attention to it.

Many glands have a well-defined pedicle in which small linear vessels can be seen.

If fewer than four glands are identified at operation, a planned, careful and methodical search must be undertaken.

When a superior gland is missing, individual ligation of the superior pole vessels (which also protect the external branch of the superior laryngeal nerve) should be performed. The upper pole of the thyroid gland should be mobilized completely, including division of the ligament of Berry. Retrothyroid and intrathyroid adenomas can be discovered only by this dissection. Bi-polar diathermy is invaluable. If still missing, an upper ectopic gland may be found within the common carotid sheath and along the vagus nerve. Access to the carotid bifurcation and the pharyngeal wall can be achieved through a cervical incision.

When the inferior parathyroid gland is missing, it should be sought in the thyrothymic ligament and thymus gland which extend from the lower thyroid pole into the anterior mediastinum. This organ has an enveloping fascia with vessels draining into the neck. It can be mobilized with gentle traction and scissor dissection. Care must be taken when the intrathoracic part of the thymus is delivered as moderate sized veins can be torn.

Sternotomy is not undertaken at a first operation as the procedures described often remove sufficient parathyroid tissue to overcome hypercalcaemia. Parathyroid hormone and calcium levels can be checked immediately, or the next day, and will give a good guide to the success of the operation.

While a superior parathyroid adenoma will descend towards the posterior mediastinum within the retropharyngeal space, an inferior gland adenoma will descend into the anterior mediastinum with the thymus.

If a superior or inferior gland is not found after extensive searching, it may be necessary to carry out an ipsilateral hemithyroidectomy.

The recurrent laryngeal nerve is part of the operative field and should be defined in most instances during parathyroid surgery. It ascends to be intimately associated with a superior parathyroid gland before entering the larynx (see Ch. 23).

ANATOMICAL POINTS DURING MINIMAL ACCESS PARATHYROIDECTOMY

Minimally invasive parathyroid (MIP) surgery involves making a 2–3 cm incision to remove an adenoma that has been localized preoperatively by nuclear scanning (sestamibi) and ultrasound. Surgeons must have a very good understanding of the anatomy to interpret these investigations and ensure that the adenoma is found. Sestamibi will only localize an adenoma to a side and thyroid pole. An upper parathyroid adenoma that the nuclear physician reports as an inferior gland may be a superior gland that plombages inferiorly behind the thyroid gland. An on table ultrasound performed by the surgeon is invaluable for the placement of the incision and for determining the anatomical planes.

The surgical technique is the same in that knowledge of the embryology and anatomy is essential and patients having a MIP must be made aware that a formal parathyroid exploration will be necessary if the lesion is not found. The smaller incision also makes it more difficult to find and protect the recurrent laryngeal nerve. Parathyroid adenomas are often deep in the neck and access via a smaller incision is more difficult.

A multi nodular goitre makes assessment more difficult and is a relative contraindication for MIP.

Minimally invasive techniques have been described using small laparoscopes. The risk of nerve damage is greater and interest in the operation has waned. Access to the parathyroid glands has been gained through incisions in the infraclavicular skin, areola and axilla. They have been used in societies where a scar in the neck is to be avoided.

25 | Excision of the submandibular gland: the anatomy of the submandibular gland and associated structures

Glyn Jamieson and Peter Devitt

The submandibular gland lies deep to the cervical fascia filling the submandibular triangle between the anterior and posterior bellies of the digastric and the inferior border of the mandible (Fig. 25.1). The gland spills out over these borders and a large proportion of it lies below the level of the mandible.

THE DIGASTRIC MUSCLE

The anterior belly of the digastric muscle arises from a fossa near the midline on the back of the mandible. The muscle belly passes backwards and downwards to its intermediate tendon which is held by a fibrous sling to the hyoid bone at the junction between body and greater cornu. This part of the muscle is supplied by the nerve to the mylohyoid muscle. The posterior belly passes backwards and upwards to its insertion on the medial side of the mastoid process (Fig. 25.1).

The digastric muscle is supplied by a branch from the facial nerve. The posterior belly crosses the internal and external carotid arteries, the hypoglossal nerve, the internal jugular vein, the transverse process of the atlas and the accessory nerve (Fig. 25.2).

THE MANDIBULAR AND CERVICAL BRANCHES OF THE FACIAL NERVE

The lowermost branches of the facial nerve are often in direct or close relationship to the submandibular gland. The mandibular branch exits from the parotid gland near the angle of the mandible and curves downwards as it runs forwards deep to the platysma and then curves upwards to cross the mandible close to the facial artery before supplying the risorius and the lower lip and chin muscles. In a majority of cases it does not lie much lower than the inferior border of the mandible, although in a minority it has been described as low as 2.5 cm below the mandible. Division of this nerve produces a noticeable facial deformity with depression of the corner of the mouth, flattening of the lower lip and drooling.

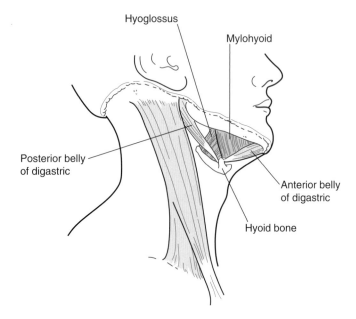

FIGURE 25.1　The submandibular triangle.

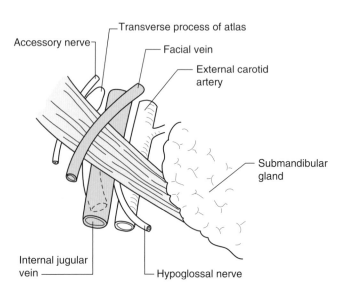

FIGURE 25.2　The posterior belly of the digastric muscle.

126

The nerve which is most often damaged in operations in this region is a division of the cervical branch of the facial nerve. The cervical branch runs deep to platysma in a downwards direction about 1–2 cm behind the angle of the mandible. Approximately 2 cm below the angle it divides, its posterior division continuing on to supply platysma and its anterior division curving forwards and upwards to provide additional supply to the muscles of the corner of the mouth.

If the anterior division of the nerve is divided, it usually causes some drooping of the corner of the mouth. As it is not the major nerve of supply, improvement in muscle function usually occurs. In most such instances the disability usually resolves within a few months.

It is unusual for this anterior branch to pass more than 3 cm below the lower border of the mandible. Thus if neck incisions are made 2 cm or more behind the angle of the mandible and 4 cm or more below it, and the incisions are taken through platysma at the same level, then neither the mandibular nor the cervical divisions of the facial nerve will be endangered.

In dissection of the gland itself the structures lying superficial to it are the facial artery and vein and the submental artery and vein (Fig. 25.3).

THE FACIAL VEIN

The facial vein descends across the face from the inner angle of the eye and crosses the border of the mandible about 2 cm in front of its angle (Fig. 25.3). It lies deep to the platysma directly on the external surface of the submandibular gland. The submental vein passes backwards across the gland to enter the facial vein. Behind the submandibular gland, the facial vein receives the anterior division of the retromandibular vein and passes downwards as the common facial vein to enter the internal jugular vein. At its termina-

tion the common facial vein overlies the carotid bifurcation. At this point a communicating branch from the anterior jugular vein (which runs along the sternomastoid muscle) often joins the facial vein near its termination.

THE FACIAL ARTERY

The facial artery arises from the external carotid artery distal to the lingual branch and passes upwards deep to the digastric muscle, to loop over the posterior belly in a sigmoid fashion. This artery then arches over the posterior portion of the submandibular gland in which it often forms a groove. It passes forwards between the gland and medial surface of the mandible until it emerges beneath the lower border and curls around the mandible to enter the face. As it curves around the mandible it is closely related to the mandibular branch of the facial nerve and it gives off its largest branch which is the submental artery which passes forwards on the mylohyoid muscle (Fig. 25.3).

The hypoglossal nerve curves forwards over the external carotid artery at about the commencement of the facial artery and courses medial to the posterior belly of the digastric muscle. This nerve usually lies below the submandibular gland, although it may be overlapped by it (Fig. 25.3).

THE MUSCLE BED OF THE SUBMANDIBULAR GLAND

Most of the submandibular gland lies immediately superficial to the mylohyoid muscle but some of the gland extends backwards beyond the muscle and so the posterior portion lies on the hyoglossus muscle (Fig. 25.1). Some of this posterior portion extends forwards with the submandibular duct deep to the mylohyoid muscle (Fig. 25.4).

The mylohyoid muscle arises from the inner surface of the mandible from the mylohyoid line and inserts into the body of the hyoid bone and from here into a midline raphe with its companion muscle from the other side. This midline raphe extends from the hyoid bone to the mandible. The nerve supply of the mylohyoid muscle is from the inferior alveolar branch of the mandibular division of the trigeminal nerve (and this branch lies on its superficial surface). The hypoglossal nerve lies deep to the mylohyoid muscle below the deep part of the submandibular gland. Likewise, the lingual nerve lies deep to the mylohyoid muscle above the deep part of the gland (Fig. 25.4).

The lingual nerve is a branch of the posterior division of the mandibular branch of the trigeminal nerve and it supplies sensation to the floor of the mouth, side of the gums and the anterior two-thirds of the tongue. This latter is from fibres of the chorda tympani which joins the lingual nerve early in its course. The lingual nerve curves forwards on the hyoglossus muscle above the deep portion of the submandibular gland and passes in a spiral manner on the

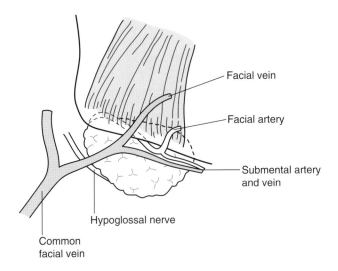

FIGURE 25.3 Structures superficial to the submandibular gland.

Facial vein

Facial artery

Submental artery and vein

Hypoglossal nerve

Common facial vein

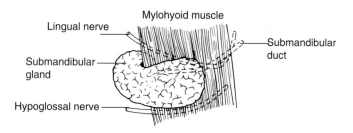

FIGURE 25.4 The submandibular gland and its deep portion.

lateral side of the submandibular duct, underneath it and upwards on the medial side (Fig 25.4). The submandibular ganglion hangs from the lingual nerve where it lies above the deep portion of the gland. In inflammatory disease, the lingual nerve can easily become adherent to the submandibular gland.

The hyoglossus muscle arises from the whole length of the greater cornu and the body of the hyoid bone and rises upwards to insert into the tongue. The hyoglossus muscle separates the lingual artery (which runs deep to it) from the hypoglossal nerve (superficial). The lingual artery gives off a sublingual branch which runs near the hypoglossal nerve. Given the close proximity of the sublingual artery to the hypoglossal nerve, the former should be preserved during excision of the submandibular gland.

THE SUBMANDIBULAR GANGLION

This is the secretomotor ganglion of the submandibular and lingual glands. Its preganglionic fibres arise in the superior salivatory nucleus and travel to the ganglion by way of the facial nerve, chorda tympani and lingual nerve. As noted it hangs from the lingual nerve above the deep part of the submandibular gland.

THE SUBMANDIBULAR DUCT

The submandibular duct runs forwards between the mylohyoid and hyoglossus muscles, and then between the sublingual gland and the genioglossus muscle before opening at the sublingual papilla. It receives some of the ducts from the sublingual gland. Its close relationship to the lingual nerve has already been noted (Fig. 25.4).

Lymphatics and the submandibular gland

The lymph nodes associated with this gland are often held in close proximity to the gland by fascial condensations in the area. Thus enlargement of one or more of these nodes can make distinction between it and enlargement of the submandibular gland very difficult.

The submandibular nodes receive drainage from the submental nodes, the oral cavity and of course the submandibular gland. They drain into the deep cervical chain of lymph nodes.

26 | Parotidectomy: the anatomy of the parotid gland and the facial nerve

Glyn Jamieson and James Katsaros

THE PAROTID GLAND

The parotid gland is a rather irregular structure because of the confined area in which it is contained. Its most clearly defined surfaces are a superficial surface and two deep surfaces, the latter formed as the gland wedges in between the external auditory canal, the mastoid process and the sternomastoid muscle behind, the zygomatic arch and temporomandibular joint above, and the ramus of the mandible in front. The first of these surfaces faces posteromedially and the second surface faces anteromedially. The gland overlaps the ramus of the mandible and the masseter muscle anteriorly and the sternomastoid muscle posteriorly.

It is contained in a tough condensation of fascia which attaches to the styloid process and mandible in front of the gland. This condensation is called the stylomandibular ligament and separates the parotid gland from the posterior aspect of the submandibular gland. The fascia also connects the posterior aspect of the gland to the external auditory canal and these connections have to be divided in mobilizing the gland.

The sternocleidomastoid muscle has been described previously (Ch. 21). Suffice it to say that it arises from the outer surface of the mastoid process and behind that from the superior nuchal line and the direction of its anterior border is roughly parallel with the styloid process – although this is about 1 cm anterior and is of course deeper.

The masseter muscle arises from the zygomatic arch and passes downwards and slightly posteriorly to insert into the angle of the mandible. Its nerve supply enters its deep surface from the mandibular division of the trigeminal nerve through the mandibular notch. Thus if one wishes to section the mandible for improvement in access to this region, the masseter can be reflected up to this level without jeopardizing its nerve supply. The parotid duct lies on the masseter muscle where the duct exits from the front of the gland and the duct dives deeply around the muscle's anterior border to open inside the cheek opposite the second upper molar tooth.

The superficial aspect of the parotid gland and related structures

The parotid gland may be covered by the platysma anteroinferiorly. There are lymph nodes superficial to the gland but most are bound to the parotid by its capsule. The posterior border of the gland lies over the sternomastoid muscle and the great auricular nerve and the external jugular vein are seen here.

THE GREAT AURICULAR NERVE AND THE EXTERNAL JUGULAR VEIN

The great auricular nerve arises from the C2, 3 nerve roots and emerges at approximately the midpoint of the posterior border of the sternomastoid muscle and passes vertically upwards lying deep to platysma (if the platysma reaches this far posteriorly) and behind the external jugular vein (Fig. 26.1). The nerve divides into an anterior and posterior division which usually lie within the dense fascia covering the parotid gland and occasionally deep to the fascia. The anterior division supplies the skin over the parotid gland and the ear lobe and the posterior division supplies the retroauricular skin. The nerve is often divided at parotidectomy and after initial numbness the residual area affected is often quite small. It may prove feasible to preserve the branches to the ear.

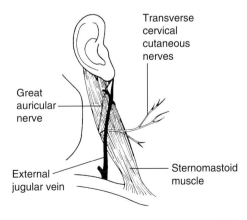

FIGURE 26.1 Structures related to the superficial aspect of the sternomastoid muscle.

The posterior auricular vein runs behind and beneath the parotid gland to join with the posterior trunk of the retromandibular vein which emerges from within the gland, and the two veins form the external jugular vein which passes vertically downwards to enter the subclavian vein.

At the point where the vein emerges from the parotid gland (sometimes as the retromandibular division, sometimes as the external jugular itself) the cervical branch of the facial nerve emerges from the parotid substance to lie superficial to the vein.

THE PERIPHERAL COURSES OF THE BRANCHES OF THE FACIAL NERVE
(Fig. 26.2)

As the facial skin is mobilized off the parotid gland, and as the anterior extent of the gland is reached care must be taken not to damage any of the branches of the facial nerve as they emerge under cover of the border of the gland.

The temporal branch emerges about 1 cm in front of the ear just below the zygomatic arch. The zygomatic division exits about 1 cm below the midpoint of the zygomatic arch (which is the point where a line from the tragus to the outer angle of the eye crosses the arch).

A line from the tragus to the outer angle of the jaw also gives the line of the buccal branch or branches, with the point of emergence of the nerve being the midpoint of this line.

The mandibular division exits in the region of the angle of the mandible and the cervical division emerges superficial to the external jugular vein. These nerves will be considered again with the facial nerve.

As the posteroinferior aspect of the gland is mobilized from the sternomastoid muscle, the posterior belly of digastric and the stylohyoid muscles are encountered.

POSTERIOR BELLY OF DIGASTRIC AND STYLOHYOID MUSCLES

The posterior belly of the digastric muscle arises from the inner aspect of the mastoid process and it is therefore deep and somewhat anterior to sternomastoid and runs a divergent path from that muscle. It runs downwards and forwards deep to the inferior aspect of the parotid gland and joins the intermediate tendon which is held by a sling to the hyoid bone. It also splits the tendon of stylohyoid muscle which is a useful way of finding this muscle. Some surgeons recommend that both of these muscles be exposed in their entirety. The advantage of doing this is that it frees up the area of emergence of the facial nerve.

The stylohyoid muscle arises by a tendon from the styloid process posteriorly, towards its base, and it passes downwards to insert into the body of the hyoid near the greater cornu's base. The tendon points directly at the stylomastoid foramen and therefore the point of exit of the facial nerve which passes forwards lateral to the base of the styloid process. The internal jugular vein is immediately deep to the proximal portion of the muscle and, deep to the vein, the transverse process of atlas is easily palpable (Fig. 26.3). The muscle is supplied by a branch of the facial nerve.

Dissection of the parotid gland posteriorly involves separating the gland away from the external auditory canal (external acoustic meatus).

THE EXTERNAL ACOUSTIC MEATUS

This cartilaginous (lateral third) and bony canal extends to the tympanic membrane and is about 4 cm in length from the tragus. The cartilaginous bony junction is about 10–12 mm from the tragus and is lateral to the plane of

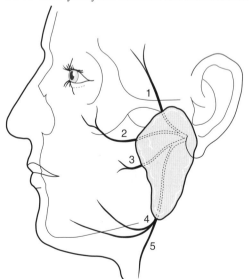

FIGURE 26.2 The branches of the facial nerve: 1, temporal; 2, zygomatic; 3, buccal; 4, mandibular; 5, cervical.

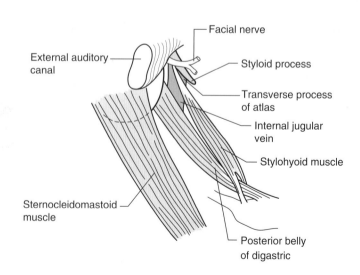

FIGURE 26.3 The posterior belly of digastric muscle and the stylohyoid muscle.

emergence of the facial nerve. A small cartilaginous extension of the external portion of the acoustic canal at the junction with the bony canal is often found and seems to point to the facial nerve, which is found approximately 1 cm inferior and 1 cm medial to the tip of the pointer.

The portion of the bony meatus running inferiorly is called the tympanic plate and the point where this joins the mastoid process posteriorly (tympanomastoid junction or suture) is usually 5–10 mm immediately lateral to the facial nerve (Fig. 26.3).

THE FACIAL NERVE AND PAROTIDECTOMY

The facial nerve emerges through the stylomastoid foramen which lies posterior to the styloid process and the nerve crosses lateral to the styloid process just above the tendon of origin of the stylohyoid muscle (Fig. 26.3). Thus, as well as running forwards, the nerve runs from deep to superficial, a direction which can be much exaggerated if the deep part of the gland is enlarged.

Dissection of the external auditory meatus opens the area above the base of the styloid process (and therefore above the facial nerve; Fig. 26.4). Dissection of the stylohyoid tendon and the digastric muscle opens the area below the facial nerve. The tissue between the two areas contains the facial nerve and the stylomastoid artery, which should be secured before division if possible (it usually lies superficial to the main trunk of the nerve). The thickness of the parotid glandular tissue varies considerably, as a result of which the depth of the nerve within the gland varies considerably.

The nerve on entering the parotid forms into a bewildering array of relationships but fortunately most, if not all, important branches maintain a relationship superficial to blood vessels in the gland. Perhaps the most common arrangement is for the nerve to split into an upper and lower division with the upper nerve providing supply to the forehead and eye muscles (temporal and zygomatic branches) and the lower division the remainder of the face, lips and platysma (buccal, mandibular and cervical branches).

We have discussed already the points of emergence of these nerves from the parotid gland (Fig. 26.2). The temporal division is usually the most anterior of the structures crossing the zygomatic arch immediately in front of the ear.

Behind the temporal branch lies the superficial temporal artery and vein and even more posteriorly lies the auriculotemporal nerve.

The buccal branch or branches of the facial nerve tend to run parallel and below or above (or both) the parotid duct.

The relationship between the mandibular branch and the cervical branch and neck incisions is discussed in relation to the surgery of the submandibular gland (see Ch. 25).

There are many connections between branches of the nerve so that division of any one or more divisions is by no means certain to produce the disability expected.

THE DEEP PORTION OF THE PAROTID GLAND

In the patient (as opposed to the dissecting room) the parotid gland is not separated into lobes with an isthmus between them. However part of the gland extends inwards and it is usually the portion deep to the ramification of the facial nerve.

The superficial temporal and maxillary veins join within the substance of the deep part of the gland to form the retromandibular vein.

Deeper still lies the external carotid artery and this is often seen when mobilizing the lower half of the gland. The external carotid artery divides within the substance of the gland into the superficial temporal and maxillary arteries. The superficial temporal artery also gives off the transverse facial artery which tends to run parallel with but above the parotid duct.

THE AURICULOTEMPORAL NERVE

This is a branch of the mandibular division of the trigeminal nerve and it traverses the parotid gland to emerge from its superior surface, behind the superficial temporal artery and vein. It communicates with the facial nerve within the gland. It supplies sensation to the external auditory meatus, the upper two-thirds of the ear and skin of the temple regions and also secretomotor fibres to the parotid gland. The preganglionic fibres travel in the glossopharyngeal nerve

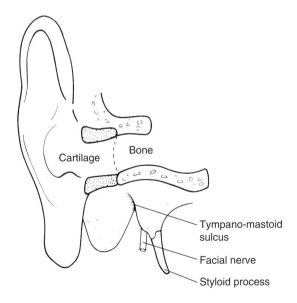

Cartilage   Bone

Tympano-mastoid sulcus

Facial nerve

Styloid process

FIGURE 26.4 The external acoustic meatus and canal and the tympanomastoid junction and its relationship to the facial nerve.

through its branch to the tympanic plexus and thence via the lesser petrosal nerve to the otic ganglion. This lies medial to the mandibular nerve, to which it contributes postganglionic fibres to the auriculotemporal nerve. Damage or division of the auriculotemporal nerve is in some way thought to be related to Frey's syndrome after parotidectomy – sweating of preauricular skin on eating.

FURTHER READING

Conley J J 1975 Surgical anatomy relative to the parotid gland. In: Conley J J (ed) Salivary glands and the facial nerve. Grune and Stratton, New York.

Keyes G R, Tenta LT 1985 Surgery of the parotid gland and the viscero-vertebral angle. Clin Plast Surg 12:323–330.

4 SURGICAL ONCOLOGICAL PROCEDURES

27 | Mastectomy; partial mastectomy; microdochectomy: the anatomy of the breast

Glyn Jamieson and Brendon Coventry

GENERAL ANATOMY

The base of the breast lies approximately between the second and the sixth ribs, the edge of the sternum medially, and the posterior axillary line laterally.

The breast base mainly overlies the pectoralis major muscle superomedially and to a lesser extent the serratus anterior inferolaterally and the external oblique muscle below and medially to this (Fig. 27.1).

It is a glandular appendage of the skin and therefore is contained within the skin and subcutaneous tissue, including the superficial fascia. It consists of 15–20 lobules of glandular tissue of varying size with varying amounts of adipose tissue between the lobules. There are also strands of connective tissue (Cooper's ligaments) connecting the pectoralis fascia on the deep surface of the breast to the superficial tissue and skin. These are most numerous in the upper

half of the breast and are probably responsible for the puckering of skin seen overlying a malignancy. The plane between the pectoralis fascia and the base of the breast is easily developed by blunt dissection, although small branches of the intercostal vessels may traverse the space larger branches are present medially and laterally (see blood supply).

Breast lobules are placed more peripherally in the breast and drain into small ductules that coalesce into larger (lactiferous) ducts individually draining each main lobule. There are some 15–20 lactiferous ducts which correspond with the lobules. Each duct has a subareolar dilatation termed an infundibulum that collects milk during lactation for suckling and each duct opens independently on the nipple. The openings of the major ducts are usually large enough to be selectively cannulated using a hollow needle which allows the duct to be X-ray imaged using radiographic contrast, producing a ductogram. A fine probe can be used to cannulate a duct at the nipple and the duct containing pathology, such as a duct papilloma, can be dissected free from the breast – a so-called microdochectomy.

Breast lobules are ill-defined and cannot usually be dissected out individually at operation because their boundaries overlap. Partial mastectomy is therefore resection of sections of breast lobules surrounding a mass, rather than excision of separate individual lobules.

While most breast tissue is superficial to the deep fascia, lobular tissue often extends along the lateral border of pectoralis major and deeply into the axilla. This is the breast's axillary tail and the glandular tissue can reach as far as the axillary vein. Separate islands of breast tissue are also not uncommon within the axilla.

The blood supply

The blood supply to each breast is mainly derived from above, i.e. from the respective subclavian artery and its extension, the axillary artery. The internal thoracic (internal mammary) artery arises from the first part of the subclavian artery and descends inside the ribs just lateral to the edge of the sternum. It gives off perforating branches which pass

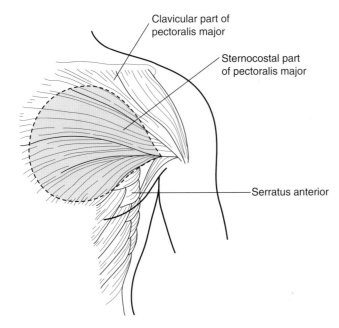

FIGURE 27.1 The muscles underlying the breast.

Clavicular part of pectoralis major

Sternocostal part of pectoralis major

Serratus anterior

through the intercostal spaces and the pectoralis major to reach the breast. The second to fourth perforating arteries are usually the largest and provide the major blood supply to the breast. The lateral thoracic artery arises from the 3rd part of the axillary artery at the lateral margin of pectoralis minor muscle and runs down the lateral border of that muscle, sending branches around the lateral border of pectoralis major into the lateral breast. Lateral branches of the intercostal vessels perforate the serratus muscle anterolaterally to supply the breast. Other branches of the intercostal arteries may also traverse the retromammary space to supply the breast medially.

There are numerous anastomoses between blood vessels in the breast permitting transposition of breast tissue flaps for reconstruction after excision. Fat necrosis may occasionally result from devascularization or from direct trauma. The blood supply to the nipple/areola complex comes from a periareolar cutaneous plexus supplied from above by superficial branches of the internal and lateral thoracic arteries, and to a lesser extent from below, by branches of the lower intercostal vessels. This anastomosis is supported by deep branches which traverse the breast to reach the nipple. Preservation of either supply will prevent necrosis of the nipple after extensive surgical incisions in this area.

The venous drainage tends to follow the corresponding arteries, except that a thoraco-epigastric vein is usually present which traverses the central axilla draining blood from the lateral breast and lower axilla.

Vascular calcification is a common finding on mammography in women over 60 years of age.

The lymphatic drainage of the breast (Fig. 27.2)

The lymphatic drainage of the breast is reflected by the pattern of spread of breast carcinoma to the axillary, internal (thoracic) mammary and supraclavicular lymph node regions (in descending order of frequency). There is a subareolar plexus of lymphatics draining the nipple and ductal system which drains predominantly to the ipsilateral axillary lymph nodes. The deep layers of the breast can also drain to the internal (thoracic) mammary lymph nodes lying along the internal mammary artery on the deep aspect of the costal cartilages about 1 cm parasternally.

The axillary lymph nodes are joined by rich lymphatic anastomotic channels and are anatomically described as Level I (inferior to the lower border of pectoralis minor muscle), Level II (behind pectoralis minor) and Level III (above pectoralis minor). Previous anatomical descriptions have included pectoral, subscapular, high axillary, lateral axillary, and infraclavicular. Lymph nodes high in the axilla communicate with supraclavicular lymph nodes at the base of the neck. Surgical access to the axillary nodes is usually via an incision obliquely across the axilla. Internal mammary lymph nodes can be accessed via a transverse incision in the medial breast to gain the intercostal space(s). Lymphatic mapping using lymphoscintigraphy is revealing more of the individual complexity of lymphatic drainage of the breast.

THE MUSCLES ASSOCIATED WITH THE BREAST

Pectoralis major

The pectoralis major muscle and fascia forms the main support for the base of the breast.

The muscle arises from three origins that can be separately seen: the medial half of the clavicle (the clavicular portion), the lateral half of the sternum and second to sixth costal cartilages (the sternocostal portion) and also from the aponeurosis of the external oblique muscle. The fibres of the three components sweep downwards, horizontally and upwards respectively to its combined tendinous insertion into the bicipital groove of the humerus.

The clavicular head is usually easily separable above from the deltoid muscle by a gap known as the deltopectoral groove in which the cephalic vein runs. When a radical mastectomy is performed – an unusual occurrence today – the clavicular head of the pectoralis major muscle can usually be retained to preserve some function.

The pectoralis major is supplied by the medial (C8) and lateral (C6, 7) pectoral nerves paradoxically innervating the lateral and medial fibres respectively.

Removal of the breast is best achieved by dissecting it from the pectoralis major muscle fascia commencing superomedially and pulling the breast inferolaterally. When the lateral border of the muscle is reached the tissue tends to dive deeply towards the axilla and is attached to clavipectoral fascia at the lateral edge of the pectoralis minor muscle

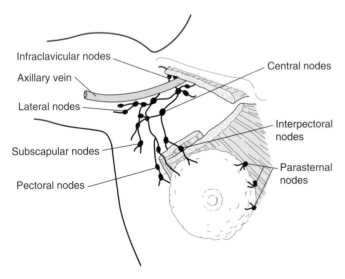

FIGURE 27.2 The lymphatic drainage of the breast.

Infraclavicular nodes

Axillary vein

Lateral nodes

Subscapular nodes

Pectoral nodes

Central nodes

Interpectoral nodes

Parasternal nodes

(the fascia splits to enclose this muscle). This attachment must be divided to separate the breast away from the thoracic wall and axilla.

Other muscles

Mastectomy for malignancy usually includes incontinuity dissection of the axilla and there are two other muscles in the axilla which are of importance because their nerve supply may be damaged during operation in this area. These are the latissimus dorsi muscle supplied by the thoracodorsal nerve (C6–8), which forms the posterior wall of the axilla, and the serratus anterior muscle, supplied by the long thoracic nerve (C5–7), which covers the medial wall. Both are described with the surgical anatomy of the axilla in Chapter 28.

28 | Block dissection of axillary lymph nodes; sentinel node biopsy: the anatomy of the axilla

Glyn Jamieson and P Grantley Gill

In the past, block dissection of the axillary lymph nodes was most frequently performed in association with mastectomy when the breast and nodal tissue were taken in continuity. Today however the procedure is often performed as a separate procedure, in conjunction with total excision of a primary breast cancer, or because of involvement from other primary tumours, typically a melanoma. An additional dimension is the concept of the sentinel draining node in breast cancer, and malignant melanoma in this part of the body.

THE AXILLA

The axilla is a more or less pyramidal area with the base formed by the convex axillary skin and the apex by the rather narrow communication in front of the first rib and behind the clavicle through which the neurovascular structures enter the axilla.

The anterior wall is made up of the pectoralis major and pectoralis minor muscles and the clavipectoral fascia (see below), the medial wall is the upper serrations of serratus anterior and the posterior wall is made up of subcapularis above and teres major and latissimus dorsi below (Fig. 28.1). The anterior and posterior wall come together in the region of the bicipital groove of the humerus so there is no lateral wall to speak of.

The axilla contains many important structures such as the infraclavicular portion of the brachial plexus, the axillary artery and vein and the axillary lymph nodes.

MUSCLES OF THE AXILLA

Pectoralis minor muscle

The pectoralis minor muscle has a variable origin from the ribs on the anterior chest wall, the most usual attachment being from the third to the fifth ribs. The muscle then ascends deep to pectoralis major to insert into the coracoid process. It lies superficial to the neurovascular structures which will enter the axilla. Pectoralis minor traditionally divides the axillary artery into three parts – the first part

proximal to. the second part behind and the third part distal to the muscle.

It is supplied by the lateral and medial pectoral nerves.

The clavipectoral fascia

At least in its upper part this is a fascial sheet worthy of its name. It arises from the clavicle enclosing the subclavius muscle and then descends to enclose the pectoralis minor and finally attaches to the floor of the axilla. Like the pectoralis minor muscle it lies anterior to the neurovascular structures of the axilla.

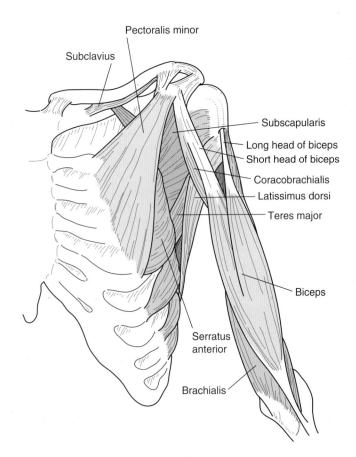

FIGURE 28.1   Some muscles of the axilla.

The serratus anterior muscle

The serratus anterior muscle arises as digitations from the outer surface of the first to eighth ribs near the costal cartilages, and the fibres pass backwards to insert along the whole of the medial border of the scapula. It holds this border of the scapula to the chest wall and it is supplied by the long thoracic nerve (see later).

The subscapularis muscle

The subscapularis muscle arises from the costal surface of the scapula and inserts into the lesser tuberosity of the humerus. It is supplied by the subscapular nerves. It steadies the head of the humerus against the glenoid cavity and assists in medial rotation of the humerus.

The teres major muscle

The teres major muscle arises near the inferior angle of the scapula and, together with the latissimus dorsi, inserts into the bicipital groove of the humerus.

It is supplied by the lower of the subscapular nerves.

The brachial plexus (Fig. 28.2)

The brachial plexus is usually formed from the ventral rami of the C5–8 and T1 nerve roots. It can be divided conveniently

into the supraclavicular and infraclavicular portion and it is the latter which most concerns us here.

The supraclavicular portion gives off branches from its roots:

❶ nerves to the scalenus muscles and longus colli (C5–8);
❷ a branch to the phrenic nerve (C5);
❸ the dorsal scapular nerve to the rhomboids (C5) and the long thoracic nerve (C5–7, see later).

The roots of the plexus then form into three trunks, C5, 6 making the upper trunk, C7 the middle trunk and C8, T1 the lower trunk. Only the upper trunk has any branches, these being the nerve to subclavius and the suprascapular nerve.

The trunks divide into an anterior and a posterior division. The posterior divisions unite to form the posterior cord of the brachial plexus, the upper two anterior divisions unite to form the lateral cord and the lowermost anterior division continues as the medial cord.

The cords and their branches are closely related to the axillary artery.

The axillary vein is anteromedial to the artery and so is medial to all the neural structures.

As the lymphatic tissue tends also to be medial to the vein it means that lymphatic tissue can be stripped from the axilla without risk of damaging nerves, with the exceptions discussed below.

In the upper part of the axilla the medial cord is behind the first part of the axillary artery and the lateral and posterior

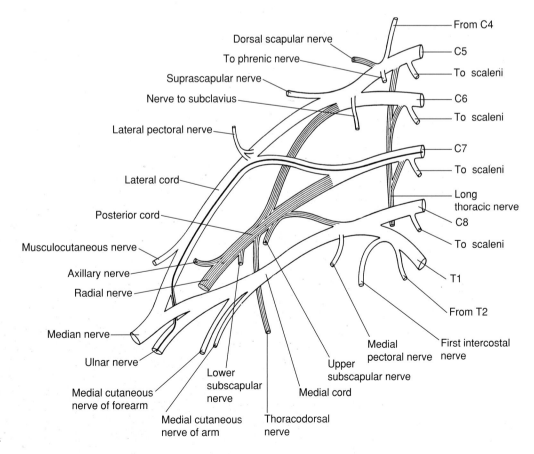

FIGURE 28.2 The brachial plexus.

cords are lateral to it. The cords assume their named relationship around the second part of the axillary artery and the branches from the cords also keep a similar relationship to the third part of the axillary artery, i.e. the branches from the lateral cord stay lateral, the branches from the posterior cord are posterior and the branches of the medial cord stay medial to the artery. The exception to the rule is the medial root of the median nerve which crosses in front of the third part of the axillary artery to join the lateral root and form the median nerve.

The branches from the infraclavicular portion of the plexus, i.e. from the cords, are listed below. Only those which have relevance to block dissection of the nodes of the axilla are considered in further detail.

❶ From the lateral cord arise the lateral pectoral nerve (C5–7), the musculocutaneous nerve (C5–7) and the lateral root of the median nerve (C5–7).
❷ From the medial cord arise the medial pectoral nerve (C8, T1), the medial cutaneous nerve of the arm (C8, T1), the medial cutaneous nerve of the forearm (C8, T1), the ulnar nerve (C7, 8, T1) and the medial root of the median nerve (C8, T1).
❸ From the posterior cord arise the upper and lower subscapular nerves (C5, 6), the axillary nerve (C5, 6), the thoracodorsal nerve (C6–8) and the radial nerve (C5–8, T1).

NERVES ASSOCIATED WITH BLOCK DISSECTION OF THE AXILLA

The lateral pectoral nerve

The lateral pectoral nerve arises either from the divisions of the brachial plexus or the lateral cord and crosses in front of the axillary artery and vein at about the level of the medial border of pectoralis minor, where the nerve penetrates the clavipectoral fascia. It supplies pectoralis major from its deep surface. It usually gives off a communicating branch to the medial pectoral nerve. This loop lies in front of the axillary artery.

The medial pectoral nerve

This arises from the medial cord more distally than the lateral pectoral nerve. It lies posterior to the axillary artery, emerges between the artery and vein, receives the communicating loop from the lateral pectoral nerve and then enters the deep surface of pectoralis minor. Some of its fibres penetrate the muscle to enter pectoralis major.

As the origin of these nerves is close to the first part of the axillary artery, division of pectoralis minor at or above the level of the axillary artery should spare the nerves – or certainly spare the lateral pectoral nerve which is more proximal in its origin than the medial pectoral nerve.

The intercostobrachial nerve

This is a cutaneous branch from the second intercostal nerve. It exits between the first and second ribs and traverses the axilla to supply a small area of skin on the medial side of the upper arm. There is frequently a second intercostobrachial nerve arising from the third intercostal nerve.

The intercostobrachial nerve exits from the chest wall 2 cm or so anterior to the line of the long thoracic nerve and it is usually divided during block dissection of the axilla, with the resultant numbness not proving a problem for most patients. In staging procedures for early breast cancers, however, this nerve is often preserved.

The thoracodorsal nerve

The thoracodorsal nerve arises between the upper and lower subscapular nerves from the posterior cord of the brachial plexus, but while these pass backwards to be out of harm's way, the thoracodorsal nerve passes downwards behind the axillary artery and vein to lie on subcapularis before the nerve enters the latissimus dorsi which it supplies. It runs with the moderately large subscapular artery in the upper part of its course and the smaller thoracodorsal artery further distally. As this nerve lies against the posterior wall of the axilla it is usually spared during block dissection of the axilla.

The long thoracic nerve

This nerve arises from the roots of C5–7 of the brachial plexus. The trunk of the nerve passes behind the axillary artery and vein and runs downwards on the serrations of serratus anterior, where it is exposed during axillary dissection and is at risk of damage.

To enter the axilla anteriorly it is necessary to divide the clavipectoral fascia at the lateral edge of pectoralis minor. This then takes the surgeon into a plane which may elevate the long thoracic nerve from the chest wall with the axillary contents. It is necessary formally to divide the fascia longitudinally in front of the nerve (on the sternal side) to allow it to drop back against the chest wall.

The nerve can also be identified as it appears from behind the axillary vein where that structure crosses the second rib.

VESSELS ASSOCIATED WITH BLOCK DISSECTION

The axillary artery

The relationship of the axillary artery to the brachial plexus has already been described, and the fact that it does not feature a great deal in a block dissection has already been mentioned.

Its branches are the superior thoracic artery and the thoracoacromial trunk (from the first part), the lateral thoracic artery (from the second part) and from the third part the subscapular and medial and lateral circumflex humeral arteries.

The axillary vein

The axillary vein is the direct continuation of the basilic vein which changes its name at the lower border of teres major muscle. At a higher point it usually receives the brachial vein or veins and the cephalic vein. It also receives the corresponding veins to the arterial branches mentioned above.

The vein initially lies medial to the axillary artery but more proximally it lies below it. Distally it is separated from the artery by the ulnar nerve and the medial cutaneous nerve of the forearm. The medial cutaneous nerve of the arm emerges between the axillary artery and vein to lie medial to the vein. More proximally the medial head of the median nerve emerges from between artery and vein. At an even higher level the medial pectoral nerve also emerges from between the artery and the vein.

THE LYMPH NODES OF THE AXILLA

As mentioned when discussing the lymphatic drainage of the breast, the apportioning of lymph nodes of the axilla into groups is arbitrary but conventional. Most of the nodes lie along the medial side of the axillary vein. Thus from proximal to distal these nodes are the apical, the central and the lateral groups. The apical nodes receive all the drainage from the other groups and give off the subclavian lymphatic trunk which drains into the thoracic duct or more directly into veins.

The central nodes are the largest set and receive efferents not only from the lowest set along the axillary vein but from a posterior wall and anterior wall set, known respectively as subscapular nodes (they lie along the subscapular vessels) and pectoral nodes (they lie along the lateral pectoral vessels) near the lateral border of pectoralis minor.

A more practical grouping of the lymph nodes used by surgeons, and accepted by pathologists, is to separate the groups into levels. Level I are those nodes below the lateral edge of pectoralis minor, level II behind it and level III above it.

Thus if all tissue covering the anterior aspect of the axillary vein from the apex to the base of the axilla is swept medially, if the tissue along the lateral margin of pectoralis minor is swept posteriorly, and if the tissue from alongside the thoracodorsal nerve and the subscapular vessels is swept anteriorly, all of the lymphatic tissue of the axilla should have been encompassed.

The operation of axillary clearance is currently defined in terms of the level of the dissection performed. The complete removal of lymphatic tissue described above to level III is usually reserved for situations where there is a proven metastatic disease in the lymph nodes. Removal of nodes to level I or II is now performed for staging early breast cancer when there is no apparent involvement by tumour.

Sentinel node

A sentinel lymph node is a node which directly receives afferent lymph from a primary tumour in the breast, or melanoma on the arm or trunk.

The anatomical location of this gland varies, but it is usually found at level I or II. Identification can only be determined by lymphoscintography, and intraoperative localization by the use of gamma probes and selective patent blue dye staining.

Less frequently it is found at level III, in the supraclavicular fossa. In the case of melanoma of the back, it may be in the quadrilateral space bounded by the scapularis muscle above, and teres major below, and the long head of triceps medially and the humeris laterally. The location of the sentinel node(s) is not dictated by the anatomical location of the primary.

FURTHER READING

Miller R E, Snyder S J 1986 A technique for identification of the long thoracic nerve during axillary dissection. Surg Gynecol Obstet 162:480–482.

29 | Radical neck dissection: the anatomy of the neck and cervical lymph nodes

Glyn Jamieson, Suren Krishnan and Daniel Hains

THE LYMPH NODES OF THE HEAD AND NECK

There are groups of outlying nodes which drain into the lymph nodes lying along the internal jugular vein. These outlying nodes are arranged as a ring around the base of the head and as vertical chains along the axis of the neck. The ring around the base of the head consists of the submental, submaxillary, parotid, retroauricular and occipital nodes. The most superficial of the vertical chains lie along the external jugular and anterior jugular veins (known as the superficial cervical and anterior cervical nodes respectively). The deeper vertical chains lie alongside the trachea (paratracheal) and behind the pharynx (retropharyngeal).

All of these groups of nodes drain into the main vertical chain which is the group known as the deep cervical nodes. These nodes lie around the internal jugular vein. The lower nodes of this group are the terminating nodes for all lymph from the head and neck and they give rise to the right and left jugular lymphatic trunks. These trunks may terminate directly into the region of the jugular vein–subclavian vein confluence or their more usual termination is into the thoracic duct on the left and the right lymphatic trunk on the right.

It is not particularly helpful to describe the various ways in which the lymphatics of the mouth, the tongue, the tonsil, etc. can drain, although clinically it probably is important to realize that the tip of the tongue and indeed any lesion near the midline can drain its lymph to either side of the head and neck. The important fact is that all of the lymphatic drainage passes to the deep cervical chain, which is the reason why these nodes have to be removed when removing the drainage nodes of head and neck regions.

The deep cervical nodes

This is a chain of nodes which are closely related to the internal jugular vein. This is unusual in that lymph nodes usually are more closely related to arteries than veins. The lymph nodes are embedded in the tissues which surround the internal jugular vein, i.e. to say in the carotid sheath, although as the chain passes downwards its nodes tend to be concentrated more posteriorly and lateral to the internal jugular

vein. Classically they were divided arbitrarily by the crossing of the omohyoid muscle into a superior and an inferior group. In the superior group there are two nodes which are individually named. The node which lies at the point where the posterior belly of digastric crosses the internal jugular vein is called the jugulodigastric node and this is the main node receiving lymphatic drainage from the tonsil.

The node which lies at the point where the omohyoid crosses the internal jugular vein is called the jugulo-omohyoid node and lymphatic drainage from the tongue (including its tip) often passes directly to this node.

More recently, work done at the Memorial Sloan-Kettering Cancer Center in New York has resulted in the classification of lymph nodes of the neck into six levels. This description is based on their clinical and surgical relevance. These levels are representative of the likely primary sites of tumour origin from the skin and its adnexa of the head and neck and the mucosa of the upper aerodigestive tract. They also have relevance to surgical treatment of the neck.

- Level I comprises the submental and submandibular nodes,
- Level II comprises the upper jugular lymph nodes,
- Level III comprises the middle jugular lymph nodes,
- Level IV comprises the lower jugular lymph nodes,
- Level V comprises the nodes of the posterior triangle associated with the spinal accessory nerve and in the supraclavicular fossa associated with the transverse cervical vessels,
- Level VI comprises the paratracheal nodes

The classical radical neck dissection involves a comprehensive clearance of five levels of lymph nodes with the removal of the internal jugular vein, the sternocleidomastoid muscle and the accessory nerve. Modifications of this operation can involve comprehensive clearance of the lymph nodes with preservation of one or all of the accessory nerve (to prevent shoulder dysfunction), the internal jugular vein (to reduce the risk of raised intracranial pressure) or the preservation of the sternocleidomastoid muscle (to prevent the cosmetic deficit of resection of sternocleido muscle). Modification of the neck dissection depends on the disease status of the neck.

The lymphatic drainage of the thyroid gland and the upper trachea drains into anterior cervical lymph nodes which lie along the anterior jugular veins and the paratracheal chain of the lymph nodes beside the trachea in the lower neck and superior mediastinum. These nodes are not part of the routine resection in a radical neck dissection, but are dissected in malignant disease of the thyroid gland.

SKIN INCISIONS FOR NECK DISSECTION

Exposure for a neck dissection requires the raising of skin flaps. The design of the incision is thus crucial since the surgeon must have regard for skin flap viability, surgical access and the necessity to provide safe skin cover for vital retained structures, such as the carotid vessels. In addition the surgeon must be sure that the incision is compatible with any likely reconstructive method and take into consideration whether previous radiotherapy is likely to have an adverse effect on wound healing.

The blood supply to the cervical skin runs in two directions: caudad from the line of the lower border of the mandible and craniad from the line of the clavicle. Theoretically therefore the safest skin incision is a transverse mid cervical incision. There have been many skin incisions described for neck dissection. Generally speaking it is best to avoid a three-point junction, particularly if the patient has previously been irradiated. Excellent exposure is afforded by a lateral 'apron flap'. This incision begins at the tip of the mastoid and extends vertically down along the anterior border of the trapezius and curves forward along a skin crease parallel to and approximately 2 cm above the clavicle. The incision is then continued along to the anterior border of the sternocleidomastoid muscle. The incision is extended upwards vertically to just below the skin. This flap has an excellent blood supply and when raised with the associated platysma muscle proves viable even in the irradiated patient.

In patients in whom there is a concern about skin viability or who already have a previous transverse skin incision, two parallel transverse skin incisions can be made. The upper incision lies along an upper skin crease approximately 5 cm below and parallel to the angle of the mandible extending from the anterior board of the trapezius to the midline and the lower skin incision lies approximately 2 cm above the clavicle and along a skin crease parallel to the clavicle from the anterior border of the trapezius to the midline. A skin and platysma flap is elevated between these incisions and the neck dissection performed under this skin bridge.

THE PLATYSMA

This is a broad sheet of muscle fibres of variable thickness and extent but often atrophic in the elderly to the point where the surgeon cannot see it. It is superficial to the deep fascia of the neck and to such structures as the anterior and external jugular veins.

It extends from the midline downwards beyond the clavicle and upwards to the mandible and beyond where some fibres blend with the facial muscles. It does not usually extend posteriorly much beyond the line of the external jugular vein.

It is supplied by the cervical branch of the facial nerve. Because of its ability to contract it should be sutured as a separate layer from the skin.

Although contrary opinion has been expressed, it is not usual to remove platysma in radical neck dissections.

When raising skin flaps in a neck dissection it is best to elevate the platysma with the skin. This increases the viability of the skin flap as the platysma supplies blood to the overlying skin. An added advantage of dissecting immediately beneath the platysma is that the plane is relatively bloodless, provided the surgeon stays superficial to the anterior and external jugular vein while raising the flaps. If the veins are ligated and raised with the platysma and skin flap an incorrect deeper plane is entered.

THE EXTERNAL JUGULAR VEIN

The external jugular vein commences at about the lower border of the parotid gland where the posterior division of the retromandibular vein and the posterior auricular vein join. It descends across the sternomastoid muscle lying on the deep fascia but deep to platysma. Just above the midpoint of the clavicle it penetrates the deep fascia and joins the subclavian vein. Its tributaries are the posterior external jugular vein which joins it about midway in its course and the transverse cervical and suprascapular veins, all of these veins joining it posteriorly, and anteriorly the anterior jugular vein.

The great auricular nerve runs in a parallel course to the vein posterior to its upper third.

THE MUSCLES

Sternocleidomastoid muscle (Fig. 29.1)

This muscle arises from the front of the manubrium sterni and the superior surface of the medial part of the clavicle and ascends obliquely backwards to insert into the outer surface of the mastoid process and the anterior part of the superior nuchal line of the skull. Because of its course across the neck it is related to many structures and it is one of the keys to the surgical anatomy of the area.

The external jugular vein courses across it from below the ear lobe to about the midpoint of the clavicle where the vein plunges deeply to join the subclavian vein.

Emerging from the posterior border at about its mid point and ascending across sternomastoid behind and parallel to the external jugular vein is the great auricular nerve, and emerging from the same point but passing transversely across the muscle is the transverse cutaneous nerve of the neck.

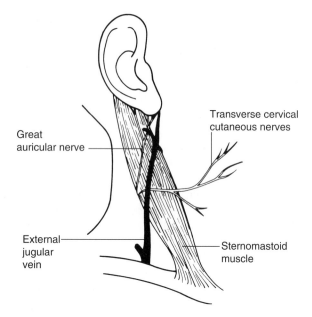

FIGURE 29.1   The sternocleidomastoid muscle.

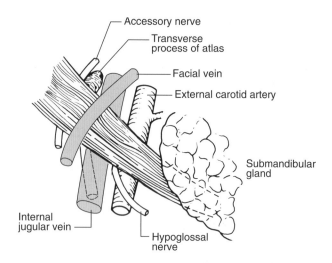

FIGURE 29.2   The posterior belly of the digastric muscle.

The accessory nerve emerges from the posterior border of the sternomastoid muscle and bears a very constant relationship to the point at which the great auricular nerve emerges (Erb's point).

This provides a useful means of identifying the accessory nerve in cases where the surgeon wishes to preserve it, e.g. the functional neck dissection.

The accessory nerve is found superior to Erb's point and within 2 cm of it in about 90% of cases.

The lower part of the parotid gland lies over the uppermost portion of the sternomastoid muscle.

Its nerve supply is from the accessory nerve, which supplies it from the muscle's deep surface about 5 cm below the mastoid process.

As the muscle lies over the carotid vessels, the internal jugular vein and the deep cervical lymph nodes, it is easy to see why it is such a key muscle in operations of this area, and many neck operations commence with an incision along the line of the anterior border of the sternocleidomastoid muscle.

This incision is necessary to enter the parapharyngolaryngeal space for operations on the vessels or the pharynx, larynx or cervical spine. The entry is made by incising the deep cervical (investing) fascia which splits to enclose the sternomastoid muscle.

The function of sternocleidomastoid muscle is shown by the movement of pushing the chin against resistance, which tenses the muscle on the opposite side. However, acting together, level rotation of the head is probably the main function of the muscles.

The digastric muscle

The digastric muscle has two muscle bellies. The anterior belly arises from a fossa near the midline on the back of the mandible. It passes backwards and downwards to its intermediate tendon which is held to the hyoid bone by a fibrous sling. This part of the muscle is supplied by the nerve to mylohyoid muscle. The posterior belly of digastric passes backwards and upwards to the medial side of the mastoid process. It is supplied by a branch from the facial nerve. The posterior belly crosses the accessory nerve, the transverse process of the atlas, the internal jugular vein, the hypoglossal nerve and the internal and external carotid arteries (Fig. 29.2).

The posterior belly is an important surgical landmark in radical neck dissection as tissues superficial to it can be confidently divided. The internal jugular vein is always deep to the posterior belly of digastric.

The omohyoid muscle

This muscle also has two muscle bellies joined by an intermediate tendon. The inferior belly arises from the superior border of the scapula near the scapular notch and passes almost transversely across the neck to the intermediate tendon which lies behind sternomastoid and overlies the internal jugular vein. The point of angulation is variable but is about the level of the cricoid cartilage. It is held down by a condensation of fascia which attaches the tendon to the clavicle. The superior belly then ascends obliquely upwards. It is close to vertical which justifies its inclusion as one of the strap muscles of the neck. It lies lateral to sternothyroid in most of its course and inserts on the body of the hyoid bone lateral to the sternohyoid insertion. It is supplied by branches from the ansae cervicalis nerve.

TRANSVERSE CERVICAL VESSELS

The thyrocervical trunk arises from the first part of the subclavian artery just medial to the overlying scalenus anterior muscle and it almost immediately breaks up into its three terminal branches. The inferior thyroid artery descends out of the field. The suprascapular artery crosses in front of scalenus anterior and the phrenic nerve and then in front of the subclavian artery and the brachial plexus. It is approximately posterior to, and parallel with, the clavicle in this part of its course.

At a level about 1 cm higher, the superficial cervical branch of the thyrocervical trunk crosses the neck. It similarly crosses in front of scalenus anterior and the phrenic nerve, and the subclavian artery and brachial plexus. These vessels are divided when carrying out a radical dissection of lymphatic tissue in the neck.

THE SPINAL ACCESSORY NERVE

The accessory nerve is the XIth cranial nerve and it exits from the jugular foramen and usually crosses posterior to the internal jugular vein, although in about a third of cases it crosses in front of the vein. It crosses the transverse process of the atlas but lies deep to the styloid process and its associated structures. It enters the deep surface of the sternomastoid muscle, supplying it, and emerges from its posterior border about the junction of the upper and middle third, superior to and within 2 cm of the emergence of the great auricular nerve. It then crosses the posterior triangle, lying on levator scapulae but separated from it by a fascial layer. The nerve disappears behind the anterior border of trapezius about 5 cm above the clavicle. It supplies the trapezius. There are usually some lymph nodes associated with the nerve which tend to drain only superficial neck structures. However higher deep jugular nodes lie very close to its course before it enters the sternocleidomastoid muscle so that preservation of the nerve in an otherwise radical neck dissection is a controversial topic. Its preservation avoids the frequently distressing shoulder droop of a standard radical neck dissection.

THE INTERNAL JUGULAR VEIN

The internal jugular vein exits from the skull through the jugular foramen and descends behind and then lateral to the carotid system to end behind the sternal end of the clavicle by joining with the subclavian vein to form the brachiocephalic vein. It is dilated near its termination into an inferior jugular bulb.

At the base of the skull where it lies behind the internal carotid artery, it is separated from the artery by the emerging cranial nerves IX–XII.

The vagus nerve lies in front of the vein between it and the carotid system.

The vein lies on the origins of levator scapulae, scalenus medius and scalenus anterior muscles, separated from them by the cervical plexus and its branches. Lower down the vein crosses the thyrocervical trunk and the first part of the subclavian artery, and on the left the thoracic duct arches behind it.

The vein is crossed superficially by the posterior belly of the digastric muscle and the tendon of omohyoid muscle. The infrahyoid strap muscles overlie it below this level and the sternomastoid muscle overlies the whole complex.

The vein receives named tributaries largely corresponding with some of the branches of the external carotid artery. However their drainage is more variable, with the lingual, superior thyroid and pharyngeal veins as likely to drain into the facial vein as directly into the internal jugular vein.

The facial vein is more constant and is considered below. The middle thyroid veins cross the common carotid artery and drain into the internal jugular vein at about the level of the crossing of the tendon of omohyoid.

None of the internal jugular vein's tributaries drain into it from the posterior direction, a fact which can be used to facilitate a neck dissection. If the dissection begins posteriorly near the anterior border of the trapezius muscle and is continued towards the midline, few vessels of significance are encountered until the internal jugular vein is exposed over almost its whole length. The vein can thus be dissected free without the encumbrance of venous tributaries requiring ligation.

In patients requiring bilateral neck dissection it is best to retain one internal jugular vein to avoid distressing postoperative facial congestion. If it is impossible to retain both veins then the second side should be left for at least three weeks to allow collateral vessels to open up. Despite such a delay, postoperative venous congestion is often severe enough to require a temporary tracheotomy.

THE FACIAL VEIN

The facial vein descends across the face from the inner angle of the eye and crosses the border of the mandible about 2 cm in front of its angle. It lies deep to platysma directly on the external surface of the submandibular gland. The submental vein passes backwards across the gland to enter the facial vein which behind the submandibular gland receives the anterior division of the retromandibular vein and passes downwards as the common facial vein to enter the internal jugular vein. At its termination the facial vein usually overlies the carotid bifurcation. A communicating branch from the anterior jugular vein sometimes runs across the sternomastoid muscle to join the facial vein near its termination.

THE MUSCLES OF THE FLOOR OF THE POSTERIOR TRIANGLE OF THE NECK (Fig. 29.3)

The splenius capitis muscle ascends from the spines of C7 and T1–3, to insert into the mastoid process and superior nuchal line deep to the sternomastoid muscle.

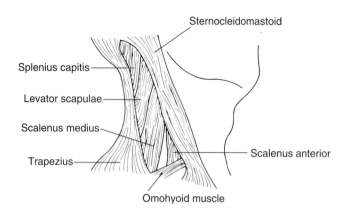

FIGURE 29.3 Muscles in the floor of the posterior triangle of the neck.

The levator scapulae muscle arises from the transverse processes of C1–4 and passes downwards to insert into the upper quarter of the medial border of the scapula.

The scalenus medius is the largest of the scalene muscles and arises from the transverse processes of C1–7 and passes downwards to insert into the first rib between its tubercle and the groove for the subclavian artery. Between it and scalenus anterior the subclavian artery and brachial plexus emerge.

The scalenus anterior arises from the transverse processes of C3–6 and passes downwards to insert into the scalene tubercle of the first rib. Near its insertion scalenius anterior separates the subclavian vein in front from the subclavian artery and brachial plexus behind. The phrenic nerve crosses the muscle's surface beneath a condensation of fascia and the two cervical arteries also tend to clamp the nerve to the muscle (suprascapular and superficial cervical arteries).

All of these muscles are supplied by branches from the cervical nerve roots.

THE HYPOGLOSSAL NERVE

This is the motor nerve to all the muscles of the tongue except palatoglossus. The hypoglossal nerve emerges from the hypoglossal canal and crosses behind the internal carotid artery to lie between it and the internal jugular vein. At about the level of the angle of the mandible it curves forwards around the occipital branch of the external carotid artery at the point where it gives off the lower sternomastoid artery. Thus the nerve is superficial to both internal and external carotid arteries, crosses the loop of the lingual artery and passes upwards on hyoglossus, deep to mylohyoid, where the nerve lies inferior to the deep portion of the submandibular gland.

It contains C1 nerve fibres, which have 'hitched a ride', and some of these are given off as it crosses the external carotid artery, as the upper root of the ansa cervicalis and the remainder as the nerves to thyrohyoid and geniohyoid.

The nerve exits behind the internal jugular vein in about 10% of cases and occasionally can cross at a lower level, a fact which is important to remember when mobilizing the carotid bifurcation.

The hypoglossal nerve is at risk of damage during neck dissection at the stage where the internal jugular vein is being separated from the carotid arteries just superior to the bifurcation. This is at a level where metastatic nodes are common. Large nodes in this area increase the difficulty of dissection, with corresponding increased risk to the hypoglossal nerve.

THE FACIAL ARTERY

The facial artery arises from the external carotid artery above the lingual branch and passes upwards deep to the digastric muscle to arch over the posterior portion of the submandibular gland in which it often forms a groove. It passes forwards between the gland and the medial surface of the mandible until it emerges beneath the lower border of the mandible and curls around it, to enter the face (Fig. 29.4). As it curves around the mandible it gives off its largest branch, the submental artery, which passes forwards on the mylohyoid muscle.

The hypoglossal nerve curves forwards over the external carotid artery at about the commencement of the facial artery and the nerve and artery usually lies below the submandibular gland, although they may be overlapped by it (Fig. 29.4).

THE MANDIBULAR AND CERVICAL BRANCHES OF THE FACIAL NERVE

The lowermost branches of the facial nerve are often direct or close relations of the submandibular gland.

The mandibular branch of the facial nerve exits from the parotid gland near the angle of the mandible and curves

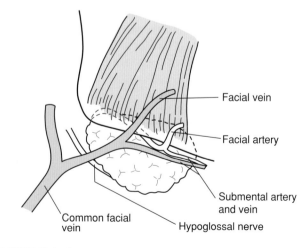

FIGURE 29.4 Structures superficial to the submandibular gland.

downwards as it runs forwards deep to the platysma and then curves upwards to supply risorius and the lower lip and chin muscles. In a majority of cases it does not lie inferior to the lower border of the mandible, although in a minority it does, and it has been described as low as 2.5 cm below the mandible. Division of this nerve produces a noticeable facial deformity with depression of the corner of the mouth and drooling.

However the nerve which is most often damaged in operations in this region is a division of the cervical branch of the facial nerve. The cervical branch also runs deep to platysma in a downward direction about 1–2 cm behind the angle of the mandible. Approximately 2 cm below the angle it divides, its posterior division continuing on to supply platysma and its anterior division curving forwards and upwards to provide additional supply to the muscles of the corner of the mouth. Division of this nerve usually shows with some drooping of the corner of the mouth. However, as it is not the major nerve of supply to the muscles, improvement in muscle function usually occurs with time and after some months disability is rarely apparent.

It is unusual for this anterior division to pass more than 3 cm inferior to the lower border of the mandible. Thus if neck incisions are made 2 cm or more behind the angle of the mandible and 4 cm or more below it, and the incisions are taken through platysma at the same level, then none of these nerves are in danger of being divided.

It should be remembered that the mandibular and cervical branches of the facial nerve run in loose areolar tissue between the platysma and the submandibular gland. When raising the skin flap it is important not to dissect too close to the platysma or the branches may be damaged.

If the deep cervical fascia which covers the submandibular gland is incised level with the lower border of the gland and raised with the skin flap, then the facial nerve branches are safe.

In dissection of the submandibular gland itself the structures lying superficial to it are the facial artery and vein and the submental artery and vein.

THE LINGUAL NERVE

The lingual nerve is in contact with the jaw posteriorly. As it lies on hyoglossus it makes a partial spiral around the submandibular duct and ends in the tongue, supplying sensation to its anterior two-thirds.

During clearance of the submandibular triangle, traction on the gland and its duct pulls the lingual nerve inferiorly.

Care must be taken to divide the duct without injuring the lingual nerve which springs away as soon as the duct has been divided.

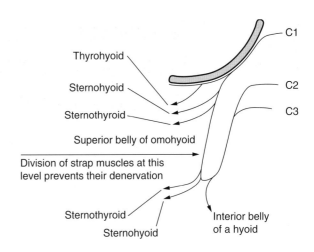

FIGURE 29.5 The ansa cervicalis and the innervation of the strap muscles.

THE ANSA CERVICALIS

The ansae cervicalis is the nerve loop which supplies the strap muscle of the neck. Its upper root comes from fibres from the C1 nerve root which travel with the hypoglossal nerve and exits from it as the hypoglossal nerve curves forwards around the occipital artery. The upper root then runs down on the anterior aspect of the internal and common carotid arteries to join the lower root at a level just above the crossing of the omohyoid muscle. The lower root usually comes from the C2, 3 nerve roots and it passes down on the lateral surface of the internal jugular vein before inclining forward to join the upper root. The distribution of its fibres to the strap muscles is shown in Figure 29.5. The lower root can emerge either behind or in front of the internal jugular vein.

THE THORACIC DUCT IN THE NECK

The thoracic duct passes upwards to the left of the oesophagus. About 3 cm above the clavicle it turns laterally behind the carotid structures, but in front of the sympathetic trunk, the vertebral artery and vein and the thyrocervical trunk. It may even curve in front of scalenus anterior before passing back downwards and ending variably in the confluence of the subclavian and internal jugular veins.

FURTHER READING

McGregor I A, McGregor F M 1986 Neck dissections in cancer of the face and mouth. Churchill Livingstone, London.
Soo K C, Hamlyn P J, Pengington J, Westbury G 1986 The anatomy of the accessory nerve and its cervical contribution in the neck. Head Neck Surg 9:111–115.

30 | Clearance lymphadenectomy of the groin: the anatomy of the femoral triangle and groin lymph nodes

Glyn Jamieson, Brendon Coventry and James Katsaros

THE FEMORAL TRIANGLE (Fig. 30.1)

The femoral triangle is important surgically because it contains the femoral artery and vein and all their branches and tributaries. It also contains the femoral nerve and its branches. The superficial and deep inguinal lymph nodes, and lymphatic channels lie amongst the vessels and nerves.

The base of the triangle is the inguinal ligament superiorly; its medial border is the *medial* border of adductor longus and its lateral border is the *medial* border of sartorius. Its floor is thus made up sequentially of adductor longus, adductor brevis, pectineus, psoas and iliacus muscles. The fascia lata makes up the roof of the triangle and is pierced by the long (great) saphenous vein entering to join the femoral vein, via the thin cribriform fascia covering the fossa ovalis. It is worth emphasizing that the boundary of a groin dissection does not correspond exactly with the boundary of the femoral triangle. The lymph node clearance is to the medial boundary and apex, but laterally is to the *lateral* border of sartorius and above it extends well beyond the inguinal ligament.

THE MUSCLES OF THE FEMORAL TRIANGLE

The adductor longus muscle (L2, 3)

This muscle arises from the body of the pubis and passes downwards as a triangular muscle inserting via an aponeurosis into the middle of the linea aspera of the femur.

It overlies adductors magnus and brevis and the anterior branch of the obturator nerve (L2, 3) lies deep to it, and supplies it.

The pectineus muscle (L2, 3)

This is a quadrangular muscle arising from the region of the pecten pubis and inserting into the femur between the lesser trochanter and the linea aspera. The anterior branch of the obturator nerve and adductor brevis lies behind it and, while it occasionally gets an accessory nerve supply from the obturator nerve, its main nerve supply is from the femoral nerve (L2–4).

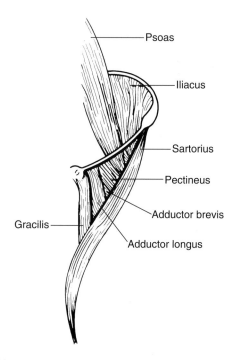

FIGURE 30.1 The femoral triangle (the margins are marked by the heavy lines).

The psoas major and iliacus muscles (L1–3)

These muscles combined are often termed the iliopsoas muscle. The psoas major arises from all the lumbar vertebrae and their transverse processes and passes downwards along the pelvic brim, behind the middle of the inguinal ligament and in front of the capsule of the hip joint to insert into the lesser trochanter. It is supplied by lumbar spinal nerves L1–3.

The iliacus arising from inside the pelvis has a tendon which blends with that of psoas major at its insertion into the lesser trochanter. It is supplied by the femoral nerve.

The sartorius muscle (L2–4)

This muscle arises from the anterior superior iliac spine and the bone immediately subjacent. It crosses the thigh obliquely and is inserted via a flat tendon into the medial surface of the tibia. It is supplied by the femoral nerve.

THE FEMORAL ARTERY

The femoral artery is sometimes termed the superficial femoral artery, The transversalis and iliopsoas fasciae condense to form a sheath around the femoral vessels (femoral sheath) which extends beneath the inguinal ligament. As a sheath it is of little surgical consequence. Medial to the femoral sheath lies a potential canal, the femoral canal, which contains lymphatic channels and lymph nodes surrounded by fat into which the femoral vein can expand and femoral hernias can develop as a protrusion of peritoneum from above. All of the tissue of the anterior aspect of the femoral sheath surrounding the artery and vein is cleared in a block dissection.

The femoral artery commences behind the midpoint of the inguinal ligament where the femoral vein lies medially to it. In the mid-thigh the femoral vein lies posteriorly to the artery and ascends on the medial side of the femoral artery.

The profunda femoris (deep femoral) vein or a branch of it lies behind the (superficial) femoral artery separating it from its own profunda femoris (deep femoral) artery branch.

The branches of the femoral artery are as follows:

❶ The superficial epigastric artery which arises in the vicinity of the inguinal ligament and passes anteriorly and superficial to the inguinal ligament.

❷ The superficial circumflex iliac artery arises at about the same level as the superficial epigastric artery and passes laterally towards the anterior superior iliac spine, approximately 1 cm below the inguinal ligament. This artery is often the supply on which a groin flap is based.

❸ The superficial external pudendal artery arises from the medial side of the proximal femoral artery and may cross superficial or deep to the long saphenous vein.

❹ The deep external pudendal artery also arises from the medial side and crosses in front of the femoral vein but behind the long saphenous vein to the medial thigh. This artery is often absent.

❺ The profunda femoris artery arises posterolaterally from the femoral artery and spirals behind the femoral artery and vein as it passes downwards lying behind the adductor longus. Soon after its origin it gives off medial and lateral circumflex arteries. These arteries not uncommonly arise directly from the femoral artery itself. The lateral circumflex femoral artery runs between the branches of the femoral nerve.

THE LONG (GREAT) SAPHENOUS VEIN AND OPENING (Fig. 30.2)

The long (great) saphenous vein commences on the foot, lies in front of the medial malleolus at the ankle (a useful cutdown site) and ascends along the medial aspect of the leg, lying very superficially. It lies just posteromedial to the knee joint and travels more deeply in the subcutaneous tissues of the thigh approximately along the medial border of sartorius muscle to reach the saphenous opening, where it then dives deep to enter the femoral vein. There is a large valve at the saphenofemoral junction preventing backflow into the long saphenous vein.

The saphenous opening is found approximately 3 cm lateral to and 3 cm below the pubic tubercle. The fascia lata has a superficial layer which forms the crescentic edge of the saphenous opening (laterally and superiorly). The edge of the saphenous opening is deficient medially and inferiorly. The long (great) saphenous vein ascends on the fascia lata from the medial aspect of the knee to join the femoral vein, via the saphenous opening. A thin (cribriform) fascia lies across the saphenous opening and the space is filled with loose fat.

THE FEMORAL VEIN

The femoral vein ascends from behind the femoral artery at the knee in the popliteal fossa to lie medially to the femoral artery in the upper femoral triangle. Its two major tributaries

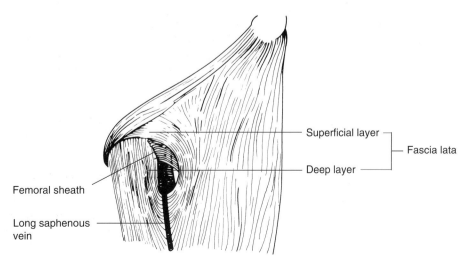

FIGURE 30.2 The saphenous opening and the fascial layers of the upper thigh.

in this region are the great (long) saphenous vein anteriorly and the profunda femoris vein posteriorly. As already mentioned, the profunda femoris vein tends to lie between the femoral and profunda femoris arteries, and is therefore at risk when these arteries are being mobilized.

The circumflex femoral veins are variable in their pattern of drainage, but more often drain directly into the femoral vein. Similarly, the cutaneous veins corresponding to the branches from the femoral artery tend to drain into the great (long) saphenous vein rather than directly into the femoral vein, although there is considerable variability.

THE FEMORAL NERVE

The femoral nerve arises from L2 to L4 and is the largest branch of the lumbar plexus. It passes downwards in psoas and emerges between the psoas and iliacus muscles, but it remains deep to the fascia over iliacus as it crosses behind the inguinal ligament. It lies directly lateral to the femoral artery and femoral sheath, but separated from them by the condensation of the iliacus fascia joining the inguinal ligament to the fascia – the iliopectineal arch. It branches high in the femoral triangle, however, before it divides into its anterior and posterior divisions it gives off twigs to iliacus and psoas muscles and also the nerve to pectineus which crosses behind the femoral sheath. The two divisions are separated by the lateral circumflex femoral artery.

The anterior division gives the intermediate femoral cutaneous nerve and nerve to sartorius (these two often arise as a single trunk) and the medial femoral cutaneous nerve. This nerve crosses in front of the femoral artery to lie medial to it distally in the apex of the femoral triangle.

The posterior division of the femoral nerve gives rise to branches to the quadriceps femoris muscle and the saphenous nerve. The saphenous nerve lies lateral to the femoral artery here, as does the nerve to vastus medialis. They both enter the adductor canal where the saphenous nerve crosses in front to lie medial to the artery, while the nerve to vastus medialis remains laterally. Below the knee the saphenous nerve then joins the long (great) saphenous vein to reach the ankle anterior to the medial malleolus.

THE INGUINAL (GROIN) LYMPH NODES

There are two groups of inguinal lymph nodes which are often named superficial and deep according to their relationship to the deep fascia. These groups are, however, contiguous being joined by lymphatic networks and are virtually inseparable anatomically. Indeed, recent information from lymphatic tracing using radionuclides has demonstrated direct drainage from the leg skin to iliac lymph nodes, bypassing the inguinal nodes.

Superficial inguinal nodes

This is much the larger of the two groups and the nodes are arranged in a T-shaped pattern, with the horizontal limb representing the nodes lying below and parallel to the inguinal ligament and the vertical limb representing the nodes lying along the great (long) saphenous vein. In general terms, the more distally placed group receives lymph from the leg while the proximal group receives lymph from the buttock, lower abdominal wall and the perineal area.

These nodes communicate with the deep inguinal nodes, but also drain to the external iliac nodes.

Deep inguinal nodes

There are several lymph nodes lying along the medial side of the femoral vein around the saphenofemoral junction and between the femoral vessels. Nodes in the vicinity of the femoral ring and near the saphenofemoral junction are probably the most constant. An enlarged node in the femoral canal was said to drain the glans penis (or clitoris/vulva) and was often the first node involved in syphilis. Depending on one's training, it is known as Cloquet's or Rosenmüller's node. The deep nodes receive the lymphatic drainage from the deeper structures of the lower thigh and leg. They tend to drain directly to obturator or medial iliac lymph nodes within the pelvis.

COMMENTS ON COMPLETE LYMPH NODE DISSECTION FROM THE GROIN

Complete lymph node dissection (block dissection) is usually performed for metastatic malignancy to the inguinal lymph nodes. As mentioned above, the limits of dissection usually exceed the femoral triangle, particularly laterally and above. Many surgeons also take the medial resection margin to the anterior border of gracilis muscle.

An oblique incision is usually made in the thigh along the line of the femoral vessels for adequate exposure. A skin ellipse is typically excised over a tumour mass with subcutaneous fat incorporating the superficial and deep inguinal lymph nodes and long saphenous vein, which is suture ligated flush with the femoral vein at the saphenofemoral junction. Lymph nodes between the femoral vessels and from the femoral canal are excised. Cutaneous branches of the femoral nerve are sacrificed if they are traversing the dissection. Deep and other superficial nerve branches are preserved. The lateral cutaneous nerve of the thigh is preserved at the lateral margin of dissection. Medially, tissue around the pubic tubercle may contain lymph nodes and is removed.

Complete inguinal lymph node dissection is often combined with incontinuity pelvic lymph node dissection, often termed 'ilio-inguinal lymph node dissection', for treatment of malignancies, such as melanoma.

ILIAC VESSELS

The common iliac arteries are formed at the L4 vertebral level and each divides at the sacroiliac joint at which point the ureter crosses on each side. The external iliac artery curves around the pelvic sidewall to reach the midpoint of the inguinal ligament to form the femoral artery. The femoral vein forms the external iliac vein beneath the inguinal ligament and ascends medially to the external iliac artery to be joined by the internal iliac vein – forming the common iliac vein that then twists posteriorly to the artery to lie to the right of the aorta at L4 level.

Just superior to the inguinal ligament the inferior epigastric artery and vein are found travelling to and from the ipsilateral rectus abdominis muscle, respectively. The inferior epigastric vein is often dual. These are divided in pelvic dissection to improve access.

In about a third of individuals an `abnormal' obturator artery arises from the inferior epigastric artery and lies either lateral (most) or medial (3% cases) to the femoral canal, where it may be injured during dissection.

Obturator, external and common iliac nodes

These are often collectively termed pelvic lymph nodes. Obturator lymph nodes lie against the obturator membrane (overlying the obturator foramen) and around the obturator nerve (L2–4). The obturator lymph nodes communicate with the iliac lymph nodes. The iliac chains of lymph nodes extend along the femoral/external iliac artery junction (under the inguinal ligament) and common iliac vessels to reach the para-aortic lymph nodes. There is a lateral iliac group of nodes, lateral to the external iliac artery, that drains the lateral thigh and lateral abdominal wall.

COMMENTS ON PELVIC LYMPH NODE DISSECTION

Dissection of the pelvic lymph nodes may be performed as part of an in-continuity dissection of the inguinal lymph nodes for treatment of melanoma or squamous skin cancers. It is also used for treatment of gynaecological and urological malignancies, usually in association with resection of adjacent pathological pelvic organs. Occasionally, pelvic lymph node dissection is performed alone. A muscle cutting incision is usually used, with or without division of the inguinal ligament. In the male the spermatic cord is mobilized, taped, retracted and preserved. The inferior epigastric vessels are usually ligated and divided for improved access. Lymph nodes are dissected laterally, anteriorly, then medially to the external iliac vessels, to include the obturator lymph nodes extending medially behind the external iliac vein. The proximal dissection is often taken to just beyond the point where the ureter crosses the common iliac artery bifurcation. The obturator and femoral nerves are identified and preserved.

FURTHER READING

Coit D, Balch C M 2003 Groin and popliteal dissection: technique and complications. In: Balch C M, Houghton A N; Sober A J; Soong S (eds) Cutaneous melanoma, 4th edn. Quality Medical Publishing, St Louis, MO.

Karakousis C P, Thompson J F 2004 Chapter 25 Groin and pelvic dissection for melanoma. In: Thompson J F, Morton D L, Kroon B B R (eds) Textbook of melanoma. Martin Dunitz, London.

31 | Retroperitoneal lymphadenopathy: the anatomy of the lymph nodes associated with the aorta and its branches

Glyn Jamieson and Murray Brennan

THE COMMON ILIAC NODES

These nodes surround the common iliac artery and are arranged predominantly in medial, posterior and lateral groupings. They receive lymph from a wide distribution. Thus they receive lymph from the lower abdominal wall and perineum, the lower limbs and the pelvis. They are in continuity with nodal groupings around the aorta.

THE AORTIC NODES

These nodes are a continuation upwards of the grouping around the common iliac artery but the concentration of groupings is different in that the major nodal groups are those that lie in front and to either side of the aorta. There may be some nodes posterior to the aorta but these are much less constant and of lesser importance than the other groups. As noted in previous chapters, there are a lot of interconnections between lymphatic tissue, and what follows is merely the most usual arrangement for lymphatic pathways.

The preaortic nodes

The nodes along the front of the aorta are grouped predominantly around the branches of the aorta and thus they are named coeliac, superior mesenteric and inferior mesenteric nodes. They receive the lymphatic drainage from all the abdominal viscera and give rise to the lymph trunk known as the intestinal trunk which helps form the cysterna chyli.

The lumbar (lateral, para-aortic) nodes

There is a chain of nodes which pass upwards on either side of the aorta and eventually form into a lumbar lymph trunk on either side, which joins with the intestinal trunk to form the cysterna chyli at about the level of L2, between the diaphragmatic crura.

On the left side the lumbar chain lies on the psoas muscle as the chain passes upwards. On the right side the nodes are distributed around the inferior vena cava: some in front, some lateral to it, some behind the cava and the aorta.

The lumbar chains receive the majority of the lymph from the common iliac nodes and therefore from the lower limbs, pelvis and lower abdominal wall. They also receive the lymph from the upper abdominal wall and genitourinary system and gonads. In block dissection of retroperitoneal nodes for tumours of the testis or lower limbs these are the most important group to clear. Obviously their clearance is considerably easier on the left compared to the right side.

GENERAL COMMENTS WITH REGARD TO RETROPERITONEAL LYMPHADENECTOMY – AORTIC BLOCK DISSECTION

The anatomical limits of dissection are the ureter and medial border of the kidney on each side laterally. This includes the adrenal gland and associated tissue on the side of the lesion for which the dissection is being undertaken. The limit above is the superior mesenteric artery and the bifurcation of the common iliac vessels is the limit below (although this may be extended downwards on the side of the lesion).

Complete removal of nodal tissue requires complete mobilization and skeletonization of the great vessels on all their aspects. This often entails division of some lumbar arteries and veins.

FURTHER READING

Bedford Waters W, Guinan P 1984 Retroperitoneal node dissection for tumours of the testis. In: Nyhus L M, Baker R J (eds) Master of Surgery. Little Brown, Boston.

32

Soft tissue resections for limb sarcomas: the anatomy of the muscle compartments of the lower and upper limbs

Glyn Jamieson and Murray Brennan

GENERAL PRINCIPLES OF SURGICAL THERAPY

Eradication of the entire extent of a soft tissue sarcoma can be achieved by a variety of treatments. All must take account of the propensity of these tumours to spread between muscle groups and along fascial septa and nerve sheaths to limits well beyond those of clinically detectable tumour. Sometimes tumour extension with 'skip' areas also occurs. Clinical evaluation must be supplemented by magnetic resonance image scanning, which frequently indicates which muscles are involved and is invaluable in planning the specific operation necessary for each individual patient.

Operations used for soft tissue tumours will be in one of three categories:

❶ *Compartmental resections* of involved muscles, nerves, vessels and aponeuroses that form the compartment (including amputation).
❷ *Soft tissue resection with limited margins, or monobloc resection*. This involves excision of tumour and involved muscle and a variable margin of soft tissue but is less than a total compartment resection.
❸ *Excision biopsy*. This leaves pseudocapsule and inevitably microscopic tumour. It is infrequently used and only in conjunction with other therapies when preservation of limb function is the aim.

Function-preserving resections are increasingly performed and a precise knowledge of limb anatomy is necessary in order to ensure complete removal of involved muscle groups as well as to preserve reasonable function following resection of whole muscle groups and/or major nerves.

Furthermore, large tumours may involve more than one aponeurotic compartment, which increases the complexity of an individual resection.

Compartmental resections are not really feasible in tumours arising in the groin, cubital fossa, popliteal fossa or the root of the neck. In the upper limb, resections are often limited by the proximity of tumour to bone, joints and major nerves and vessels because of the absence of muscle bulk in the upper limbs.

THE THIGH (Fig. 32.1)

There are three major muscle compartments of the thigh and they are enclosed by the deep fascia of the thigh – the fascia lata. This is of variable thickness and is thickest laterally where it forms the iliotibial tract. The fascia lata gives off two septa which separate the muscles of the thigh into two compartments. The lateral intermuscular septum is thicker than the medial intermuscular septum; both septa insert into the linea aspera of the femur.

The compartments of the thigh are distinct anatomical units so that their lymphatic drainage tends to be separate and tumours which arise in the area tend to involve only muscles and structures of the compartment in which they have arisen. This is why all of the muscles and contents of a particular compartment may have to be resected en bloc.

The adductor compartment muscles

The gracilis muscle

This is the most superficial of the muscles. It arises from the lower part of the pubic body and ramus and ischial ramus (Fig. 32.2) and passes downwards to curve around the medial femoral condyle as a flat tendon which inserts into the upper tibia immediately behind the sartorius insertion. It is supplied by the obturator nerve and it is a hip flexor and adductor. It overlies the adductor magnus.

The pectineus muscle

This is a flat, quadrangular muscle which arises from the pecten pubis and the adjacent bone (Fig. 32.2) and it passes obliquely to insert into the femur between the lesser trochanter and the linea aspera. It is supplied by the femoral nerve and in 10% of cases it receives additional supply from the obturator nerve. It is one of the muscles of the floor of the femoral triangle (see Ch. 30) and it is an adductor of the thigh.

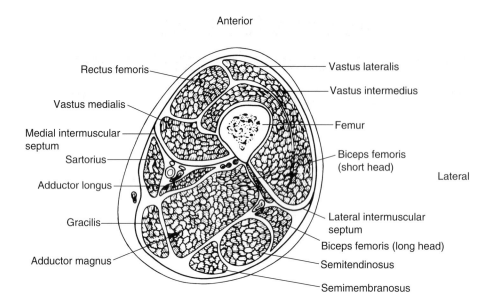

FIGURE 32.1 Cross-section of the left thigh, diagrammatic representation of CT scan view.

The adductor longus muscle

This muscle arises from the front of the pubis between the medial end of the origin of pectineus and the upper end of origin of gracilis. It is the most anterior of the adductor muscles in the thigh and it fans out from its origin to insert into the linea aspera in the middle third of the femur (Fig. 32.3).

It lies between the vastus medialis anteriorly and the adductor magnus posteriorly; the medial intermuscular septum also lies between these two muscles. All four structures are blended near the femur and there is no plane of separation between them.

The adductor longus is regarded as forming the floor or posterior wall of the adductor canal (see Ch. 30). It is supplied by the anterior division of the obturator nerve.

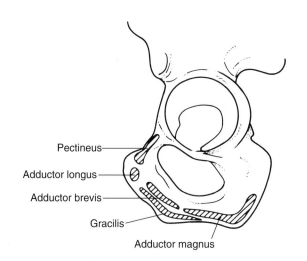

FIGURE 32.2 The origins of the adductor compartment muscles.

Adductor brevis muscle

This muscle arises from the pubis immediately deep to gracilis and it is inserted into the femur in a line from the lesser trochanter to the linea aspera, again immediately deep to gracilis. It may be partially fused with adductor magnus.

The profunda femoris vessels lie in front of it, as does the anterior branch of the obturator nerve which supplies it. The posterior branch of the obturator nerve lies behind it (Fig. 31.3).

The adductor magnus muscle

This is the largest of the adductor muscles and it arises from the inferior pubic ramus, the ischial pubic ramus and the ischial tuberosity (Fig. 32.2). The pubic fibres pass almost horizontally into the lower part of the gluteal tuberosity (adductor minimus) and then the descending fibres are inserted into the linea aspera and medial supracondylar line. The fibres from the ischial tuberosity insert as a tendon into the adductor tubercle of the medial femoral condyle (Fig. 32.3). The muscle has tendinous arches in its insertion, through the proximal four of which pass perforating arteries from the profunda femoris artery. The distal arch is called the adductor hiatus and the femoral vessels pass through it.

The adductor magnus is supplied by the obturator nerve, except for the part arising from the ischial tuberosity which is supplied by the sciatic nerve. The profunda femoris vessels below adductor brevis are anterior to the muscle and the sciatic nerve lies posterior to it, as does the hamstring group of muscles (Fig. 32.1).

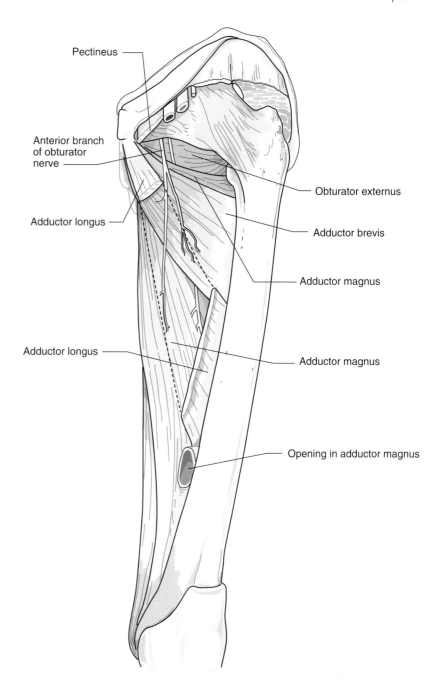

FIGURE 32.3 The adductor muscles, left thigh.

The quadriceps compartment muscles (Fig. 32.4)

Quadriceps femoris is the muscle mass which is the extensor compartment of the leg. It consists of four parts. The first part is the rectus femoris which arises from the ilium and the other three parts are the vasti which arise from the femur. The muscle mass covers almost all of the front and the sides of the femur.

❶ Rectus femoris arises by two tendons, one from the anterior inferior iliac spine and the other above the acetabulum (Fig. 32.5). Its superficial fibres are bipennate and it inserts via the patellar tendon.

❷ Vastus lateralis is the largest of the vasti. It arises by a broad aponeurosis from the front of the femur below the greater trochanter, then its origin spirals around the shaft laterally and down to the proximal half of the linea aspera. It inserts via the patellar tendon (see below).

❸ Vastus medialis also arises from the front of the femur below the lesser trochanter. Its origin spirals around the shaft medially and downwards to involve all of the linea aspera and the proximal part of the medial supracondylar line. It also takes its origin from adductor longus and magnus and the medial

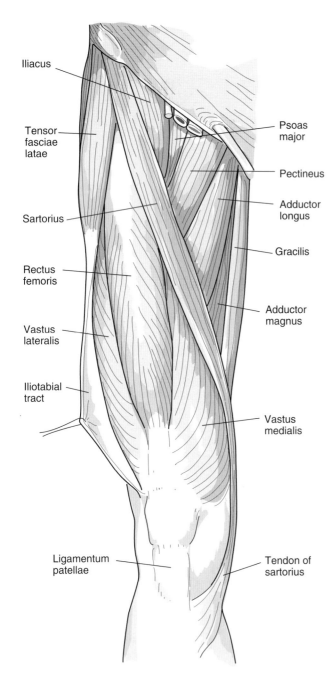

FIGURE 32.4 The quadriceps compartment muscles, right thigh.

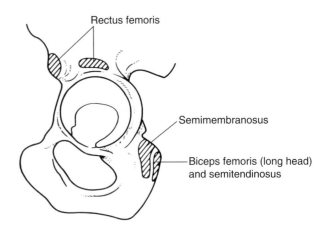

FIGURE 32.5 The origins of the rectus femoris and the hamstring muscles, left side.

medial sides, blending with fibres of the capsule of the knee joint. These fibres insert into the sides of the tibial tuberosity and are called the lateral and medial patellar retinacula. The ligamentum patellae inserts into the tibial tuberosity.

The quadriceps femoris muscle is supplied by branches of the femoral nerve.

The posterior femoral compartment muscles – the hamstrings (Fig. 32.6)

The three hamstring muscles span the hip and knee joint, extending the hip and flexing the knee.

❶ Biceps femoris arises by two heads. One, the long head, is from the inferior aspect of the ischial tuberosity (in common with the origin of semitendinosus; Fig. 32.5) and the other, the short head, is from the linea aspera and lateral supra condylar line between the insertion of adductor magnus and the origin of vastus lateralis. It also arises from the lateral intermuscular septum. Its belly lies posterior to the sciatic nerve (Fig. 32.1) and it inserts via a tendon which splits around the fibular collateral ligament and attaches to the head of the fibula. The common peroneal nerve lies immediately medial to the tendon of biceps, between it and the lateral head of gastrocnemius. The long head of the muscle is supplied by the tibial component of the sciatic nerve and the short head by the common peroneal component.

❷ Semitendinosus arises from the ischial tuberosity, in common with the long head of biceps, and its muscle belly ends about halfway down the thigh, where it gives way to a tendon which runs down on the muscle belly of semimembranosus and then curves around the medial femoral condyle to insert into the tibia immediately behind the insertion of sartorius and fused with that of gracilis (Fig. 32.7). At its insertion

intermuscular septum. Its lowermost fibres are horizontal and give the rounded bulge above the knee joint. It inserts via the patellar tendon

❹ Vastus intermedius arises from the proximal two-thirds of the anterior and lateral surface of the femur. This is the deepest of the muscles to insert via the patellar tendon.

The quadriceps patellar tendon is the strong tendon through which all of the quadriceps muscles insert into the base of the patella. Some of their fibres continue over it into the ligamentum patellae and some fibres sweep to lateral and

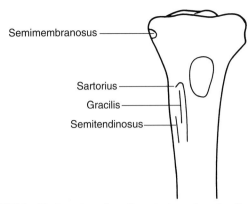

FIGURE 32.7 The insertions of gracilis, sartorius and semitendinosus on the tibial shaft and semimembranosus higher on the tibial condyle, left thigh.

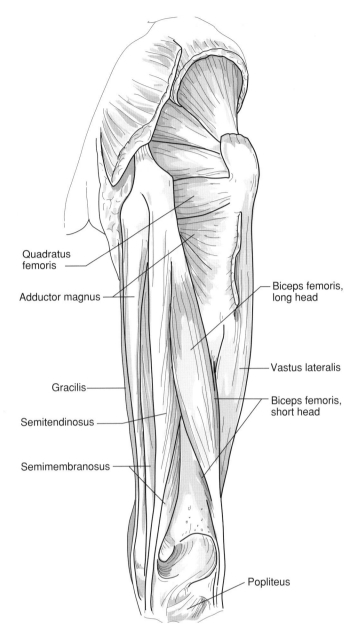

Quadratus femoris

Adductor magnus

Gracilis

Semitendinosus

Semimembranosus

Biceps femoris, long head

Vastus lateralis

Biceps femoris, short head

Popliteus

FIGURE 32.6 The hamstring muscles, right thigh.

its tendon is often fused with that of gracilis. Semitendinosus is supplied by the tibial part of the sciatic nerve.

❸ Semimebranosus is attached to the ischial tuberosity in front of the biceps/semitendinosus origin (Fig. 32.5) and it also arises from an aponeurosis associated with these muscles. Its insertion is also somewhat complex, giving a strong slip of insertion into the posterior and lateral aspect of the medial tibial condyle and other slips passing in various directions from this insertion and blending with the capsule of the knee joint. It is supplied by the tibial component of the sciatic nerve. In the lower part of its course the muscle belly overlies, i.e. is posterior to, the popliteal vessels.

The femoral artery and vein in the thigh

The femoral artery and vein descend from anterior to posterior on the medial side of the thigh, running through the adductor muscles of the thigh in what is referred to as the adductor canal (Fig. 32.1). This is a somewhat triangular tunnel which is bounded anteriorly by the medial intermuscular septum and outside it the vastus medialis, posteriorly by adductor longus above and adductor magnus below and medially by sartorius. The sartorius is separated from the vessels by a strong fascial layer which joins the medial intermuscular septum. The canal also contains the long saphenous nerve lying anterior to the artery and further medially the nerve to vastus medialis before it penetrates that muscle. The femoral vein crosses behind the artery to lie lateral to it in the distal reaches of the canal.

Branches from the artery in the thigh are muscular only and in health usually are small. However they can enlarge considerably if supplying a tumour.

The profunda femoris artery and vein in the thigh

These lie posterolaterally to their femoral counterparts at their origin and then pass downwards towards the medial surface of the femur. They lie deep to adductor longus (which therefore separates them from the femoral vessels) on adductor brevis and then adductor magnus and terminate as the fourth perforating vessels.

They give off muscular branches, including the first to third perforating vessels, which traverse the tendinous arches in adductor magnus.

The sciatic nerve in the thigh

The sciatic nerve lies behind adductor magnus and is crossed posteriorly by the biceps femoris muscle. It gives off branches to the hamstrings and divides into its tibial and common peroneal components above the knee joint.

THE LEG

The anterior leg; muscles: the extensor group
(Fig. 32.8)

This is the muscle mass lying lateral to the subcutaneous surface of the tibia, between the tibia and fibula and anterior to the interosseous membrane. The muscles are the tibialis anterior, the extensor hallucis longus, the extensor digito-

rum longus and peroneus tertius. As shown in Figure 32.8b, these muscles arise from the lateral surface of the tibia and medial surface of the fibula. They also arise from the fibrous septa of this region, i.e. the interosseous membrane between tibia and fibula, the anterior intermuscular septum and the overlying deep fascia which is here quite thick.

The tendons from the muscle pass deep to the extensor retinaculae at the ankle (Fig. 32.9) and insert in various ways: the tibialis anterior into the base of the first metatarsal; the extensor hallucis longus into the base of the distal phalanx of the hallux; the extensor digitorum longus via four tendons into the base of the middle phalanges of the lateral four toes and by two side slips into the bases of

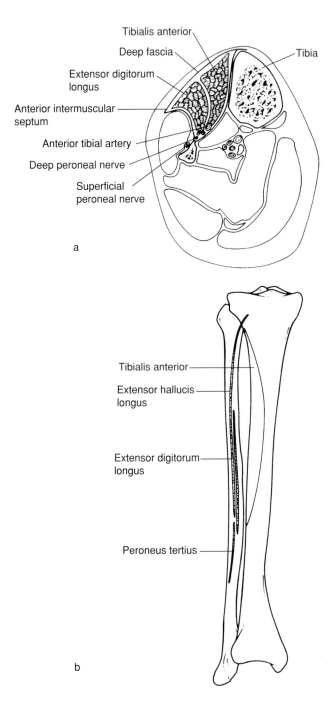

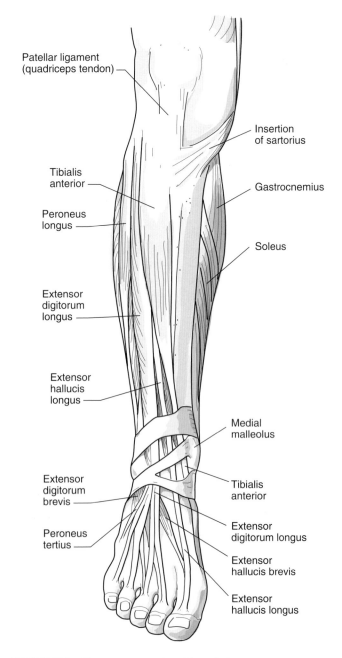

FIGURE 32.8   (a) The extensor muscles of the right leg – cross-section at about the junction of the mid and upper thirds. (b) Origins of the extensor muscles – right leg.

FIGURE 32.9   The extensor muscles of the right leg.

the distal phalanges, and the peroneus tertius into the base of the fifth metatarsal.

All of the muscles are supplied by the deep peroneal nerve. Their main action is extension of the foot as well as subsidiary actions such as inversion (tibialis anterior) and eversion (peroneus tertius). The anterior tibial artery and deep peroneal nerve lie in this compartment. The artery lies on the interosseous membrane and further laterally the nerve lies related to the fibula, although it often comes to lie in front of the artery in the middle of the leg and then lateral again further distally.

The strength of this osseoaponeurotic compartment is demonstrated by the pressure increases which can occur following swelling of the muscles, e.g. after excessive exercise or following ischaemia when normal blood supply is restored. The pressure increases with swelling and can be great enough to impair the flow through the anterior tibial vessels, leading to ischaemic necrosis of the muscles. The pressure increases are ameliorated by dividing the deep fascia along its length over the compartment.

The lateral leg muscles

These are the two muscles arising from the lateral surface of the upper two-thirds of the fibula and also from the interosseous membrane and anterior and posterior intermuscular septa (Fig. 32.10a). The peroneus longus arises proximally and therefore lies on peroneus brevis as the two pass downwards. Their tendons pass behind the lateral malleolus, with brevis maintaining its anterior relation to longus. The brevis tendon is attached to the base of the fifth

metatarsal and the longus tendon bowstrings across the undersurface of the foot to insert into the base of the first metatarsal and adjacent medial cuneiform bone. The muscles are supplied by the superficial peroneal (musculocutaneous) nerve and they evert the foot and aid in flexion of it.

As the peroneal nerve winds around the neck of the fibula it passes through a gap in the origin of the peroneus longus.

The superficial peroneal nerve lies in this compartment, initially deep to peroneus longus, but it emerges between that muscle and extensor digitorum longus to pierce the deep fascia and give branches of supply to the skin of the lower leg.

The posterior leg muscles: superficial group (Figs 32.11 and 32.12a)

These are the soleus, plantaris and gastrocnemius muscles. They are all flexors of the foot and gastrocnemius is also a flexor of the knee. They are supplied by the tibial nerve.

The gastrocnemius muscle arises by two heads from the femoral condyles (Fig. 32.12b). Sometimes one or other head is absent and sometimes the medial head can be displaced laterally in its origin. This can push the popliteal artery medially, causing popliteal artery entrapment, one of the few causes of lower limb claudication in the young (see Ch. 38 and Fig. 38.1). The soleus arises from the posterior aspect of the head of the fibula and the upper quarter of the shaft, the soleal line on the tibia (Fig. 32.12b) and the fibrous arch which passes between the two origins and through which the neurovascular bundle passes to the leg. Plantaris is a vestigial muscle arising from the posterior surface of the

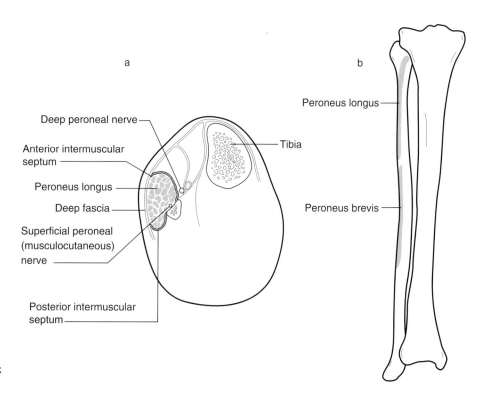

a

Deep peroneal nerve

Anterior intermuscular septum

Peroneus longus

Deep fascia

Superficial peroneal (musculocutaneous) nerve

Posterior intermuscular septum

Tibia

b

Peroneus longus

Peroneus brevis

FIGURE 32.10 (a) The right lateral leg muscles; (b) the origins of the right lateral leg muscles.

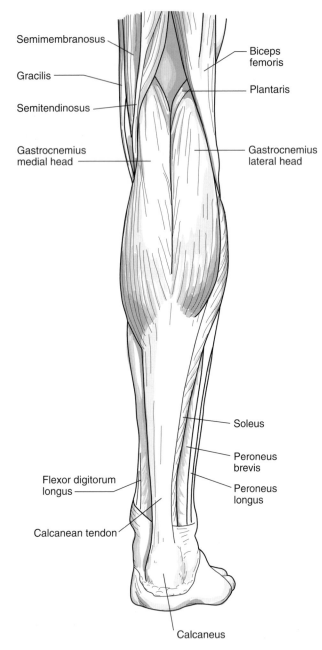

FIGURE 32.11 Posterior leg muscles of the right calf – superficial group.

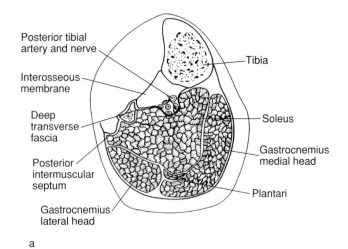

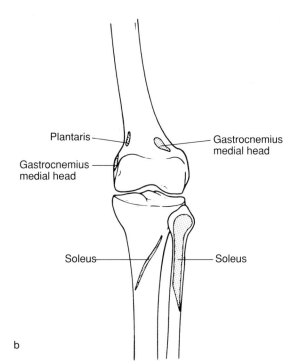

FIGURE 32.12 (a) Cross-section of upper third of right calf showing the superficial group of posterior leg muscles. (b) Origins of posterior leg muscles – superficial group.

femur and its long tendon lies between soleus and gastrocnemius (Fig. 32.12a). All of these muscles insert into the tendocalcaneus which begins in about mid calf but receives muscle fibres from soleus all the way to the ankle region. The tendon inserts into the mid posterior region of the calcaneus.

Although the neurovascular structures lie on the deep surface of soleus they are not actually part of this compartment as they are deep (anterior) to the deep transverse fascia of the leg.

The common peroneal nerve is related to the lateral head of gastrocnemius, lying between it and the biceps tendon.

The posterior leg muscles – deep group
(Figs 32.13 and 32.14a)

The popliteus muscle is a small flat muscle arising from the lateral condyle of the femur and it inserts into the posterior surface of the tibia above the soleal line (Fig. 32.14b). It forms the distal-most floor of the popliteal fossa. The more major muscles of this group arise as a sheet from the posterior surface of the two long bones and the intervening interosseous membrane (Fig. 31.14b), with flexor hallucis longus lateral, tibialis posterior central and flexor digitorum longus medial. The tendon of hallucis is inserted into the base of the distal phalanx of the great toe, and the tendon of digitorum longus is attached to the base of the distal

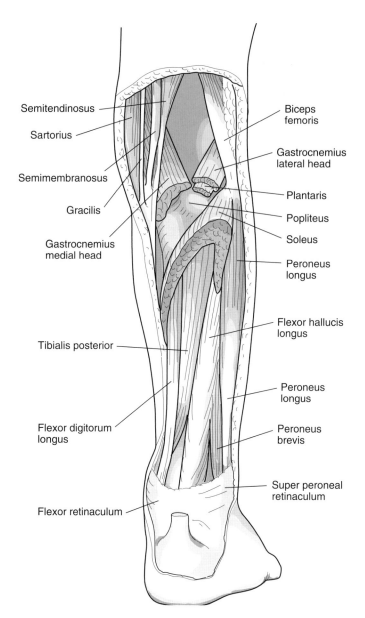

FIGURE 32.13 The deep group of right posterior leg muscles.

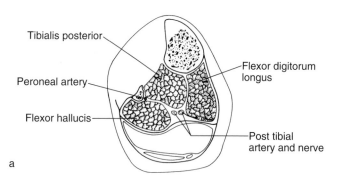

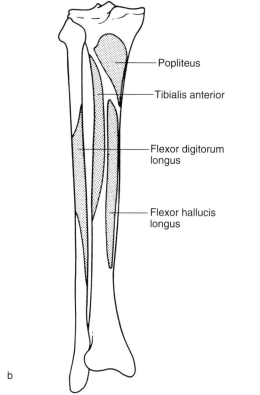

FIGURE 32.14 (a) Transverse section through the right calf about halfway down the leg showing the deep muscles. (b) Origins of the deep group of posterior leg muscles.

phallanges of the lateral four toes. The tibialis posterior is the most deeply placed of the three and ends by a tendon inserting into the tuberosity of the navicular bone.

These three muscles are the flexors of the ankle joint and their tendons all pass posterior to the medial malleolus before reaching their insertions. All four muscles in the group are supplied by the tibial nerve.

The tibial nerve and posterior tibial vessels pass through this compartment. The tibial nerve initially lies posterior to the popliteal artery in the distal popliteal fossa and as it passes into the deep compartment in front of the soleal arch it lies medial to the vessels. It then crosses superficial (posterior) to the vessels to lie lateral to them during most of its course in the leg. It lies on tibialis posterior deep to soleus and the deep transverse fascia. In the lower leg it is subcutaneous and lies midway between the tendocalcaneus and

the medial malleolus, where it divides into the lateral and medial plantar nerves. It supplies all the muscles of the superficial and deep posterior compartments.

The sural nerve, which arises from the tibial nerve, passes between the heads of gastrocnemius to perforate the deep fascia and pass down the leg medial to the small saphenous vein.

The posterior tibial artery passes down lying on tibialis posterior with the same general relations as the tibial nerve.

The peroneal artery arises about 2 cm beyond the popliteal bifurcation and passes laterally in the deep compartment to lie along the lateral side of the fibula between tibialis posterior and flexor hallucis longus. It can actually be embedded in the latter muscle.

THE ARM

The anterior compartment of the arm

These muscles are separated from the posterior compartment muscles by the quite well characterized medial and lateral intermuscular septa (Fig. 32.15).

The coracobrachialis and short head of biceps both arise from the coracoid process and the long head of biceps arises from the superior aspect of the glenoid cavity. The coracobrachialis inserts into the middle of the shaft of the radius and the biceps tendon inserts into the upper radius into the medial tuberosity (Fig. 32.16). The biceps tendon gives off the bicipital aponeurosis which sweeps medially to blend with the fascia of the forearm. The brachialis muscle arises from the anterior aspect of the lower half of the humeral shaft and inserts into the coronoid process of the ulnar (Fig. 32.16).

These muscles are flexors of the shoulder joint and the elbow joint and biceps is a powerful supinator of the forearm.

They are supplied by the nerve which travels through their compartment – the musculocutaneous nerve, which arises from the lateral cord of the brachial plexus.

Neurovascular components of the anterior compartment

The brachial artery and the median nerve lie initially behind the coracobrachialis muscle and then lateral to it and deep to the medial edge of the biceps muscle (Fig. 32.15). The ulnar nerve perforates the medial intermuscular septum to exit from the anterior compartment and lie in the posterior compartment. In the anterior compartment, the ulnar nerve lies behind the brachial artery.

The musculocutaneous nerve travels through the coracobrachialis muscle to lie between the biceps and brachialis muscles and it supplies the muscles of the compartment.

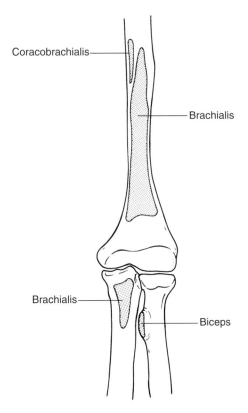

FIGURE 32.16 Insertions and origins of some anterior compartment arm muscles.

The radial nerve enters the anterior compartment from behind by perforating the lateral intermuscular septum in the lower third of the upper arm. The nerve then lies under the brachialis muscle.

The posterior compartment of the arm

The muscle of the posterior compartment is the triceps muscle (Fig. 32.17). The long head arises from the inferior aspect of the glenoid cavity; the lateral head arises from a linear origin which slopes from lateral to medial on the upper humeral shaft and from most of the posterior aspect; below where the lateral head arises, the medial head originates. The triceps inserts into the olecranon and it is the major extensor of the forearm.

The long head passes deep to the teres minor muscle which crosses it at right angles. Lateral to the triceps muscle and above the crossing of the teres minor muscle, the axillary nerve passes backwards.

The radial nerve crosses the compartment posteriorly, winding around the posterior aspect of the humerus between the lateral and medial heads of triceps to lie beneath the lateral head until it exits from the posterior compartment by perforating the lateral intermuscular septum. The ulnar nerve enters the compartment and lies in front of the medial head of the triceps.

The muscle is supplied by the radial nerve.

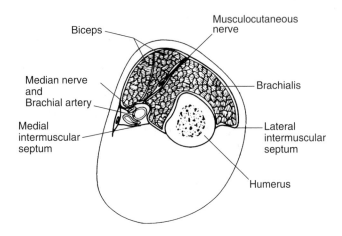

FIGURE 32.15 Transverse section through the left arm showing the anterior compartment.

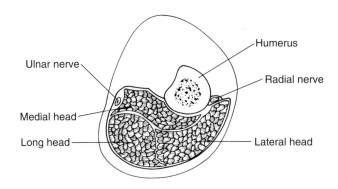

FIGURE 32.17 Cross-section through the posterior compartment of the arm showing the three heads of triceps.

The anterior compartment of the forearm – superficial group of muscles
(Figs 32.18 and 32.19a)

These muscles are mainly a flexor group (except for pronator teres). They arise largely from the humerus from the common flexor origin on the medial epicondyle but they all have other origins. The pronator teres arises from humerus above and the ulna below (Fig. 32.19b); the flexor carpi radialis also takes origin from the fascia of the region and intermuscular septa, palmaris longus likewise and the flexor carpi ulnaris has a second head of origin from the upper two-thirds of the ulna's medial margin, by an aponeurosis

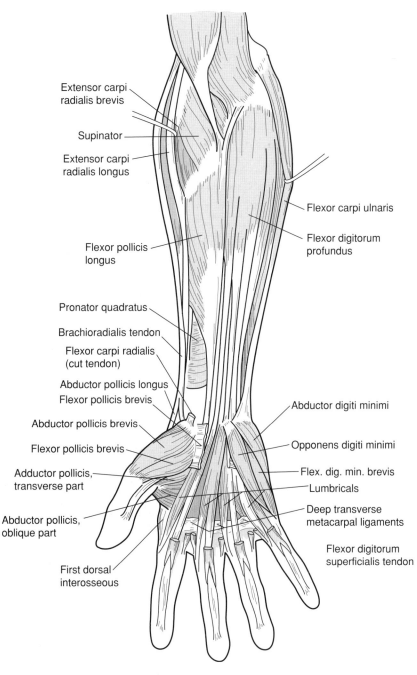

FIGURE 32.18 Superficial muscles in the anterior compartment of the right forearm.

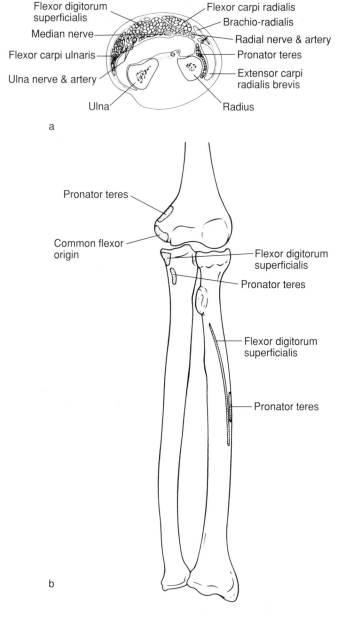

FIGURE 32.19 (a) Transverse section through left mid forearm showing the superficial group of muscles in the anterior compartment. (b) Some anterior compartment muscle origins.

ulnar nerve. As Figure 32.19a indicates, there are many important neurovascular relations with the muscles.

The median nerve enters for the forearm between the two heads of pronator teres and comes to lie deep to flexor digitorum superficialis by passing between the two heads of origin of that muscle. It emerges from under superficialis and the tendon of palmaris longus near the wrist, lying between superficialis and radialis as it passes under the flexor retinaculum (see Ch. 42).

The ulnar nerve enters the forearm between the two heads of flexor carpi ulnaris and lies under that muscle through the forearm. It lies medial to the ulnar artery.

The ulnar artery enters the forearm by passing posterior to pronator teres and flexor digitorum superficialis and lies lateral to the ulnar nerve which it accompanies.

The radial nerve lies under brachioradialis in the forearm. The radial artery crosses the biceps tendon to enter the forearm and descend lying medial to the radial nerve.

The anterior compartment of the forearm – deep muscles (Fig. 32.20a)

The deep muscles of the anterior compartment consist of flexor digitorum profundus, flexor pollicis longus and pronator quadratus muscles. They all arise from the shafts of the long bones, digitorum and quadratus from the ulna and pollicis from the radius. The digitorum and pollicis also arise from the interosseous membrane, as shown in Figure 32.20b. The flexor digitorum inserts as four tendons into the fibrous flexor sheaths on the front of the fingers, forming these with superficialis tendons. The flexor pollicis longus muscle inserts into the base of the distal phalanx and the pronator quadratus muscle inserts into the shaft of the radius (Fig. 32.20b). These muscles are supplied by the median nerve, except for the ulnar half of the profundus muscle which is supplied by the ulnar nerve. The median nerve and ulnar nerve and artery pass downwards lying on the profundus muscle, but actually in the superficial part of the anterior compartment. The anterior interosseous branch of the median nerve runs down deep to the muscles.

The posterior compartment of the forearm – superficial muscles (Fig. 32.21a)

Extensor carpi ulnaris and extensor digitorum with extensor digiti minimi are truly posterior, while extensor carpi radialis longus and brevis and brachioradialis are really lateral rather than posterior (Fig. 32.21b).

The muscles all arise from the humerus or inter-muscular septa of the arm, except for ulnaris which has additional attachment to the back of the ulna from the aponeurosis which also gives origin to flexor ulnaris and profundus.

The brachioradialis muscle arises laterally from the proximal two-thirds of the lateral supracondylar line, the extensor carpi radialis longus muscle arises from the distal third of the supracondylar line and then all the others arise from

from which extensor carpi ulnaris and flexor digitorum fundus also take origin. The flexor digitorum superficialis has an upper head arising from the common origin and the ulna and a lower head arising from the shaft of the radius (Fig. 32.19b).

Pronator teres inserts into the shaft of the radius; flexor carpi radialis inserts into the base of the second metacarpal, palmaris longus into the flexor retinaculum, flexor carpi ulnaris into the pisiform bone and flexor digitorum superficialis into the sides of the shaft of the middle phalanges of each of the digits.

All of the muscles are supplied by the median nerve, except for the flexor carpi ulnaris which is supplied by the

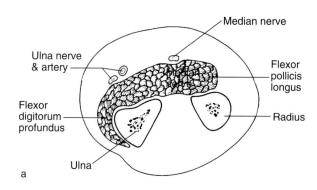

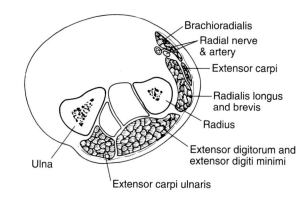

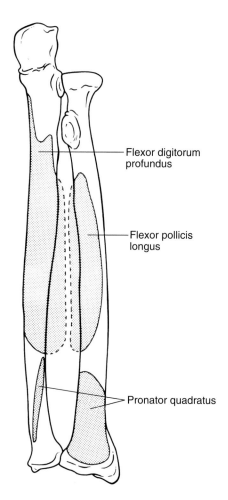

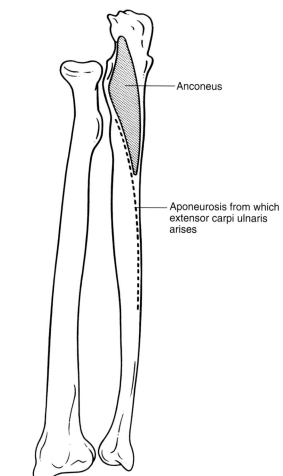

FIGURE 32.20 (a) Cross-section through left mid forearm showing the deep muscles of the anterior compartment. (b) Some origins and insertions of the deep muscles of the anterior compartment.

FIGURE 32.21 (a) Cross-section through left forearm at about mid forearm level, showing the superficial muscles of the posterior compartment. (b) Some origins of posterior compartment muscles – the superficial group.

the bottom of the line from the common extensor origin on the front of the lateral epicondyle. The small anconeus muscle arises from the back of the lateral epicondyle and inserts into the back of the upper humerus (Fig. 32.21b). All the other muscles form tendons inserting beyond the wrist joint, except for brachioradialis which inserts into the base of the radial styloid process. The extensor digitorum longus muscle inserts into the base of the 2nd metacarpal, the extensor digitorum brevis muscle inserts into the base of the 3rd

metacarpal, the extensor ulnaris muscle into the base of the 5th metacarpal and the extensor digitorum and extensor digiti minimi muscles insert via the dorsal digital fibrous expansions into the bases of the phalanges.

All the muscles are supplied by the radial nerve, either from the main trunk (brachioradialis and anconeus) and the remainder via the posterior interosseous branch.

These muscles extend the joints which they cross.

The posterior compartment of the forearm: deep muscles (Figs 32.22 and 32.23a)

Unlike the superficial group, which arises mainly from the humerus, this group arises from the posterior surfaces of the forearm bones and the intervening interosseous membrane (Fig. 32.23b). Supinator is the exception, as it has a head arising from the lateral epicondyle and it inserts into the posterior surface of the upper quarter of the radius.

The abductor pollicis longus muscle inserts into the base of the first metacarpal, the extensor pollicis longus muscle into the base of the distal phalanx of the thumb and the extensor pollicis brevis muscle inserts into the base of the proximal phalanx of the thumb.

The extensor indicis muscle inserts into the dorsal digital expansion of the index finger.

The muscles carry out the actions implicit in their names and are supplied by the posterior interosseous nerve.

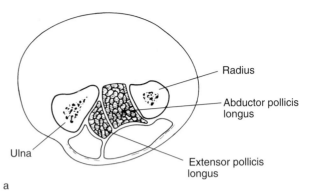

a

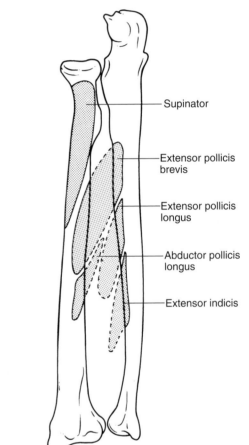

b

FIGURE 32.23 (a) Cross-section through the left forearm at about mid arm level showing the deep muscles of the posterior compartment. (b) Some origins of the deep muscles of the posterior compartment.

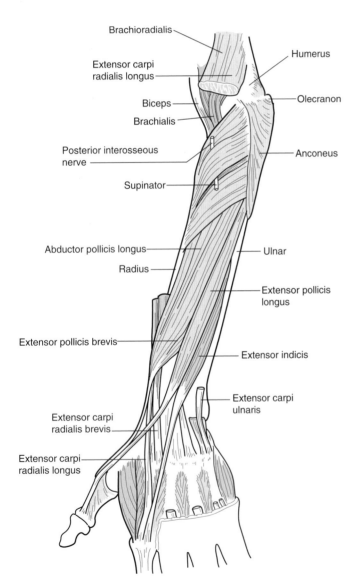

FIGURE 32.22 Deep muscles of the posterior compartment of the left forearm.

The radial nerve in the posterior compartment

The radial nerve lies in the anterior compartment of the lower arm behind brachialis, then brachioradialis and then extensor carpi radialis. In front of the lateral epi-condyle it divides into its two terminal branches. The superficial terminal branch (usually still called the radial nerve) runs down the forearm under brachoradialis lying lateral to the radial artery. The deep terminal branch (the posterior interosseous nerve) reaches the posterior compartment by winding around the radius between the two heads of origin of the supinator muscle. In the proximal part of its course it lies between the superficial and deep extensors but then passes deep to extensor pollicis longus.

SURGICAL CONSIDERATIONS

In the thigh

The thigh is the commonest single site for soft tissue sarcoma, and its fleshy nature makes compartmental resection frequently possible. The tumours may involve adjacent compartments and lie adjacent to, displace or invade the femoral vessels, the sciatic nerve, the femur and capsule of the hip joint.

Displacement of the sciatic nerve may lead to its confusion with the semitendinous tendon, as may its high division in the buttock into its two major branches.

The superficial femoral artery and vein may supply large branches from its posterior aspect to large tumours in the adductor muscles, while the perforating branches of the deep femoral vessels are encountered during division of the adductor magnus on the femur. The medial circumflex femoral vessels are often very large in medial tumours and must be carefully secured.

The availability of thick skin in adequate amounts and of muscle tissue for pedicle transfer, facilitates healing and prevents problems arising from exposure of vessels or vascular grafts in the event of necrosis.

Consideration in the leg and forearm

The fleshy areas of the calf, anterior and peroneal compartments of the leg lend themselves to en bloc resection of muscle groups, as do the flexor and extensor muscle groups of the forearm. However, if tumour involves adjacent compartments or lies close to major vessels, nerves or joints, as in the popliteal and antecubital fossae, then surgery must be modified to suit the circumstances, according to the general principles outlined at the beginning of the chapter. Thus resection of the fibula may be necessary for extensive tumour involving the lateral/anterior compartments, or narrower margins of excision accepted with the intention of using adjuvant radiotherapy. In the distal part of the limb the limited amount of skin available may be a potential problem where arteries and nerves may be exposed in the event of wound breakdown following surgery or radiotherapy. Special attention to wound closure is therefore required.

Amputation

Aponeurotic compartments and the muscles associated with them extend across joints and thus the potential exists for microscopic extension across major joints and well above clinically evident tumour. Stump recurrences following apparently adequate amputation are both the consequence and evidence of this. Thus amputations performed for soft tissue sarcoma must take this into account and be placed in the muscle and fascial compartments above those related to the tumour.

FURTHER READING

Rosenberg S A, Suit H D, Baker L H, Rosen G 1982 Sarcomas of the soft tissue and bone. In: De Vita V T, Hellman S, Rosenberg S A (eds) Cancer: principles and practice of oncology. J B Lippincott Philadelphia.

ARTERIAL AND VENOUS SURGERY

33 Operations involving the thoracic aorta and its branches: the anatomy of the thoracic aorta

Glyn Jamieson and Robert Fitridge

The arch of the aorta begins at about the level of the second right costal cartilage, where the aorta lies in front of the trachea. It then arches upwards to the left of the trachea and downwards to become the descending aorta at about the level of the second left costal cartilage. The arch reaches to about the mid manubrium sterni level.

The brachiocephalic artery

This artery arises from the aorta as it lies in front of the trachea, about 2–3 cm below the centre of the sternal notch. It passes upwards and to the right of the trachea and ends behind the right sternoclavicular joint by dividing into the right subclavian and right common carotid vessels.

The left brachiocephalic vein crosses in front of the artery just above the artery's origin and the inferior thyroid vein or veins often descend in front of it. The only named branch from it is the inconstant thyroidea ima artery which if present ascends to the isthmus of the thyroid gland in front of the trachea.

The common carotid arteries will be considered later (see Ch. 34).

The first part of the right subclavian artery

The right subclavian artery tends to lie behind the right common carotid at its origin. It then curves to the right, lying on the suprapleural membrane, until it disappears behind the scalenus anterior, where it lies on the first rib.

It is crossed by the vagus nerve just beyond the subclavian artery origin and then the termination of the jugular vein and its vertebral tributary. The vagus nerve gives off the recurrent laryngeal nerve on the first part of the subclavian artery. The nerve passes back under the artery and ascends in the tracheo-oesophageal groove, while the vagus continues down behind the right main bronchus and then passes along the oesophagus.

The first part of the left subclavian artery

The next major branch of the arch of the aorta is the left common carotid artery (see Ch. 34), followed by the left subclavian artery.

The left subclavian artery differs from the right in having a thoracic course where it lies behind the left common carotid artery with the trachea and oesophagus medially and the left lung and pleura laterally. Its cervical course is similar to the right subclavian artery, except that the left recurrent laryngeal nerve has no close relationship to it and the thoracic duct crosses behind it. On the left side the vagus passes between the left brachiocephalic vein and subclavian artery and along the lateral side of the arch, and then along the oesophagus. The left recurrent laryngeal nerve comes off the vagus on the side of the arch, passes to the side of the trachea and ascends in the groove between the trachea and oesophagus. The left phrenic nerve is more medially placed than on the right side and often leaves the scalenus anterior and crosses the first part of the left subclavian artery.

The second part of the subclavian artery

Each subclavian artery usually ascends to a point about 2 cm above the level of the clavicle behind the scalenus anterior, although this height is variable.

The trunks of the brachial plexus lie above and behind the artery here and the scalenus anterior muscle separates it from the subclavian vein anteriorly, which is also at a lower level because of the obliquity of the thoracic inlet.

The third part of the subclavian artery

This descends to the outer border of the first rib where it changes its name to the axillary artery. The external jugular vein pierces the deep fascia and crosses the artery to enter the subclavian vein which lies at a lower level than the artery. This means that not only the subclavian vein but its tributaries (suprascapular vein, transverse cervical vein, anterior jugular vein) lie in front of the subclavian artery. The artery lies on the first rib, which it grooves, and the brachial plexus continues to lie above and behind it.

The branches of the subclavian artery

❶ The vertebral artery is the most important branch and it arises from the posterior and superior aspect of the first part of the subclavian artery. It lies behind the common carotid artery and it ascends for about 3 cm, before disappearing from the field by entering the foramen of the transverse process of C7. Although the stellate ganglion tends to lie behind it, if the inferior cervical ganglion has not fused with the first thoracic ganglion then the inferior cervical ganglion lies in front and communications between the two tend to embrace the artery. (The cervical sympathetic trunk lies in front of the artery regardless of the manner of fusion of the ganglia.) The inferior thyroid artery crosses in front of the vertebral artery and on the left side the thoracic duct also crosses in front of it.

❷ The internal mammary artery arises from the inferior surface of the subclavian artery. It crosses behind the termination of the subclavian vein and passes down behind the upper six costal cartilages about 1 cm from the lateral edge of the sternum. Early in its course the phrenic nerve crosses in front of it.

❸ The thyrocervical trunk arises from the superior surface of the first part of the subclavian artery opposite the internal thoracic artery origin. The trunk gives rise to the inferior thyroid artery (see Ch. 23), the suprascapular and superficial (transverse) cervical arteries (see Ch. 29).

❹ The costocervical trunk arises from about the junction of the first and second parts of the subclavian artery posteriorly, and gives rise to the superior intercostal artery which descends between the pleura and the neck of the first rib and the deep cervical artery which ascends into the neck.

❺ The dorsal scapular artery is the only branch to arise from the third part of the subclavian artery. It passes laterally through the brachial plexus.

ANOMALIES AND VARIATIONS OF THE ARCH OF THE AORTA AND ITS BRANCHES

The commonest variation is for the brachiocephalic artery and the left common carotid artery to arise as a single and usually short common trunk.

Double aortic arch usually presents in childhood because it forms a complete ring around the oesophagus and trachea and causes obstructive symptoms early. Very occasionally the anomaly is seen in the adult. Right aortic arch is also an uncommon anomaly but can be present in the adult and it is often associated with situs inversus. In this situation the left subclavian artery crosses behind the oesophagus and the other branches lie in front of the trachea. The descending aorta then crosses to the left side behind the oesophagus.

The commonest anomaly of the aortic arch – occurring in perhaps 1% of individuals – is an aberrant right subclavian artery arising from the fourth part of the aortic arch. This vessel usually passes posterior to the oesophagus and can cause compressive symptoms. (dysphagia lusoria). The aberrant right subclavian artery often originates from a Kommerell's diverticulum.

THE THORACIC AORTA

The descending thoracic aorta is the most accessible part of the aorta and its major relations are all large and easily visualized. It commences at the level of T4 and lies initially to the left of the midline. It inclines to lie in the midline as it descends and it passes through the aortic hiatus in the diaphragm at about the level of T12, in the midline.

The oesophagus initially lies to its right but inclines to the left so that it lies progressively in front of the aorta and then to its left side.

The root of the left lung lies in front of the aorta above and the left atrium lies in front below.

The descending aorta gives off a variable number of bronchial, oesophageal, pericardial and mediastinal branches as well as nine pairs of posterior intercostal arteries and the subcostal arteries. The main significance of these arteries for the vascular surgeon is the branches they give to the spinal column.

The spinal cord obtains its blood supply locally from spinal arteries, i.e. from the vertebral, deep cervical, intercostal and lumbar arteries. In most patients these vessels anastomose and removing segmental supply produces no untoward effects. However it is not uncommon for one of the arteries of supply to the cord to be larger than the others. This is usually a lower intercostal or upper lumbar artery, and it is dignified with the impressive name of arteria radicularis magna. It arises more frequently from a left-sided artery and in a small proportion of cases it provides the major supply to the cord below its level. If it is divided, excluded or clamped for a long period it can lead to paraplegia.

EXPOSURE OF THE AORTA AND ORIGINS OF BRANCHES OF THE AORTIC ARCH

For elective exposure of the right or left subclavian arteries distal to their origin from the aorta a supraclavicular incision usually suffices – with or without division of the clavicular fibres of the origin of the sternocleidomastoid muscle. However, it is important to be able to gain control of the origins of the great vessels from the aorta particularly when managing trauma.

Generally, median sternotomy is required for adequate exposure of the origins of the brachiocephalic, right subclavian and both proximal carotid arteries. The sternotomy may be extended along the anterior border of the sternomastoid if necessary. The proximal left subclavian artery lies posteriorly and is difficult to access through this approach and most authors advocate a 'trap door' extension from the median sternotomy through the 4th interspace (just below the nipple). If only proximal control is required for a left subclavian injury in the root of the neck and there is no mediastinal injury, a left anterolateral thoracotomy can be performed through the fourth interspace.

Access to the descending aorta is obtained via a left posterolateral thoracotomy performed through the 4th to 6th interspace depending on the proximal level of the thoracic aorta which requires exposure.

FURTHER READING

Roos D B 1977 Chapter 66, The management of neurovascular diseases involving the upper extremity: overview. In: Rutherford R B (ed.) Vascular surgery. W B Saunders, Philadelphia.

Valentine J R , Wind G G 2003 Anatomic exposures in vascular surgery, 2nd edn. Lipincott, Philadelphia.

34 | Carotid endarterectomy: the anatomy of the carotid artery and related structures

Glyn Jamieson and Robert Fitridge

THE COMMON CAROTID ARTERY

The common carotid artery initially differs on the right and left sides with the right common carotid artery commencing posterior to the right sternoclavicular joint at the bifurcation of the brachiocephalic artery. The left common carotid artery arises from the arch of the aorta partly in front of the trachea and it ascends to lie behind the left sternoclavicular joint. The left brachiocephalic vein crosses in front of it in its ascent.

The cervical course of the common carotid artery

The common carotid artery ascends from behind the sternoclavicular joint to the level of the upper border of the thyroid cartilage where it divides into external and internal carotid vessels. The bifurcation can be below or above the level of the cartilage. A high bifurcation is more common than a low one. It is crossed by the tendon joining the two bellies of omohyoid muscle. Below this point it is relatively deep behind the sternomastoid muscle and lying on longus colli muscle; it is overlapped somewhat by the lobe of the thyroid gland. The oesophagus lies medial to it; the internal jugular vein lies laterally and between the artery and vein posteriorly lies the vagus nerve. These three structures are described as being enclosed within a sheath, but this is little in evidence in the living.

The superior limb of the ansa cervicalis descends superficial to the common carotid artery and joins its inferior limb which appears between the common carotid artery and the internal jugular vein.

The distal common carotid artery superior to the omohyoid muscle tendon is more superficial and is deep to the anterior margin of the sternomastoid muscle. The artery is crossed by a muscular branch from the superior thyroid artery to the sternomastoid muscle. It is crossed also by the middle thyroid and superior thyroid veins – the latter crosses it quite close to the bifurcation of the artery. The facial vein usually crosses the bifurcation itself. Dividing the facial vein is virtually the gateway to the carotid bifurcation.

THE EXTERNAL CAROTID ARTERY

The external carotid artery emerges from the bifurcation, initially seemingly the innermost of the two vessels, but it soon gives off branches which is one of its major distinguishing features. It passes upwards and backwards at a point midway between the tip of the mastoid process and the angle of the mandible and divides within the parotid gland into its two terminal branches, the superficial temporal and maxillary arteries. In its ascent it is crossed by the lingual vein and the hypoglossal nerve and the posterior belly of digastric. It is separated from the internal carotid artery by the styloid process and its related structures. Its branches in the neck are:

❶ The ascending pharyngeal artery which arises medially near the bifurcation and ascends on the pharynx deep to the internal carotid artery.

Then arise three arteries from the front of the external carotid artery in the vicinity of the greater cornu of the hyoid bone. These are:

❷ The superior thyroid artery which arises from the anterior surface of the carotid bifurcation (and it is sometimes difficult to tell if it is actually arising from the common or the external carotid). It passes downwards to the superior pole of the thyroid gland.
❸ The lingual artery which loops upwards and forwards to disappear behind the hyoglossus muscle.
❹ The facial artery which arches upwards to groove the posterior surface of the submandibular gland.

There are two branches arising posteriorly. These are:

❺ The occipital artery which arises opposite the origin of the facial artery and passes backwards. It is of surgical significance as it is around this artery that the hypoglossal nerve winds forwards.
❻ The posterior auricular artery.

THE INTERNAL CAROTID ARTERY

This is expanded at its origin as the carotid bulb and it usually seems to lie more external, i.e. lateral, than the external carotid at its origin. The carotid vessels are often rotated in orientation which can mislead the surgeon. The internal carotid artery ascends to the cranial base and enters the skull through the carotid canal. It passes through the lateral wall of the cavernous sinus and terminates by dividing into the anterior and middle cerebral arteries.

The internal jugular vein becomes gradually posterior to it as the base of the skull is reached and passes through the jugular foramen. The IXth–XIIth cranial nerves all exit the skull between the vein behind and the artery in front.

The internal carotid artery has no branches in the neck, but it gives off the ophthalmic artery in the carotid canal, which has great surgical significance in a diagnostic sense in carotid disease, as embolization to this vessel causes the typical temporary blindness of carotid vascular disease (amaurosis fugax).

The facial vein

The facial vein descends over the masseter muscle posterior to the facial artery. Just below the mandible it receives the anterior division of the retromandibular vein to form the common facial vein (Fig. 34.1). It passes obliquely backwards deep to the sternomastoid muscle but superficial to the loop of the lingual artery, the hypoglossal nerve and the bifurcation of the common carotid artery. Along the anterior border of the sternomastoid muscle, the vein often receives a moderately large tributary which connects it to the anterior jugular vein. Dissection of the vein back to its entry into the internal jugular vein and then division of the vein 'opens the door' to the carotid bifurcation.

The hypoglossal (XIIth) nerve

The nerve is motor to all the muscles of the tongue except palatoglossus. It emerges from the hypoglossal canal and

crosses behind the internal carotid artery to lie between it and the internal jugular vein. At about the level of the angle of the mandible it curves forwards around the occipital branch of the external carotid artery and so lies superficial to both internal and external carotid arteries. It then crosses the loop of the lingual artery and inclines upwards on hyoglossus but deep to mylohyoid where it is inferior to the deep portion of the submandibular gland.

It contains C1 nerve fibres which have 'hitched a ride' and some of these are given off as it crosses the external carotid, as the upper root of the ansa cervicalis, and the remainder as the nerves to thyrohyoid and geniohyoid muscles.

The nerve exits *behind* the internal jugular vein in about 10% of cases and occasionally can cross at a lower level, so that it is important to watch out for it in mobilizing the carotid bifurcation.

The glossopharyngeal (IXth) nerve

The glossopharyngeal nerve exits the skull through the jugular foramen lying between the internal jugular vein and the internal carotid artery. The nerve curves forwards superficial to the internal carotid artery (but deep to the external carotid artery) and at a level about 2 cm above the hypoglossal nerve. It is therefore at less risk than the XIIth nerve during carotid endarterectomy. The branch to the carotid sinus from the IXth nerve descends on the internal carotid artery and is often divided during mobilization of the carotid bifurcation. This division is safely achieved by removing the tissue which lies between the external and internal carotid artery immediately above the bifurcation of the common carotid artery.

The superior laryngeal nerve passes deep to the vessels and is generally not seen during carotid endarterectomy. Very occasionally it courses superficial to the carotid vessels.

Exposure of the carotid vessels

While the overwhelming majority of procedures are performed upon the carotid bifurcation for atherosclerosis, neck trauma or more complex carotid procedures require more extensive exposure of proximal or distal vessels and can thus be more challenging for the surgeon.

Particularly in managing trauma, the neck may be divided into three zones:

Zone I extends from the root of the neck up to 1cm above the clavicle.
Zone II extends from the upper part of zone I to the angle of the mandible.
Zone III extends from the angle of the mandible to the skull base.

Access to zone I lesions usually requires a median sternotomy in addition to the standard anterior sternomastoid incision.

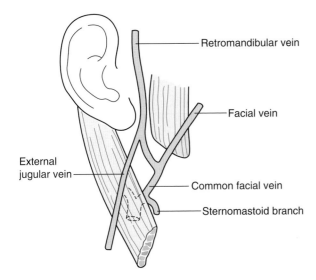

FIGURE 34.1   The facial vein.

Exposure of the carotid bifurcation (zone II)

A longitudinal incision is made along the anterior border of the sternomastoid at least 2 cm behind the angle of the mandible to avoid injury to the mandibular and cervical branches of the facial nerve. Some surgeons advocate a transverse cervical incision. However this is associated with a higher risk of injury to the mandibular branch of the facial nerve and tends to limit the exposure of the internal carotid artery.

The external jugular vein is encountered lying on the superficial surface of the sternomastoid muscle level. The great auricular nerve emerges behind the middle of the sternomastoid muscle and runs upwards and forwards close to the posterior aspect of the external jugular vein. This nerve should be preserved if possible because division results in numbness of the ear lobe, which is a source of annoyance to the patient.

As mentioned already, the key to exposure of the bifurcation of the common carotid artery is division of the facial vein near to its termination in the internal jugular vein.

During carotid endarterectomy, the dissection usually proceeds as far as the XIIth nerve. However further dissection may be required if the internal carotid is diseased at this level or there is a high carotid bifurcation. The XIIth nerve is best found by following the descendens hypoglossi nerve cranially to the point where is leaves the XIIth nerve. Dissection along the posterior aspect of the descendens hypoglossi leads to the XIIth nerve with the least risk of damaging it. Once the trunk of the XIIth nerve has been identified it can be dissected anteriorly as necessary for adequate exposure of the internal carotid artery. Division of the sternomastoid and/or occipital branches of the external carotid artery and associated veins allows the hypoglossal nerve to be gentle pushed forward giving a further 1–2 cm exposure of the internal carotid artery.

If it is necessary to expose the internal carotid artery even further towards the base of the skull, the dissection should focus on the posterior belly of the digastric muscle.

If further exposure is required, the posterior belly of the digastric can be safely divided, ensuring that the XIIth nerve is seen and protected.

If it is considered that access to the upper part of the extracranial internal carotid artery is needed the incision is usually extended superiorly and curved behind the earlobe, then there are two manoeuvres which may be undertaken to aid exposure. First, a transnasal endotracheal tube allows the position of the angle of the mandible to lie more anteriorly and this improves access. Second, the ramus of the mandible may be moved forwards by subluxing the temporomandibular joint.

FURTHER READING

Monson D O, Saletta J D, Freeark R J 1969 Carotid-vertebral trauma. J Trauma 9(12):987–999.

Operations on arteries of the upper limb: the anatomy of the arteries of the arm

Glyn Jamieson and Robert Fitridge

THE AXILLARY ARTERY (Fig. 35.1)

The subclavian artery changes its name to the axillary artery at the outer border of the first rib. The artery then passes behind pectoralis minor lying on the serratus anterior muscle and then the subscapularis muscle. Pectoralis major overlies the axillary artery throughout its course, except for the last 5 cm where the artery is subcutaneous.

Pectoralis minor traditionally divides the artery into three parts. The first part of the artery has the least relationship with the brachial plexus, with the medial cord lying behind the artery. The lateral and posterior cords of the brachial plexus lie lateral to the vessel. The lateral cord gives off the lateral pectoral nerve which crosses the first part of the axillary artery and often gives off a branch to the medial pectoral nerve which arises further laterally. The lateral pectoral nerve courses forwards but its branch is usually a direct relation of the axillary artery. (The branch can be divided but the lateral pectoral nerve should be maintained if possible.) None of the cords are generally seen or exposed when the first part of the artery is exposed to perform an axillofemoral bypass. The axillary vein lies superficial and inferior to the artery at this level.

The other structures encountered in front of the artery when exposing it here (Fig. 35.1) are the termination of the cephalic vein and various venous tributaries of the thoraco-acromial trunk.

The first part of the axillary artery gives off the small superior thoracic artery and just under the medial edge of pectoralis minor the thoracoacromial trunk which curls around the edge of the muscle.

As the artery passes laterally, the cords of the brachial plexus embrace it and lie medial, posterior and lateral to it according to their names. The branches of the cords also maintain their relationship to the artery according to their cord of origin, except for the medial head of the median nerve which crosses from medial to lateral in front of the artery towards the distal end of its course. The third part of the artery gives off the lateral thoracic artery just beyond the lateral border of pectoralis minor and near its termination are given off the large subscapular artery and the lateral and medial circumflex vessels.

While these six described branches are the commonest pattern, it occurs in only a minority of cases with less or more branches being commoner. When less, it is usually because two branches arise from a common trunk.

The axillary artery sometimes divides proximally into two limb arteries but this virtually never occurs as high as the first part, which is another reason for choosing the first part of the artery for an axillofemoral or axilloaxillary graft.

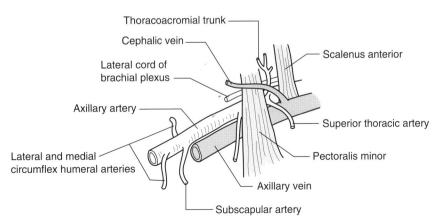

FIGURE 35.1 Some relations of the axillary artery.

As the artery crosses the inferior border of teres major it changes its name to the brachial artery.

THE BRACHIAL ARTERY

Although the brachial artery is described as being subcutaneous throughout its course, it is overlapped by biceps to a great degree so that its subcutaneous position is more of a myth than a fact (Fig. 35.2) However it is easy to remain medial to biceps when exposing the artery so that no muscles have to be divided to expose the artery. It runs down on triceps to the cubital fossa (see below) and there it divides into its terminal branches, the radial and ulnar arteries.

The artery lies medially in the arm area to begin with, but more distally it spirals in front of the humerus, always lying on brachialis to reach the front of the elbow joint about midway between the epicondyles.

Proximally the three major nerves maintain their brachial plexus relationships to the artery with the radial nerve posterior, the median nerve lateral and the ulnar nerve medial. However the radial and ulnar nerves fall away from the artery and during most of its course it is only the median nerve which has a close relationship with the artery. This nerve commences lateral and crosses anteriorly to be medial to the artery.

The branches of the axillary artery do not have much surgical significance, other than the large profunda brachii branch which travels with the radial nerve and is an important collateral vessel when occlusion of the brachial artery occurs distal to the profunda brachii.

The brachial artery in the cubital fossa (Fig. 35.3)

The brachial artery lies on the brachialis muscle and the tendon of the biceps dives lateral to the artery, while the bicipital aponeurosis passes medially superficial to the artery. The artery usually bifurcates about 1 cm distal to the skin crease of the elbow.

The ulnar branch, usually the larger of the terminal branches, passes medially between the two heads of pronator teres. The radial artery is the direct continuation of the brachial artery but is the smaller of the terminal branches at

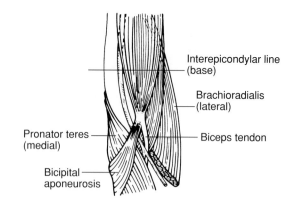

FIGURE 35.3 The brachial artery in the cubital fossa.

this point. It passes down under brachioradialis and is easily palpable at the wrist.

The median nerve remains medial to the brachial artery in the antecubital fossa. The only structures of note anterior to the artery are the bicipital aponeurosis and in front of this the median cubital vein.

The radial artery at the wrist (Fig. 35.4)

The radial artery emerges medial to the tendon of brachioradialis and lateral to the tendon of flexor carpi radialis where the artery lies on pronator quadratus and then the radius. It is here that it is usually exposed for the purpose of constructing an arteriovenous fistula. Further distally it crosses the anatomical snuff box deep to the tendons of the abductor pollicis longus muscle and the extensor pollicis brevis and longus muscles. The origin of the cephalic vein crosses it here, making it a convenient site for formation of

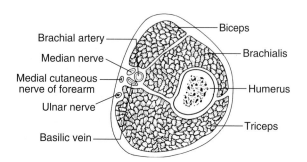

FIGURE 35.2 The brachial artery and its relations in mid arm.

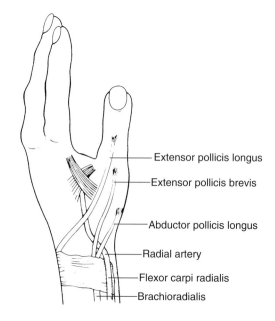

FIGURE 35.4 The radial artery in the hand.

an arteriovenous fistula. The terminal branch or branches of the radial nerve also lie superficial to it here.

By the time the wrist is reached the radial artery is larger than the ulnar artery. The ulnar artery lies lateral to the pisiform bone and is subcutaneous, and although most clinicians do not make a habit of palpating it, its pulse can usually be readily felt.

The radial artery is predominantly used for creating forearm arteriovenous fistulae for a number of reasons. It is larger than the ulnar artery at the wrist level, the cephalic vein is more superficial in the forearm than the basilic vein and the position of the cephalic vein is more convenient for self cannulation of the fistula.

36 | The surgery of abdominal aortic aneurysms; renal artery surgery: the anatomy of the abdominal aorta and its branches

Glyn Jamieson and Peter Morris

The abdominal aorta passes through the aortic hiatus in the diaphragm at approximately the level of T12 and extends to L4 before it divides. It lies on the anterior spinal ligament and its only posterior relations of surgical significance are the cysterna chyli above and the left lumbar veins (which pass behind the aorta to reach the inferior vena cava) and the left sympathetic trunk.

Proximally, the floor of the lesser sac lies anterior to the aorta and it is through here and above the coeliac axis that the aorta can be mobilized for rapid clamping, if necessary, in cases of ruptured aortic aneurysm. The aorta at this point lies between the crura of the diaphragm and it can also be approached by splitting the crural fibres to its left. (It should be remembered that the thoracic duct lies behind the aorta at this level.) However, it is easier to compress the suprarenal aorta through the lesser sac with the left hand or a blunt instrument with a curved cross piece on the end (snake catcher) whilst the neck of the aneurysm is cleared and clamped.

The neck of the pancreas crosses the aorta above, although the pancreas is partly separated from it by the superior mesenteric artery origin. Below this, the uncinate process of the pancreas and then the third part of the duodenum lie in front of the aorta. The extent to which the third part of the duodenum covers the aorta is variable. The aorta is easily found here by dividing the peritoneum alongside the third part of the duodenum. The fourth part of the duodenum can be mobilized by continuing the dissection alongside the duodenum and dividing the ligament of Treitz (suspensory ligament of the duodenum), which usually contains some small blood vessels. Mobilization to this extent provides better access to the left renal vein and its junction with the inferior vena cava and also the origin of the right renal artery. Its major lateral relation is the inferior vena cava on its right side, which is closely applied to the aorta, but is separated from it by a thin layer of fibrous tissue.

The unpaired visceral branches

The coeliac axis

The coeliac axis typically arises within 2 cm of the aorta's emergence through the diaphragm. It projects forwards and downwards for about 12 mm before dividing into its three terminal branches of left gastric, common hepatic and splenic arteries.

It is surrounded by the coeliac nerve plexus and whether it is this tissue or the median arcuate ligament which sometimes constricts the origin of the coeliac axis is a moot point. This tissue is very dense and has to be divided by sharp dissection in order to dissect free the origin of the coeliac axis.

It is difficult to gain access to the coeliac axis. It is probably best approached through a left thoraco-abdominal incision which remains extraperitoneal so that the spleen and pancreas are swept forwards off the aorta. If exposure of the aorta is required at a higher level the diaphragm may be divided down to the aorta. This then provides exposure to the whole of the lower thoracic and abdominal aorta, but exposure of the right common iliac artery is difficult from this approach. However in thin patients the coeliac axis can be approached from the midline transperitoneally. Mobilization of the superior aspect of the pancreas can improve this anterior exposure.

The superior mesenteric artery

The superior mesenteric artery arises from the front of the aorta about 10 mm below the coeliac axis. It is separated from the aorta by the uncinate process of the pancreas and the left renal vein. It can be approached either retroperitoneally as for the coeliac axis or transperitoneally beneath the pancreas and in front of the left renal vein. The trunk of the superior mesenteric artery is usually about 3–5 cm long and it has no significant branches (although an accessory right hepatic artery arises from it in about 10% of cases). It is the structure which limits the mobility of the small bowel and duodenum as they are displaced to the right during aortic surgery. The artery lies to the left of its corresponding vein, and its pulsation can be felt in the root of the mesentery. To expose it here, it is necessary to divide the peritoneum and perivascular neural and lymphatic tissue which surrounds the artery as it lies in front of the left renal vein. This dissection can be carried proximally as far as the aorta, if indicated, for endarterectomy or bypass procedures. The branches of the superior mesenteric artery are considered in Chapter 11.

The inferior mesenteric artery

The inferior mesenteric artery arises from the left side of the front of the aorta about 3–4 cm above the aortic bifurcation. It can usually be ligated close to its origin, or bypassed with impunity, although the vascularity of the left colon should always be checked visually at the end of any such operation. It is considered in detail in Chapters 13 and 14.

The paired visceral branches

The middle suprarenal arteries

The middle suprarenal arteries are small vessels to the suprarenal gland arising immediately above the renal arteries. They can cause troublesome bleeding if they are avulsed during mobilization of a renal artery.

The renal arteries

The renal arteries are large branches which have a sloping origin at, or just below, the level of the superior mesenteric artery.

It is useful to know this as the renal arteries are usually approached transperitoneally and it is often difficult to gain access to their origins. Thus if the operator has dissected the anterior surface of the aorta, proximal to the crossing of the left renal vein, and found the point of origin of the superior mesenteric artery then he or she will probably be at the level of the renal arteries which arise from the posterolateral surface of the aorta.

Anatomy books seem to be divided in their opinion as to which renal artery is likely to be more proximal in its origin. It is probably the right renal artery – at any rate for the surgeon it always seems more proximal, perhaps because it is more difficult to gain access to it.

After the left renal vein has been mobilized, the left renal artery can be mobilized along its whole length, by dissecting its various surfaces. The left adrenal vein is easily damaged during such dissection, and care must be taken to avoid it as it drains into the superior aspect of the left renal vein. Indeed it is probably safer to ligate and divide it, as this allows a sling to be placed around the left renal vein, so it can be lifted with impunity off the aorta and the origin of the renal artery.

Access to the right renal artery is more difficult because the inferior vena cava overlies its origin and proximal course. It is necessary to mobilize the left renal vein and the segment of inferior vena cava into which it runs in order to gain access to the origin of the right renal artery. Once the origin and proximal portion of the artery are freed, the distal portion is approached by mobilizing the duodenum (Kocher's manoeuvre) and the inferior vena cava behind the duodenum.

Accessory renal arteries either from above or below the renal artery take-off are quite common. They have a normal relationship to the ureter if they cross it, i.e. they lie in front of it. On the right they usually pass in front of the inferior vena cava. Any arteries of significant size which arise from the lateral aspect of the aorta should be assumed to be accessory renal arteries and therefore they should be protected.

The gonadal arteries

The gonadal arteries are somewhat variable in origin and course. They arise from the anterolateral aspect of the aorta, quite high up but 1–3 cm distal to the origin of the renal arteries. The right gonadal artery crosses anterior to the inferior cava.

The parietal branches

The inferior phrenic arteries

The inferior phrenic arteries are extremely variable in origin and arise as often from the coeliac trunk as from the aorta.

The lumbar arteries

There are usually four pairs of lumbar arteries and it is usually the distal two pairs which are encountered in infrarenal aortic surgery. The arteries pass posterior to the structures they cross: thus they are posterior to the inferior vena cava and cysterna chyli (for the right lumbars) and the sympathetic trunks.

The origins of the vessels are directly posterior, and their right and left origins usually lie close together. The fourth pair, and occasionally the third, sometimes arise from a common trunk.

The median sacral artery

The median sacral artery is a small vessel arising posteriorly from the aorta, just above the aortic bifurcation, and passing directly inferiorly.

EXPOSURE OF THE ABDOMINAL AORTA

The lower abdominal aorta is retroperitoneal and it can be approached transperitoneally. It is usual to mobilize the third and fourth parts of the duodenum off the aorta. When the peritoneum is divided vertically alongside the third and fourth parts of the duodenum the inferior mesenteric vein forms a barrier to continued division. Although it can be divided, it is close to the upper limit of direct vision anyway as the inferior border of the pancreas comes into view.

There is a large amount of tissue, of lymphatic and nervous origin, surrounding the aorta,. It has to be divided in order to dissect close to the aortic wall, but dissection should always be minimized in the male, to avoid post-operative sexual dysfunction.

The other structure of note during this dissection is the left renal vein which usually crosses across the front of the aorta, quite proximally underneath the pancreas. As discussed above, mobilization of the left renal vein provides access to the aorta up to the superior mesenteric artery and renal artery origins.

As well as the posterior lumbar arteries, which limit dissection posterior to the aorta, it should be remembered that the left lumbar veins pass behind the lower aorta on their way to the interior vena cava.

THE COMMON ILIAC ARTERIES

As the termination of the aorta lies slightly to the left of the midline, the right common iliac artery is slightly longer than the left common iliac artery.

The right common iliac artery crosses the formation of the inferior vena cava so that it tends to overlie the termination of the left common iliac vein (Fig. 36.1). This sometimes causes a relative narrowing of the termination of the left common iliac vein, and this is sometimes advanced as the reason why iliofemoral thrombosis is more common on the left side than on the right side. The veins are usually intimately adherent to the aortic bifurcation and dissection of the one from the other is a hazardous procedure. Venous damage in this region is difficult to control as bleeding comes from both the inferior vena cava and the right and left common iliac veins. For this reason most surgeons avoid such a dissection, if possible.

The left common iliac artery on the other hand is not related to any venous structure posteriorly near its origin with the left common iliac vein lying medial, but becoming posterior. The left artery is behind the root of the mesosigmoid and the superior rectal artery.

Both arteries are crossed near their termination by the ureters. The common iliac arteries have no major branches but both give small unnamed branches to muscles, peritoneum, ureters, etc. The common iliac arteries divide into the external and internal iliac arteries in front of the sacroiliac joints.

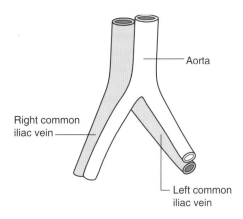

FIGURE 36.1 The aortic bifurcation and its relationship to the iliac veins.

Aorta

Right common iliac vein

Left common iliac vein

THE EXTERNAL ILIAC ARTERIES

The external iliac arteries commence in front of the sacroiliac joints and course along the pelvic brim on psoas major to pass deep to the midpoint of the inguinal ligament. This point is slightly below and lateral to the mid-inguinal point, which is the surface marking of the deep inguinal ring. They initially tend to lie on the external iliac vein but by the time the inguinal ligament is reached the vein is a direct medial relation.

The ureters cross anteriorly at about the origins of the external iliac arteries and the genitofemoral nerves lie in front of the vessels.

In the female the gonadal vessels cross in front, distal to the ureteric crossing. In the male the gonadal vessels lie in front on their way to the internal inguinal ring and the ductus deferens crosses in front of the vessels also.

Each external iliac artery gives two moderate-sized branches just before it exits into the thigh. The inferior epigastric artery arises from the external iliac artery's anterior surface and passes forwards medial to the internal inguinal ring. The deep circumflex iliac artery arises from the external iliac artery's lateral side and passes deeply along the inguinal ligament towards the anterior superior iliac spine. These vessels are accessible by dissecting the common femoral artery and then the distal external iliac artery from below the inguinal ligament.

When the common and external iliac arteries are approached extraperitoneally, structures such as the ureter and gonadal vessels tend to stay with the peritoneum as it is swept off the vessels.

THE INTERNAL ILIAC ARTERY

The internal iliac artery is usually from 2 to 4 cm long and it passes downwards and posteriorly towards the greater sciatic foramen where it divides into an anterior and posterior trunk.

The artery lies anterior to its corresponding vein and behind the ureter (and ovary in the female). The obturator nerve lies on the pelvic wall lateral to it.

While the trunk of the artery is accessible the branches are less so. When the internal iliac artery is being prepared for anastomosis end-to-end to the renal artery of a donor kidney, these branches are individually ligated so that the full length of the internal iliac artery will be available for the anastomosis. Its branches do not have any other surgical significance other than their importance as collateral pathways to the thigh. When dealing with an aneurysm of the internal iliac artery, the origins of the branches can be sutured from within the aneurysm sac.

Although the usual origin of the obturator artery is the anterior trunk of the internal iliac artery, in about 20% of cases it arises from the inferior epigastric artery. This artery then passes variably in relation to the femoral ring, probably most often in front of the ring.

37

Operations on the common femoral artery, profunda femoris artery and leg vessels: the anatomy of the femoral artery and its branches, the popliteal fossa, and the popliteal artery and its branches

Glyn Jamieson, Jesper Swedenborg and Spero Raptis

THE COMMON FEMORAL ARTERY

The external iliac artery crosses behind the midpoint of the inguinal ligament and its name changes to the femoral artery. By tradition vascular surgeons tend to refer to the artery above the profunda femoris branch as the common femoral artery and distal to this branch as the superficial femoral artery.

The common femoral artery and its major branches, especially profunda femoris, are the centrepoint of most arterial reconstructions involving the lower limb. They serve as the outflow for aortic reconstructions and the inflow for femorodistal reconstructions. Apart from a few overlying lymph nodes the common femoral artery is entirely subcutaneous, making it one of the most accessible of all arteries, a fact of some convenience in many emergency situations, and to interventional radiologists.

The common femoral artery lies within the femoral triangle (see Ch. 30) which is bounded by the inguinal ligament above, the medial border of sartorius muscle on the outer side and the medial border of adductor longus on the inner side (Fig. 37.1).

The sartorius and adductor longus muscles are key muscles of the arterial anatomy of the whole inner thigh and a precise knowledge of these muscles is a help in understanding arterial operations in this area.

The sartorius muscle arises from the anterior superior iliac spine and the area just below and it crosses the thigh from lateral to medial to end as a flat tendon which inserts into the upper tibia in front of the insertions of the gracilis and semitendinosus muscles. It is a flat muscle and it is the longest muscle in the body. This length allows it to be mobilized on its proximal blood supply and used as a bolstering component or replacement muscle in certain operations.

The muscle lies on a thick layer of deep fascia in the mid thigh and the femoral artery lies beneath the muscle in this region.

The muscle is a flexor of the thigh and knee and also helps externally rotate the femur. It is supplied by the femoral nerve.

The adductor longus muscle arises from the front of the pubis between the medial end of the origin of the pectineus muscle and the upper end of the origin of the gracilis muscle. It is the most anterior of the adductor muscles in the thigh and it fans out from its origin to insert into the linea aspera in the middle third of the posterior surface of the femur.

The muscle lies between the vastus medialis muscle anteriorly and the adductor magnus muscle posteriorly. The medial intermuscular septum lies between the vastus medialis muscle and the adductor longus muscle and adductor brevis and the three muscles are blended near the femur where there is no plane of separation between them.

The adductor longus muscle is regarded as forming the floor or posterior wall of the adductor canal (see below). It is an adductor of the thigh and it is supplied by the anterior divisions of the obturator nerve.

A knowledge of the surface anatomy of some of these structures is useful. The sartorius muscle can be represented by a line drawn from the anterior superior iliac spine to the medial condyle of the femur. The common femoral and superficial femoral artery can be represented by a line drawn from the midpoint of the inguinal ligament to the medial condyle of the femur.

The floor of the femoral triangle has been likened to a trough, with the iliopsoas muscle the lateral sloping side and pectineus and adductor longus muscles the medial slope. The femoral artery is in the middle at the bottom of the trough, the femoral nerve is on its lateral side (but embedded beneath the iliopsoas fascia) and the femoral vein

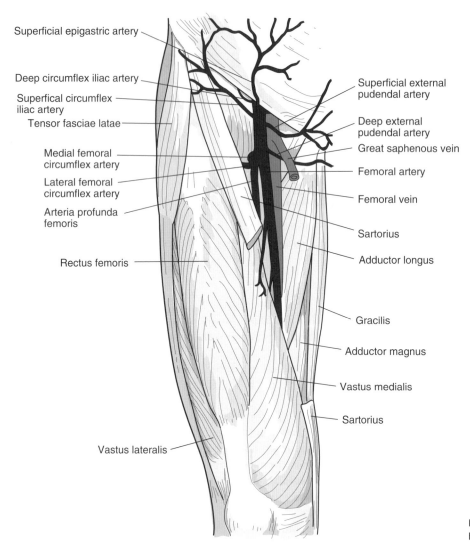

Superficial epigastric artery

Deep circumflex iliac artery

Superfical circumflex iliac artery

Tensor fasciae latae

Medial femoral circumflex artery

Lateral femoral circumflex artery

Arteria profunda femoris

Rectus femoris

Vastus lateralis

Superficial external pudendal artery

Deep external pudendal artery

Great saphenous vein

Femoral artery

Femoral vein

Sartorius

Adductor longus

Gracilis

Adductor magnus

Vastus medialis

Sartorius

FIGURE 37.1   The femoral artery and its branches.

is on the medial side. The first part of the profunda femoris artery and the superficial femoral artery are within the triangle, but thereafter the profunda artery lies behind the adductor longus muscle and is outside the triangle.

As the common femoral artery is subcutaneous, the only structures which need to be divided in exposing it, after dividing the skin, are the superficial and deep fascia and occasionally some lymph nodes. There is some fascial tissue in front of the artery which is thickest near the inguinal ligament and this fascial condensation is dignified with the name of the femoral sheath. Immediately under the inguinal ligament the fibres of this sheath tend to run transversely whereas close to the artery they run longitudinally with the artery. It is worth remembering this point during scissors dissection of the artery. The femoral sheath is very loosely bound to the artery and it is quite distinct from the artery's adventitia. This means the sheath is easily separable from the artery with scissors dissection. However, in re-operations the sheath is intimately adherent to the adventitia and blunt dissection at this stage can easily create a plane between the intima and adventitia of the artery.

The branches of the femoral artery

Two vessels usually arise in the vicinity of the inguinal ligament. The first is the superficial epigastric which passes anteromedially in front of the inguinal ligament and the other which is usually smaller passes laterally towards the anterior superior iliac spine. It is the superficial circumflex iliac artery.

The external pudendal arteries are variable but may be two in number (superficial and deep). They arise from the medial side of the common femoral artery and pass medially either in front of or behind the great saphenous vein. The deep external pudendal artery usually crosses behind the great saphenous vein at the point where it joins the deep femoral vein.

The origin of the profunda femoris artery is somewhat posterior as well as lateral so that its origin is not always obvious, particularly as the level of origin is variable relative to the inguinal ligament. The surgeon can get a clue to the origin from the fact that the common femoral suddenly narrows down and the point of change in size corresponds with the origin of the profunda femoris artery.

One or other of the lateral or medial circumflex femoral arteries arises from the common femoral artery in about 50% of cases (usually the lateral circumflex femoral artery). In the remaining cases they arise from the profunda femoris artery. The medial circumflex artery arises from the posterior wall of the vessel, almost invariably from the main trunk itself but occasionally from the origin of the profunda femoris artery. This tends to run straight backwards and in towards the medial side.

Surgical considerations in regard to the common femoral artery

The most constant site for application of a clamp at the beginning of the femoral artery is under the inguinal ligament, usually just above or between the deep circumflex iliac artery and the inferior epigastric which really are branches from the external iliac artery and which arise very constantly just behind the inguinal ligament. The deep circumflex iliac artery is often more cephalad so that it is possible to apply a straight clamp between the two vessels from the lateral side. To free the external iliac artery, one needs to retract the inguinal ligament in a cephalad direction or even divide the lower fibres of the inguinal ligament, which tends to be a rounded structure made of the transverse running fibres of the external oblique aponeurosis. These fibres, the recurved part of the inguinal ligament, can be divided with impunity, without destroying the integrity of the ligament. Structures above this (including the peritoneum) can be retracted upwards so that it is possible to free 2–3 cm of the external iliac artery for application of a clamp from below without dividing the abdominal muscle wall. Passing across the artery from lateral to medial is the vein accompanying the deep circumflex iliac artery, on its way to the external iliac vein, and it is recommended that this circumflex iliac vein be divided.

The artery can be recognized by its pulsation and also by the pattern of venules which are seen in its wall.

The small branches of the femoral artery, the superficial circumflex iliac and the superficial external pudendal can usually be preserved, but the superficial epigastric artery tends to come straight off the front of the common femoral artery and often has to be divided. More distally, the deep external pudendal artery is not usually encountered. This artery is more likely to be divided in ligation of the great saphenous vein because of the artery's intimate proximity to the fossa ovalis.

The veins accompanying these arteries and running to join the great saphenous vein are best ligated between ligatures lest their bleeding obscure the operative field. One of these veins, the anterior femoral cutaneous vein, is often quite large and is a useful vein to use if a short conduit or patch is needed.

The femoral nerve

The femoral nerve lies lateral to the common femoral artery on a deeper plane, beneath the iliopsoas fascia, and sometimes with some fibres of the iliopsoas between it and the artery. The main nerve breaks up early into its terminal branches and so the trunk is not really at risk. However, cutaneous branches emerge and cross in front of the artery and are easily damaged during extensive dissection of the vessel. This is particularly so after re-explorations of the common femoral artery or the profunda femoris; about 50% of patients complain after surgery of either numbness or hyperaesthesia on the inner side of the thigh.

The inguinal lymph nodes

The superficial inguinal lymph nodes are the largest of the inguinal nodes. In the young they are small and of no consequence but in the elderly it is common for them to be enlarged. Although the nodes tend to accompany the veins and therefore lie medial to the region of dissection of the artery, in chronic inflammatory states the nodes tend to enlarge laterally in front of the femoral artery.

It is usually possible to avoid the lymph nodes by exposing the artery either high up, immediately under the inguinal ligament, or dissecting much further down nearer to the bifurcation. However it is impossible to avoid the nodes if dissecting the whole length of the artery, as the nodes lie in between these two positions.

It is a matter of preference whether to dissect from the lateral side to mobilize the nodes medially or to cut between the nodes on to the artery. The former method decreases the risk of postoperative lymphocele, but is difficult if an in situ bypass using the saphenous vein is to be performed.

THE PROFUNDA FEMORIS ARTERY

The profunda femoris artery arises from the posterolateral aspect of the common femoral artery and passes down towards the medial surface of the femur. There is considerable variation in the length of the common femoral artery before it divides into superficial and deep femoral vessels (range 1–8.5 cm; mean 5.2 cm).

Sometimes when the division is high the profunda artery appears to come from the posterior wall of the parent vessel, or even the medial wall, and it may run for a short period on the medial side of the femoral vessel before drifting more laterally.

The profunda femoris artery lies first on the pectineus muscle, then on the adductor brevis muscle before passing between adductor brevis and adductor longus ultimately to become embedded in the tendon of adductor magnus, by which time it is almost posterior to the linea aspera of the femur (Figs 37.2 and 37.3). It is enveloped throughout its length by the fascia enveloping the vastus medialis and the anterior aspect of the adductor muscles sweeping from the sartorius to the linea aspera.

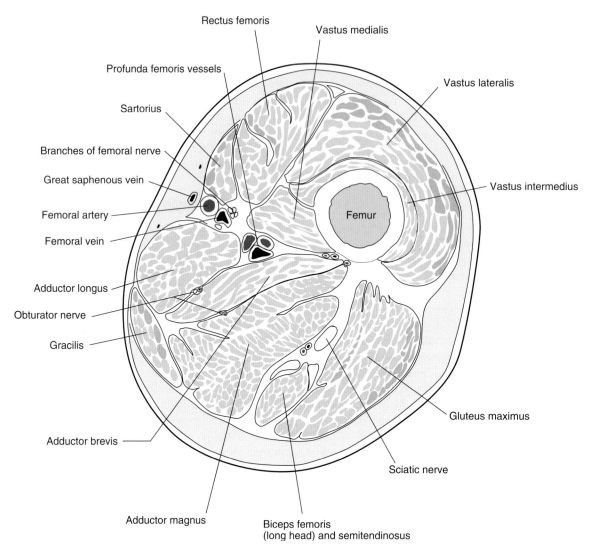

FIGURE 37.2 Cross-section of the left thigh at about the level of the apex of the femoral triangle showing the relationship of the superficial femoral and profunda femoris arteries.

As the artery passes deep into the thigh, it lies first behind the superficial femoral vein which separates it from the superficial femoral artery. The profunda femoris vein crosses in front of the profunda artery to join the femoral vein on the medial side. Henry 1973 points out that this relationship of femoral artery, femoral vein, profunda femoris vein and artery is maintained throughout, but the whole complex spirals in an anticlockwise direction as the profunda artery shifts laterally approaching the femur, ultimately to be placed behind the linea aspera almost to the middle of the thigh, whereas the femoral artery maintains an almost subcutaneous course until it passes through the adductor hiatus to become the popliteal artery. This relationship is apparent when viewing a cross-section of the thigh at the apex of the femoral triangle, where it is obvious that the two arteries lie in the coronal plane lying on adductor longus (Fig. 37.2). Note that the profunda artery is not far from the linea aspera and further down in the distal section

of the profunda femoris the vessels lie behind the linea aspera. They can be reached by separating the tendinous attachment of adductor longus from this bony ridge (Fig. 37.3).

The artery is in reality longer than most surgeons' concept of it, averaging 30 cm in length. Vascular surgeons generally are only interested in the proximal 3 or 4 cm of the artery.

The lateral circumflex artery arises from the first centimetre or so of the profunda artery in about 50% of cases. The medial circumflex artery arises from the profunda artery less often but when it does, it arises near to the profunda origin and passes straight back and medially. It can be a troublesome artery to control when it causes back-bleeding on opening the orifice of the profunda femoris.

The profunda femoris artery gives off several large branches which pass laterally into the muscles and are therefore called the muscular branches. The largest of these

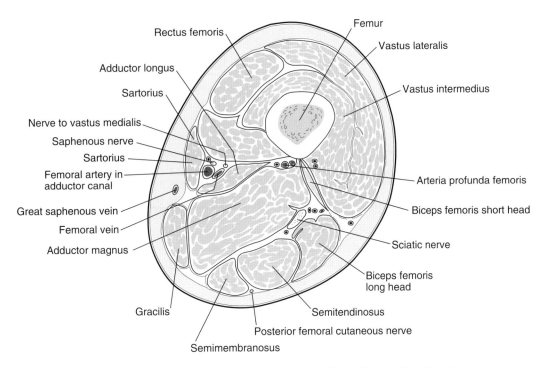

FIGURE 37.3   Cross-section of the left mid thigh showing the relationship of the superficial femoral and profunda femoris arteries.

are the proximal three perforating arteries which travel through adductor brevis and fibrous arches in adductor magnus.

Surgical considerations of the profunda femoris artery

The profunda femoris artery is best considered in three sections. The proximal section is that portion in the femoral triangle, the middle section that portion lying behind the adductor longus muscle and the distal section that portion which lies behind the linea aspera embedded in the insertion of the adductor magnus muscle.

The first section usually has the origin of the vital lateral circumflex artery. It is best approached from its anterior aspect as it leaves the femoral triangle by a downwards continuation of the approach to the common femoral artery. The origin of the artery can be recognized behind the large profunda femoris vein and lateral circumflex vein, which therefore hide the artery from the front and which need to be divided. The sartorius muscle is retracted laterally. The posterior aspect of the profunda artery should be examined for a late origin of the medial circumflex artery, as this can cause back-bleeding which is profuse when uncontrolled.

The middle section of the profunda femoris artery gives off the first and second perforating arteries. The profunda artery is still quite large at this point, about the size of the infragenicular popliteal artery. It is possible to approach the middle section by a continuation of the anterior approach, but the dissection is hampered by the bulk of vastus medialis

protruding into the wound. Figure 37.3 shows the impracticality of an approach in the sagittal plane. This approach is especially difficult in re-operations where the tissue planes are scarred.

The medial approach to the middle section of the profunda femoris is the one we recommend. The key structures in this approach are the sartorius and adductor longus muscles. The approach is made with the thigh in external rotation and with slight abduction of the hip and flexion of the knee. The approach is then directed to the depression created between the adductor muscles and the sartorius muscle. An incision is made in the mid portion of this depression. The femoral artery vein and nerve bundle should be anterior and the profunda located within the glistening dense fascia that runs from the adductor longus to vastus medialis. It is necessary to divide some of the tendinous fibres of insertion of adductor longus and some branches of the profunda vein which lie on the artery (Fig. 37.3). The surgeon must be aware of the lateral drift of the vessel and not seek it immediately behind the femoral bundle. If muscle fibres are encountered then the dissection is too medial and the surgeon should seek the tendinous fibres of insertion of adductor longus to the linea aspera, which is located by palpation.

In the distal section the profunda artery is reduced to about the size of the tibioperoneal trunk. The same medial approach is mandatory, separating the adductor longus muscle from the vastus medialis muscle and dividing fibres of the adductor magnus insertion to linea aspera, in which the artery is embedded.

THE SUPERFICIAL FEMORAL ARTERY

This is best recognized by the transition to a much narrower vessel after the profunda femoris artery has been given off. The artery is covered by the fascia passing from the adductors to the vastus medialis muscle (the roof of the subsartorial canal), and the sartorius muscle which angles across from lateral to the medial and posterior aspect of the leg. The medial intermuscular septum and vastus medialis lie anterior to it and the artery lies on adductor longus above; lower in the leg it lies on adductor magnus. In its subsartorial position the vein lies initially behind the artery but comes to lie lateral to it. The long saphenous nerve and the nerve to vastus medialis both lie lateral to it initially and the vastus nerve maintains that position until it enters its muscle. The long saphenous nerve however crosses anterior to the artery to lie on its medial side.

In its upper portion the artery is reached by retracting the sartorius in a lateral direction, in its lower reaches the muscle is retracted in a medial and posterior direction. In its middle portion the most direct and least destructive approach is simply to split the fibres of sartorius (Figs 37.2 and 37.3).

The artery gives off only minor branches until it reaches the adductor hiatus where it gives off the genicular branch which traverses the adductor hiatus on the medial side of the artery. At this point it becomes the popliteal artery.

THE FEMORAL VEIN

The femoral vein lies behind the femoral artery as it proceeds to the groin where it comes to lie medial to the artery. The major vein may be duplicated in the lower region before it is joined by the profunda vein, the two veins being joined by numerous branches which cross the artery. These can be a hindrance in access to the artery, especially if there has been previous thrombosis of the vein with recanalization. The first major tributary of the vein is the profunda vein. Most of the subcutaneous branches join the great saphenous vein before it enters the femoral vein. Communications with the great saphenous vein in the thigh are discussed in Chapter 41.

THE POPLITEAL FOSSA

The popliteal fossa is a diamond-shaped area bounded by two hamstrings above and the heads of gastrocnemius below. Thus medially are semitendinosus and semimembranosus and the medial head of gastrocnemius and laterally are biceps femoris and the lateral head of gastrocnemius. The floor is made up of the posterior surface of the lower end of the femur and the capsule of the knee joint above, and the posterior surface of the tibia with popliteus and its overlying fascia more distally. The roof of the popliteal fossa, is the deep fascia of the leg.

The common peroneal nerve is far lateral in the fossa, staying close to biceps tendon. The major contents are the tibial nerve, the popliteal vein and the popliteal artery which lie in this order from superficial to deep. The tibial nerve commences lateral to the vessels and crosses superficial to them to lie medially in the lower part of the fossa. The popliteal vein also crosses superficial to the artery from lateral to medial. The vein is always closely applied to the artery and as it is often double with numerous communications between the two veins, tends to envelop the artery.

When viewed from a posteromedial approach (which is the usual approach of the vascular surgeon to the popliteal fossa) the nerve is well posterior (superficial), so that it is not usually seen, and the vein lies posterior (superficial) to the artery also.

The descending genicular artery is given off just before the adductor hiatus and it emerges with the saphenous nerve and runs posterior to sartorius so that it is usually not in danger with exposure of the popliteal artery. However, a branch of the saphenous nerve, the infrapatellar nerve, emerges from the lower end of the adductor canal and tends to travel across the operative field. If it is divided the area in front of and below the patella is left numb.

THE POPLITEAL ARTERY

As has been stated already, the popliteal artery is the deepest of the neurovascular structures in the popliteal fossa. From the point of view of the surgeon operating from the usual posteromedial approach, proximally the artery is closest to the surgeon (because it is medial to the vein and nerve) but distally it is furthest away from the surgeon (because it is now lateral to the vein and nerve). But at all times the vein and nerve are nearest to the roof of the popliteal fossa and the artery remains accessible throughout.

Very occasionally the popliteal artery is separated from the nerve and vein by the medial head of gastrocnemius. This can cause the artery to be displaced medially, and can be associated with popliteal arterial disease in the young, when it is known as the popliteal artery entrapment syndrome (Fig. 37.4).

In the distal limit of the popliteal fossa the artery divides into the anterior and posterior tibial vessels.

The branches of the popliteal artery tend to come off from its proximal half. It is perhaps for this reason that atheromatous disease is usually more severe in the proximal half with the distal half of the vessel usually being free of severe atheroma.

Apart from small unnamed and unimportant muscular and cutaneous branches the main branches are the superior genicular arteries (medial and lateral), the middle genicular artery and the inferior genicular arteries (medial and lateral), all arising from the proximal half of the artery.

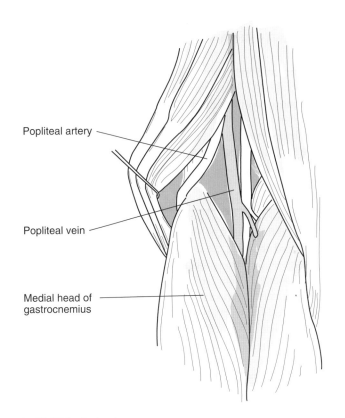

FIGURE 37.4 Popliteal artery entrapment.

Labels on figure:
- Popliteal artery
- Popliteal vein
- Medial head of gastrocnemius

Exposure of the popliteal artery

Above the level of the knee joint the popliteal artery is exposed by incising along the anterior border of sartorius and retracting the muscle posteriorly. If greater exposure distally is required then the medial head of gastrocnemius is divided.

Below the level of the knee joint the popliteal artery is exposed by making an incision along the medial border of the upper tibia and dividing the insertions of sartorius, gracilis and semitendinosus.

When opened thus the muscle which lies deep to the artery is popliteus, and the muscle it disappears beneath is the arching origin of soleus. The vein(s) tend to be closely applied to the artery while the tibial nerve lies posterolaterally and is not usually seen.

THE TIBIOPERONEAL TRUNK

The tibioperoneal trunk begins at the origin of the anterior tibial artery and continues for a length of 2–3 cm. It lies on the tibialis posterior and passes underneath the fibrous arch of the tibial origin of soleus. This must be divided to expose the tibioperoneal trunk. It is often surrounded by multiple large veins which follow the posterior tibial and peroneal arteries and frequently interconnect, making venous bleeding a common problem when exposing this portion of the artery. The nerve lies posterolaterally and is easily separated

from the trunk. The artery is covered by the soleus (posterior) and lies on the tibialis posterior (anterior).

It gives off the posterior tibial artery as the main vessel and this continues inferiorly between flexor digitorum longus and flexor hallucis longus and is covered by soleus. The peroneal artery is a smaller branch and runs anteriorly (deep) towards the interosseous membrane and lies in a fibrous tunnel between the interosseus membrane and flexor hallucis longus.

The tibioperoneal trunk is usually exposed along with the distal popliteal artery by extending the skin incision inferiorly along the medial border of the tibia. The popliteal vein is mobilized distally until a large venous tributary is found, joining it from the medial side (this is the anterior tibial vein). Division of this tributary exposes the origin of the anterior tibial artery and the tibioperoneal trunk.

THE POSTERIOR TIBIAL ARTERY

After giving off the peroneal artery, the posterior tibial artery continues down the leg between the superficial and deep group of muscles, i.e. it lies deep to soleus.

The tibial nerve commences medial to the artery but crosses it superficially and lies lateral to it through most of its course.

In the mid lower leg the artery is exposed by an incision slightly posterior to the tibia. The soleus muscle is detached from the tibia and it is retracted posteriorly. The space between the soleus muscle and the flexor digitorum muscle is entered and the posterior tibial vessels are found on the posterior surface of the tibialis posterior muscle. The dissection can be extended deeper to the medial surface of the fibula, where the peroneal artery in the mid-leg is found. Both arteries are surrounded by networks of veins, which have to be carefully divided in order to avoid venous bleeding.

Behind the lateral malleolus it lies in a special compartment with the posterior tibial nerve deep to the flexor retinaculum. The flexor hallucis longus tendon lies deep to it and flexor digitorum longus tendon lies superficial to it, although somewhat in front so that the artery is superficial here with its accompanying nerve deep (lateral) to it (Fig. 37.5). This point of accessibility is usually palpable midway between the medial malleolus and the right point of the heel (medial tuberosity of calcaneus).

THE PERONEAL ARTERY

The peroneal artery arises soon after the bifurcation of the popliteal artery. It arises from the posterior tibial artery and runs along a fibrous tunnel associated with the medial crest of the fibula, between tibialis posterior and flexor hallucis longus. It is sometimes embedded in the latter muscle. Its origin can be approached as for the approach to the

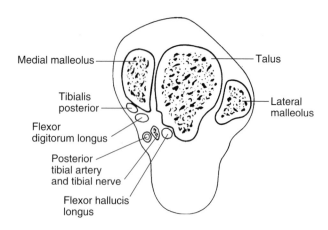

FIGURE 37.5 Cross-section through the left ankle joint showing the relationships of the tibial artery.

tibioperoneal trunk. Its mid portion can also be exposed either from the lateral side or from the medial side as described above.

The lateral approach is made through a longitudinal incision in the middle third of the leg directly over the fibula. The underlying muscular fibres of peroneus longus and soleus are split to expose the fibula. The periosteum is elevated and the fibula divided and removed. The peroneal artery is easily found on the surface of flexor hallucis longus. Numerous veins tend to surround the artery. The anterior tibial artery can also be identified by this approach, lying more anteriorly on extensor hallucis longus (Fig. 37.6).

THE ANTERIOR TIBIAL ARTERY

The anterior tibial artery passes anteriorly between the two heads of tibialis posterior, above the upper border of the interosseous membrane, medial to the neck of the fibula, and it then runs down the leg lying on the interosseus membrane. It becomes superficial in front of the ankle joint where it lies midway between the malleoli as the dorsalis pedis artery (Fig. 37.7).

It is accessible at its origin, in the mid lower leg and when it lies in front of the ankle joint. The deep peroneal nerve is lateral to it.

Between the knee and the ankle the anterior tibial artery is approached through the anterior compartment. Slight flexion of the knee facilitates the procedure. The incision is made approximately 2–3 cm laterally to the tibial border. After division of the crural fascia a plane is developed by blunt dissection between the tibialis anterior muscle and the extensor digitorum longus muscle. The former is retracted medially and the latter laterally. In the groove between these two muscles the artery, vein and nerve can be found on the interosseus membrane. Further down in the leg the plane between the tibialis anterior muscle and the extensor hallucis longus muscle is used.

All approaches to the lower leg arteries in the mid-leg are being used for bypasses, either with reversed vein or with the in situ technique.

At its point of emergence subcutaneously just above the ankle joint the tendon of tibialis anterior lies medially and the tendon of extensor hallucis longus lies laterally. The extensor hallucis longus muscle crosses in front of the artery in front of the ankle joint to lie on the medial side of the dorsalis pedis artery.

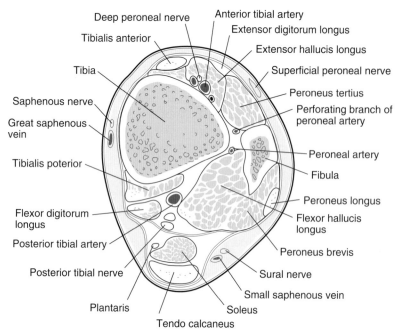

FIGURE 37.6 The peroneal and anterior tibial arteries – access by removal of the shaft of the fibula.

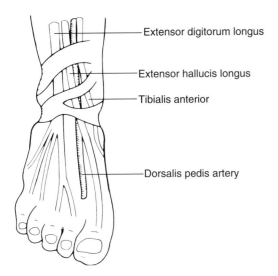

Extensor digitorum longus

Extensor hallucis longus

Tibialis anterior

Dorsalis pedis artery

FIGURE 37.7 The anterior tibial (tibialis anterior) artery in front of the ankle joint.

While its branches may be of clinical importance in collateral circulation they are not of operative importance.

THE DORSALIS PEDIS ARTERY

This is the continuation of the anterior tibial artery in the foot. It passes under the extensor retinaculum between the tendons of flexor hallucis longus and posterior to flexor digitorum longus to the second toe. It lies superficially and is found by longitudinal incision over the dorsum of the foot between the first and second metatarsals.

REFERENCE

Henry A K 1973 Extensile exposure, 2nd edn. Churchill Livingstone, Edinburgh.

FURTHER READING

Depalma R G, Malgieri J J, Rhodes R S, Clowes A W 1980 Profunda femoris bypass for secondary revascularization. Surg Gynecol Obst 151:387–390.
Nunez A A, Veith F J, Collier P et al 1988 Direct approaches to the distal portions of the deep femoral artery for limb salvage bypass. J Vasc Surg 8:576–581.
Tiefenbrun J, Beckerman M, Singer A 1975 Surgical anatomy in bypass of the distal part of the lower limb. Surg Gynecol Obstet 141(4):528–533.

38 | Cervical and lumbar sympathectomy; thoracic endoscopic sympathectomy: the anatomy of the sympathetic chain

Glyn Jamieson and Frank G Quigley

The sympathetic nervous system is very complex and there is much about both its anatomy and physiology which remains unknown.

The preganglionic fibres

These arise in cell bodies in the lateral column of the grey matter of the spinal cord in all of the thoracic spinal segments and the first two or three lumbar spinal segments. The fibres pass via the ventral nerve root and exit as the white ramus communicans to enter the ganglion or the sympathetic chain between the ganglia. The preganglionic fibres terminate in one of four main ways.

- ❶ By synapse in the ganglion which they enter; the postganglionic fibres pass back into the spinal nerve through the grey ramus communicans (Fig. 38.1a).
- ❷ They may either ascend or descend to a higher or lower ganglion than the ganglion of entry, and then exit after synapse through that ganglion's grey ramus (Fig. 38.1b).
- ❸ They may ascend or descend and exit from the sympathetic chain to synapse in ganglia of the coeliac or aortic plexuses, for example (Fig. 38.1c).
- ❹ They may exit from the sympathetic chain to synapse with cells in the adrenal medulla.

The postganglionic fibres

Most of these pass back into the spinal nerve through the grey ramus communicans. They supply vasoconstrictor nerves to blood vessels, secretomotor fibres to sweat glands and motor fibres to the arrectores pilorum of the skin.

Unlike the other postganglionic sympathetic fibres, those supplying the eccrine sweat glands are cholinergic in nature and are inhibited by atropine and other anti-cholinergics. The eccrine sweat glands are distributed over the whole body but are most numerous on the palms and soles. They secrete a hypotonic solution of sodium chloride and serve primarily a thermoregulatory function.

Their action is inhibited by sympathectomy. The apocrine sweat glands found in the mammary areolar region, external auditory meatus, axillae and pelvic areas are not influenced by sympathetic innervation.

Those fibres accompanying motor nerves to muscles may be vasodilatory and in other regions they seem more inhibitory than excitatory, e.g. alimentary tract, bronchial muscle, etc.

The sympathetic trunks

These are two irregular nerve trunks extending from the base of the skull to the coccyx, containing ganglia at irregular intervals. The sympathetic trunk in the cervical region lies in front of the cervical transverse processes; in the thorax it lies in front of the heads of the ribs; in the abdomen anterolateral to the lumbar bodies, in the pelvis it lies medial

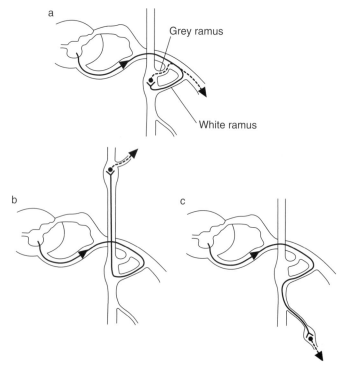

FIGURE 38.1 The three methods of termination of sympathetic preganglionic fibres. See text for details.

to the anterior sacral foramina and it terminates in front of the coccyx by joining with its fellow to form the ganglion impar.

There are typically three cervical ganglia, 11 thoracic ganglia, four lumbar and four sacral ganglia.

THE CERVICAL SYMPATHETIC TRUNK

The preganglionic fibres to the three cervical sympathetic ganglia all arise from the upper thoracic outflow and ascend in the cervical sympathetic trunk to reach the cervical ganglia. The cervical ganglia give grey rami to each of the cervical nerves.

The superior cervical ganglion gives off the internal carotid nerve which travels into the skull with the internal carotid artery and amongst other branches supplies the dilator pupillae of the eye by passing along the ophthalmic nerve.

The superior cervical ganglion lies behind the internal carotid artery just above the carotid sinus; the small middle ganglion lies at about the level where the inferior thyroid artery crosses the trunk and the inferior ganglion is variable in position. It is present as a distinct entity in about 20% of cases when it lies in front of the vertebral artery and sends loops on either side of the vessel back to the first thoracic ganglion which lies posterior to the vertebral artery on the neck of the first rib. In the remaining cases it is fused with the first thoracic ganglion to form the stellate ganglion, which also lies in front of and below the neck of the first rib. Some ascending preganglionic fibres pass from the first thoracic or stellate ganglion, below the subclavian artery and then in front of it as they ascend to the middle cervical ganglion. These fibres are called the ansa subclavia.

The major outflow for the head and neck is thought to come from the T1 level, with its fibres passing to the T1 ganglion (or stellate ganglion) through the white ramus of T1. If this ganglion is left intact then Homer's syndrome does not occur when the sympathetic trunk is divided below this level (Fig. 38.2).

The upper limb derives its sympathetic innervation predominantly from the second and third thoracic level and partly from the first, fourth and fifth thoracic levels. In dividing the sympathetic chain between the stellate or first thoracic ganglion and the second thoracic ganglion nearly all the ascending axons of the sympathetic nerves supplying the upper limb will be divided. To achieve a complete upper limb sympathectomy the grey post-ganglionic rami passing from the stellate ganglion to the brachial plexus must also be divided along with the nerve of Kuntz. The nerve of Kuntz is an intrathoracic nerve of variable size and location that passes from the second intercostal nerve to the T1 nerve root above, bypassing the sympathetic chain between the T2 ganglion and the stellate ganglion. In practice an adequate sympathectomy, especially when being done for hyperhidrosis,

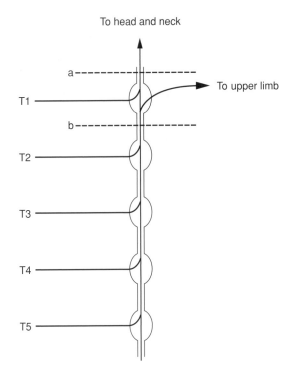

FIGURE 38.2 Division of the sympathetic chain at a will denervate the head and neck, while division at b will denervate the upper limb, but leave head and neck innervation intact.

is obtained by ablating the T2 ganglion without disturbing the stellate ganglion.

Division of the sympathetic chain at this point also results in a partial sympathetic denervation of the head and neck. The percentage or amount of denervation of the head and neck is variable and unpredictable but while it almost never results in a clinically obvious Horner's syndrome it appears to be adequate to alleviate hyperhidrosis of the head and neck and to diminish facial flushing.

There are a number of operative approaches to ablate the sympathetic outflow to the upper limb. Possibly the least invasive and the most acceptable to patients is the percutaneous endoscopic approach developed by Kux. Using this approach the sympathetic chain is identified beneath the parietal pleura over the necks of the second and third ribs and the chain can be diathermied at this point. Although the stellate ganglion lies immediately above and posterior to the parietal pleura, the neck of the first rib is virtually invisible from within the chest so that as long as the sympathetic chain is only diathermied on or below the prominent neck of the second rib there is little risk of damaging the stellate ganglion. To achieve a complete upper limb sympathectomy a transthoracic or supraclavicular approach may be used but both are associated with a greater risk of Horner's syndrome, haemorrhage and damage to the brachial plexus, phrenic nerve and thoracic duct.

The ideal endoscopic approach for access to the sympathetic chain on the neck of the second and third ribs while allowing the best cosmetic result is via the third interspace in the midaxillary and anterior axillary lines with the patient in a semi sitting position to allow the collapsed lung to fall forward and down away from the chain. In more obese patients the chain can be difficult to visualize beneath the pleura, but can usually be palpated on the neck of second and third ribs with an insulated diathermy probe.

THE LUMBAR SYMPATHETIC TRUNK

This is the continuation of the thoracic sympathetic trunk (see Ch. 20) which passes under the medial arcuate ligament to lie along the anterolateral surfaces of the lumbar vertebrae, at the medial margin of the psoas muscle.

On the right side it lies behind the inferior vena cava and although theoretically the lumbar veins pass behind it, occasionally one or more passes in front of it. Care has to be taken therefore when elevating the sympathetic trunk during lumbar sympathectomy not to damage the veins. The distal trunk passes behind the common iliac arteries to become the pelvic sympathetic trunk.

The lumbar sympathetic trunks are usually easily visible but may lie in a groove between the psoas muscle and the vertebral column or occasionally behind some fibres of the psoas muscle. The thickness of the inter-ganglionic portion of the lumbar sympathetic chain varies from that of a piece of cotton to a cord 6 mm in diameter.

The number and situation of the lumbar ganglia are extremely variable and often differ from one side of the body to the other. They vary from one to eight on each side and opinion seems to be divided as to whether three or four is the most typical number. The most constant and largest of the ganglia lies at about the disc between lumbar vertebrae two and three, but this level is virtually impossible to determine with assurance at operation. If there is a ganglion associated with the fourth lumbar vertebra it usually lies behind the common iliac artery. Thus in dissecting the trunk free the surgeon should commence behind the common iliac artery and dissect upwards for 4 or 5 cm, or higher if that proves feasible.

Since the outflow from the lateral columns to the sympathetic trunks occurs no lower than L3 and usually no lower than 1–2 it is clear that removal of the trunk below this level should denervate the lower limb. Nevertheless the effects of such a sympathectomy are extremely variable for reasons more than just inadequacy of operation. However it is unusual for the foot not to be sympathetically denervated and as the operation is carried out mainly for rest pain, when direct arterial surgery is not possible, then the operation can be expected to help in such situations.

As well as denervating the lower limb, the pelvic sympathetic outflow is also interrupted by lumbar sympathectomy. The sympathetic nerves associated with ejaculation are concentrated in the white ramus from the first lumbar nerve and so in a lumbar sympathectomy for pathology in the lower limb it should be helpful to leave the first lumbar ganglion intact if possible.

When carrying out lumbar sympathectomy at the time of an abdominal operation the trunk is approached anteriorly by dissection immediately lateral to the inferior vena cava and aorta respectively. When using the more common posterolateral retroperitoneal approach the trunk is found by following the anterior surface of the psoas muscle medially on to the anterolateral aspect of the vertebral bodies. Damage to the ureter, another longitudinally running structure, can be avoided by ensuring that the ureter is swept forward with the peritoneum.

Although bilateral lumbar sympathectomy sometimes leads to retrograde ejaculation in males, it does not occur as often as might be expected on theoretical grounds, with interruption of the sympathetic inflow to the pelvis.

FURTHER READING

Kux M 1978 Thoracic endoscopic sympathectomy in palmar and axillary hyperhidrosis. Arch Surg 113:264–266.

39 Operations for thoracic outlet syndrome: the anatomy of the first rib and cervical rib

Glyn Jamieson and Larry Ferguson

THE FIRST RIB

The first rib derives its surgical importance from the numerous vital structures related to it at the thoracic outlet. The rib slopes obliquely downwards and forwards, presenting flat anterior and posterior surfaces and sharper inner and outer margins. The small head of the first rib articulates with the upper part of the body of the T1 vertebra and a short narrow neck runs superiorly and posteriorly from the head to the tubercle of the rib, which articulates with the transverse process of the T1 vertebra. The shaft of the bone runs inferiorly and medially and its anterior surface is marked by roughened areas of muscular origin and insertion. The anterior end of the rib is attached to its costal cartilage and to the clavicle by the strong costa clavicular ligament and the subclavius muscle.

The most prominent landmark on the first rib is the scalene tubercle, marking the site of insertion of the scalenus anterior muscle (Fig. 39.1) which arises from the transverse processes of the third to the sixth cervical vertebrae.

The subclavian vein crosses the first rib anterior to the scalene tubercle with the subclavian artery and inferior root of the brachial plexus grooving the rib posterior to the tubercle. Behind and below the arterial groove the bone is roughened on its outer aspect by the origin of serratus anterior muscle and posteriorly by the site of insertion of scalenus medius muscle which arises from the transverse processes of all the cervical vertebrae. The neck of the first rib is crossed from below upwards by the root of the first thoracic nerve laterally with the supreme intercostal artery and stellate ganglion lying more medially on the neck (Fig. 39.2). Because of the oblique slope of the rib the costal end is several centimetres lower than the vertebral end. This is the reason why the pleura extends superior to the anterior aspect of the rib and holds the structures crossing the neck against the neck of the rib.

CERVICAL RIB

A persistence of a separate costal element of the seventh cervical vertebra, as a cervical rib, occurs in about 1% of

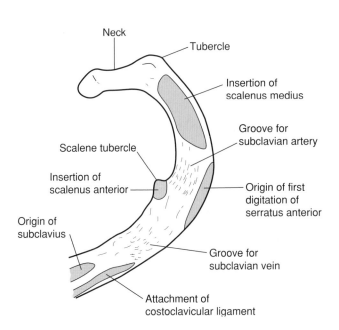

FIGURE 39.1   Some markings on the first rib.

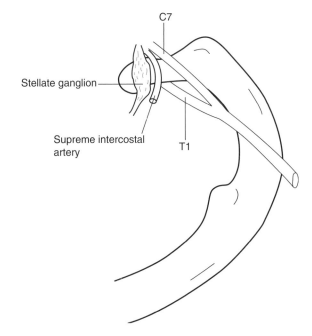

FIGURE 39.2   Some important relations of the neck of the first rib.

individuals (Fig. 39.3). Cervical ribs are often bilateral. In about 10% of individuals the persisting rib causes symptoms by compressing the neurovascular structures related to it.

Occasionally the rib is complete and articulates with the sternum but this is very uncommon. More usually it either articulates with the superior surface of the first rib or terminates in a fibrous band which then joins the first rib. These bands are sometimes characterized into different types:

Type I – tip of cervical rib to inner edge of first rib behind the scalene tubercle.

Type II – tip of costal element of C7 to the same point on the first rib.

Type III – originates from the neck of the first rib and inserts into the inner edge of the rest of the rib – this may be no more than a condensation in the suprapleural membrane.

Type IV – is a band passing from scalenus medius beneath the brachial plexus and subclavian artery to insert behind the scalene tubercle.

Type V – is the scalenus minimus muscle which corresponds with a few muscle fibres in the suprapleural membrane.

All of these described bands are divided by a scalenotomy operation, except type III which may or may not be divided.

THE SCALENE MUSCLES AND ANTERIOR SCALENOTOMY

The scalene muscles descend from the transverse processes of the first six or seven cervical vertebrae to insert in the first two ribs. The posterior scalene muscle arises from the fifth and sixth vertebrae and is not easily separable from the middle scalene muscle except that it passes beyond the first rib to insert into the second rib. The middle scalene is the largest of three muscles arising from the sixth or seventh cervical vertebra and passing down to insert into the first rib behind the subclavian artery and brachial plexus. These structures separate the middle scalene from the scalenus anterior,

which arises from the cervical transverse processes of C3–6 and inserts into the first rib in front of the subclavian artery but behind the subclavian vein. The lateral border of sternomastoid is an approximation of the lateral border of scalenus anterior, which is also where the brachial plexus and subclavian artery emerge from behind the anterior scalene.

The anterior scalene muscle can be divided to open out the area through which the subclavian artery and the brachial plexus pass.

There is a pad of fibrofatty tissue containing lymph nodes lying in front of the muscle, behind the clavicular fibres of sternomastoid (see below).

The thyrocervical trunk of the subclavian artery typically arises alongside the medial border of the scalenus anterior muscle and two of its branches run transversely in front of the scalene muscle, just above the clavicle. Deep to all is a fascial condensation, beneath which the phrenic nerve crosses the muscle from lateral to medial.

On the left side the thoracic duct lies in the lower part of the field as it curves in to its termination at the junction of the subclavian and internal jugular veins.

It is best to expose the phrenic nerve by excising the scalene fat pad prior to dividing the muscle.

SURGERY OF THE THORACIC OUTLET

The most common indications for thoracic outlet decompression are symptoms of nerve, arterial or, less commonly, venous compression. The neurological symptoms are typically caused by involvement of the inferior root of the brachial plexus causing pain down the ulnar aspect of the arm or weakness of the small muscles of the hand. More common, however, is arterial obstruction which can take the form of either intermittent claudication in the muscles of the arm (particularly with the arm elevated), or manifestations of embolization in the digits. Venous compression is uncommon causing swelling and, if severe, cyanosis of the hand and forearm. This can lead to a subclavian vein thrombosis.

The thoracic outlet can be decompressed from either a supraclavicular or transaxillary approach, the method used being generally determined by the personal preference of the surgeon and familiarity with the technique involved. The traditional procedure for treating the thoracic outlet syndrome was an anterior scalenotomy done through a supraclavicular approach, but most authors now believe that this does not produce a satisfactory result and that resection of the first rib is preferable. The safest and most effective method for excising the first rib is by a transaxillary approach, but if a cervical rib is present or if it is felt that a subclavian endarterectomy may be needed, then the supraclavicular route should be used. Some surgeons perform a combined procedure starting above the clavicle to allow inspection of the subclavian artery, then complete the decompression by excising the first

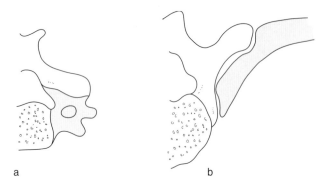

FIGURE 39.3 (a) Normal cervical vertebra with the costal element shaded. (b) Costal element has developed into a rib in normal thoracic vertebra.

rib through the axilla. Cervical sympathectomy can be performed with equal facility by either route but endoscopically it is usually undertaken via a transthoracic approach.

THE SUPRACLAVICULAR APPROACH TO THE THORACIC OUTLET

An incision is made 1 cm above and parallel to the medial half of the clavicle. Platysma and the clavicular head of sternomastoid muscle are divided and the external jugular vein, if encountered, is also divided between ligatures. The omohyoid muscle is identified running parallel to and just above the clavicle deep to the sternomastoid and this muscle is divided between artery forceps to display the scalene pad of fat and lymph nodes lying on the anterior scalene muscle. Care must be taken not to damage the thoracic duct as the fat pad is dislocated superiorly to reveal the fascia overlying the scalenus anterior. The deep cervical branch of the thyrocervical trunk may have to be divided during this manoeuvre. The phrenic nerve is dissected off the anterior surface of scalenus anterior muscle and is protected. The brachial plexus is separated from the lateral aspect of the muscle and the scalene tubercle of the first rib is palpated deep behind the clavicle. The scalenus anterior muscle is then divided using small scissor cuts so as to avoid damage to the subclavian artery which occasionally runs within the muscle. The deepest layer of scalenus anterior is occasionally a tough aponeurosis which may have to be divided by sharp blade dissection to expose the subclavian artery. The artery is mobilized over 3–4 cm with division of the thyrocervical and internal mammary arteries if necessary.

The preceding steps are required whether cervical rib resection, first rib resection or cervical sympathectomy is being undertaken – but from this stage on the procedure will vary. To proceed with first rib resection, the subclavian artery is mobilized superiorly to allow disconnection of the suprapleural membrane and reflection of the parietal pleura off the posterior thoracic wall. This allows identification of the sharp inner border of the first rib with the prominent scalene tubercle anteriorly. The T1 nerve root is palpated by rolling it against the neck of the first rib and more medially the sympathetic trunk is identified. All tissue on the inner aspect of the first rib is dissected from it and the outer border of the rib is cleared also. The rib is then divided with bone cutters as far anteriorly and posteriorly as possible: care is taken to avoid damage to the T1 nerve root. Jagged bone ends should be removed with rongeurs. The lungs are fully inflated by the anaesthetist to ensure there is no pneumothorax and the wound is closed with a suction drain in situ.

Because of the great variation in the anatomy of cervical ribs, when such a rib is being excised it must be identified and dissected free from all surrounding tissues and excised as far posteriorly as possible. A thorough search must be made for associated fibrous bands, all of which are divided.

TRANSAXILLARY APPROACH (Fig. 39.4)

The patient is positioned in a 60° anterolateral thoracotomy position with an arm rest in place to support the affected arm. At times during the procedure it helps greatly to have the arm retracted strongly superiorly. A transverse incision is made over the third rib in the axilla and the incision is deepened to the rib cage, the thoracodorsal vein being tied in the midline. Once the third rib has been identified the dissection is carried superiorly by blunt dissection along the outside of the rib cage until the first rib can be palpated. The axillary fascia at the apex of this subcutaneous tunnel must be divided by blunt dissection or spreading with the scissors. The first rib is identified by palpating the scalene tubercle through the scalenus anterior muscle and it is then palpated anteriorly as far as the clavicle and posteriorly to the scalenus medius muscle. The subclavian artery is palpated and along with the vein is displaced superiorly by blunt dissection. The tendon of the subclavius muscle is divided to allow clearance of the anterior end of the rib. Care must be taken to avoid damage to the subclavian vein at this point.

A right-angled forceps is passed round the scalenus anterior muscle which is retracted laterally and divided with the scissors. All fibrous bands on the inner concavity of the first rib are divided by a combination of blunt and sharp dissection. The T1 nerve root is protected as scalenus medius is lifted off the posterior aspect of the first rib using a periosteal elevator. The intercostal muscle between the first and second ribs is then divided, completing circumferential clearance of the first rib. The rib is divided as far posteriorly as possible using bone cutters (care being taken not to damage the T1 nerve root) and, using bone-holding forceps, it is possible then to disarticulate the rib anteriorly from its costal cartilage. Jagged bone ends are trimmed and after a check for pneumothorax the wound is closed with suction drainage.

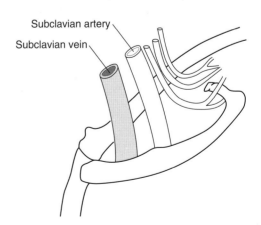

FIGURE 39.4 Relationship of structures crossing the first rib when viewed from an axillary approach.

FURTHER READING

Roos D B 1977 Thoracic outlet and carpal tunnel syndromes. In: Rutherford R B (ed.) Vascular surgery. WB Saunders, Philadelphia.

40 Lower limb amputations: the anatomy of mid-thigh and below-knee amputations

Glyn Jamieson and Michael Berce

As this is not a surgical text no detailed description of amputations will be given. However it may prove useful to the surgeon to have a cross-sectional picture of the anatomy of the areas through which most amputations are made.

BELOW-KNEE AMPUTATION

This is usually carried out approximately 10 cm (or one hand's breadth) below the tibial tubercle. The anterior skin incision is made longer than the level of division of the tibia which is itself longer than the level of division of the fibula. A diagrammatic cross-section of the anatomical structures divided at operation is shown in Figure 40.1.

Long posterior myocutaneous flaps have become popular for covering the stump. The blood supply to such flaps is derived mainly from two sources: first, vessels accompanying the various cutaneous nerves, e.g. the saphenous nerve, the sural nerve, the sural communicating nerve and the lateral cutaneous nerve of the calf. Second are perforating vessels from the gastrocnemius muscle. No blood supply comes from the soleus muscle which is therefore best excised from the flap.

The anterior tibial vessels are found on the interosseous membrane after dividing all the extensor group of muscles anteriorly down on to the membrane.

The long saphenous vein lies medially in the subcutaneous plane and is commonly encountered during the medial incision of the posterior skin flap.

The peroneal artery is perhaps the most likely of the three main vessels to be patent – it runs along the medial border of the fibula deep to the tibialis posterior (as seen in an anterior approach) and it can be damaged along with its accompanying veins during freeing up of the fibula prior to its transection.

Having divided the tibia and fibula, the peroneal and posterior tibial vessels are found in the same plane between soleus and the flexor group of muscles. Soleus should be excised at the same level as (or slightly longer than) the bone but gastrocnemius is left at the same length as the posterior skin flap. Care should be taken to avoid dissecting the plane between the gastrocnemius and the posterior skin flap with

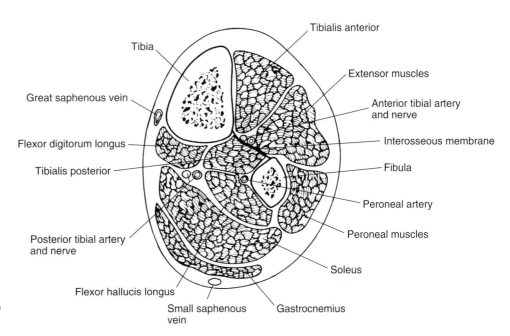

FIGURE 40.1 Below-knee amputation: cross-section through left leg about 10 cm below tibial tubercle.

Labels on figure:
Tibia
Tibialis anterior
Extensor muscles
Great saphenous vein
Anterior tibial artery and nerve
Interosseous membrane
Flexor digitorum longus
Fibula
Tibialis posterior
Peroneal artery
Peroneal muscles
Posterior tibial artery and nerve
Soleus
Flexor hallucis longus
Gastrocnemius
Small saphenous vein

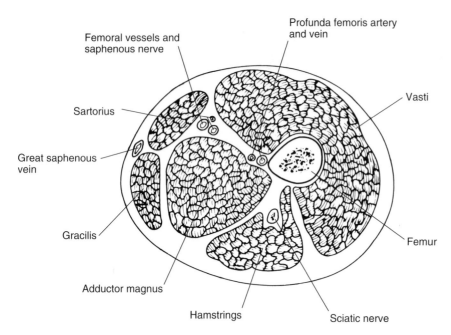

FIGURE 40.2 Above-knee amputation: cross-section through the left thigh at about mid thigh level.

the subsequent disruption of feeding blood vessels from gastrocnemius to the skin.

The small (short) saphenous vein is found in the posterior skin flap in the midline, superficial to the fascia. It is accompanied by the sural nerve.

The most important component of the closure of the stump is to join the superficial fascia over the tibia, tibialis anterior and extensor muscles to a 'double bite' of the fascia over gastrocnemius and its tendons.

ABOVE-KNEE AMPUTATION

The bone incision for a formal mid thigh amputation is made 10 cm (or one hand's breadth) above the upper border of the patella. However clinical circumstances may dictate a higher level of division of the femur anywhere up to the level of the lesser trochanter. A diagrammatic cross-section of the mid thigh is shown in Figure 40.2.

Skin flaps in the thigh are as well perfused anteriorly as they are posteriorly, by communicating vessels from the underlying muscles. Consequently equal-sized flaps are fashioned 10 cm below the level of bone division.

The great (long) saphenous vein is found medially in the subcutaneous plane and is formally divided during the skin incision.

Anteromedially lies sartorius which is easily identified, as a narrow strap like muscle, deep to which the superficial femoral vessels are sought.

The deep femoral artery at the mid thigh level is usually small, having already given off its main perforating branches and it lies between the vasti and the adductor magnus muscles close to the medial surface of the femur. Once the femur has been divided the sciatic nerve is found on the deep surface of adductor magnus. The nerve commonly has a patent artery running within it.

The superficial fascia is a definite layer that allows closure of the stump, reinforced laterally by the ileotibial tract.

FURTHER READING

Gray D W R, Ng R L H 1990 Anatomical aspects of the blood supply to the skin of the posterior calf: technique of below knee amputations. Br J Surg 77:662–664.

41 | Operations involving veins of the upper and lower limbs: the anatomy of the superficial and deep veins of the upper and lower limbs

Glyn Jamieson and Robert Fitridge

SUPERFICIAL VEINS OF THE UPPER LIMB

There is a considerable variation in the superficial veins of the upper limb but the commonest pattern is that which is described below.

The cephalic vein

This vein begins on the dorsum of the hand and winds around the lower end of the radius in the roof of the anatomical snuff box or just proximal to it to reach the flexor surface of the forearm. The vein ascends on the radial side of the forearm and in the vicinity of the elbow crease it gives off the median cubital vein (Fig. 41.1).

The cephalic vein continues upwards on the lateral side of the biceps muscle and then in the groove between the deltoid and pectoralis major muscles to pierce the deep (clavipectoral) fascia several centimetres below the clavicle. It then passes deep to pectoralis major to enter the axillary vein just below the level of the clavicle. It often receives a branch from the external jugular vein, the branch crossing anterior to the clavicle.

The cephalic vein is a useful vein for arterial bypass operations if the great saphenous vein cannot be used for any reason. It contains valves and so must be reversed when put in position. Care must be taken when using the proximal cephalic vein for bypass or fistula surgery as the vessel tends to become particularly thin-walled just prior to passing into the deltopectoral groove. The distal end of the cephalic vein may be anastomosed to the distal radial artery either in the anatomical snuff box or just proximal to the wrist joint. The advantage of the snuff box site is that the vein lies directly superficial to the radial artery, so that the anastomosis can be performed with very little mobilization of the vessels.

The median cubital vein

This vein arises from the cephalic vein and ascends obliquely across the cubital fossa, lying on the bicipital aponeurosis to join the basilic vein. Just distal to the lower edge of the bicipital aponeurosis it receives a large branch

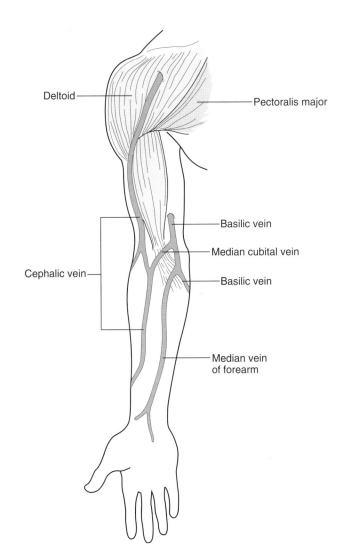

FIGURE 41.1   The superficial veins of the upper limb.

from the deep veins of the forearm. This branch enters posteriorly at an acute angle in the direction of flow. The median cubital vein is an excellent low-pressure conduit for the construction of arteriovenous shunts or fistulae, particularly as the brachial artery lies immediately beneath it, separated only by the bicipital aponeurosis.

The basilic vein

The basilic vein winds around the medial side of the forearm to reach the flexor surface in its upper third. Here it receives the median vein of the forearm and medial to the biceps tendon it receives the median cubital vein (Fig. 41.1). It continues upwards medial to the biceps muscle and pierces the deep fascia at about the mid upper arm level. It then lies on the medial side of the brachial sheath. The sheath contains the brachial artery surrounded by two brachial veins, the median nerve lying superficial to the artery and the ulnar nerve posteriorly. The basilic vein changes its name to the axillary vein at the lower border of teres major.

DEEP VEINS OF THE UPPER LIMB

Venae comitantes of the forearm are usually double and run with the arteries with which they correspond in the forearm. At the level of the elbow joint the ulnar and radial veins form two brachial veins which ascend around the brachial artery. They join the axillary vein in a variable manner, with the medial one often joining the basilic vein before it has become the axillary vein.

The axillary vein

The axillary vein is the continuation of the basilic vein which changes its name at the lower border of the teres major muscle. It ascends at first medial to the axillary artery and more proximally it lies medial and inferior to the axillary artery until it reaches the first rib where it becomes the subclavian vein.

Distally it is overlapped somewhat by the biceps muscle, but in most of its course it is a subcutaneous structure with only the medial cutaneous nerve of the arm lying medial to it. Brachial plexus structures lie lateral to the vein, between it and the axillary artery. From distal to proximal these are first the medial cutaneous nerve of the forearm and the ulnar nerve, then the medial cord of the brachial plexus and proximally the medial pectoral nerve.

It receives all of the tributaries corresponding with branches of the axillary artery and also the brachial and cephalic veins. The axillary vein is often cannulated for venovenous bypass in liver transplant operations.

The axillary vein/subclavian vein is commonly cannulated for measurement of central venous pressure or for parenteral access. If a cannula is inserted below the mid point of the clavicle and directed towards the jugular notch the vein is usually encountered.

SUPERFICIAL VEINS OF THE LOWER LIMB

There are two main superficial veins of the lower limb. Beginning with veins along the medial side of the foot, the great (long) saphenous vein forms and passes in front of the medial malleolus. It ascends on the medial side of the leg to enter the femoral vein at the saphenofemoral junction. The veins on the lateral side of the foot join to pass behind the lateral malleolus and ascend in the midline of the calf as the small (short) saphenous vein which enters the popliteal vein in the popliteal fossa.

These two venous systems usually communicate with each other. The superficial venous systems also communicate with the deep venous system via perforating veins. The valves in the veins joining the superficial to the deep system are directed inwards so that blood can only flow from the superficial to the deep system, except on the dorsum of the foot where the valves direct flow from deep to superficial.

Great saphenous vein

This vein arises on the medial side of the foot and it usually lies about midway between the tip of the medial malleolus and the tendon of tibialis anterior, both of which are easily palpable. It then passes along the medial border of the tibia inclining posteriorly to pass the knee joint just behind the medial condyles of the tibia and the femur. It continues upwards inclining anteriorly and ends by passing through the fossa ovalis at a point about 3–4 cm lateral and below the pubic tubercle. The superficial external pudendal artery usually lies on the curved lower free border of the foramen ovale behind the saphenofemoral junction and immediately beneath the great saphenous vein. The artery may lie superficial to the great saphenous vein in about 30% of limbs when it usually has to be divided to display adequately the saphenofemoral junction at operation.

The position of the saphenofemoral junction is relatively constant. Rarely the great saphenous vein will join the femoral vein as low as mid thigh level, will be absent altogether, or there will be a bifid great saphenous vein with two saphenofemoral junctions. The saphenous nerve lies in close proximity to the vein (usually in front) in the calf, generally joining the vein about 12 cm below the knee crease.

The great saphenous vein is not uncommonly bifid or even trifurcate in at least part of its course. If the vein is found to bifurcate during dissection or harvesting for bypass, the main vein is almost always the deeper of the two branches and is more likely to remain invested in a fascial sheath and will have fewer tributaries.

The tributaries of the vein are extremely variable, although the importance of such variations in surgical terms has probably been overemphasized.

Tributaries of the great saphenous vein (Fig. 41.2)

Larger than usual tributaries usually join the great saphenous vein just below the knee joint – an anterolateral vein in front and a posterolateral one from behind. The posterior arch vein usually joins the great saphenous a few centimetres further distally in the leg.

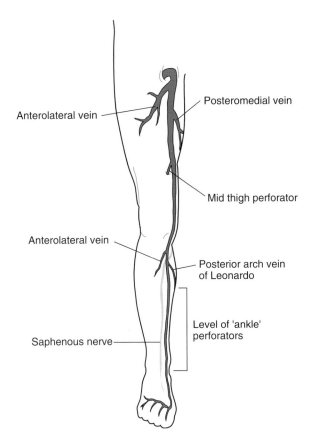

FIGURE 41.2 Superficial veins of the lower limb.

In the region of the knee joint some form of communication between the great saphenous and the small saphenous vein is very common.

In the thigh there is usually an anterolateral and a posteromedial tributary which joins the great saphenous vein just below its termination. The posteromedial tributary can sometimes be larger than the great saphenous vein itself and may be mistaken for the main vein.

A recent consensus statement for lower limb venous terminology has recommended adoption of the term anterior accessory great saphenous vein to described any venous segment in the thigh or calf lying anterior and parallel to the great saphenous vein and posterior accessory great saphenous vein for venous segments lying posterior and running parallel to the great saphenous vein (Coggiati et al 2002).

The small tributaries near the termination of the great saphenous vein are the superficial circumflex iliac, the superficial epigastric and the superficial and deep external pudendal veins. Their methods of termination are highly variable and of no surgical significance if certain points are borne in mind. In operations for varicose veins the ligation of the great saphenous must be at its junction with the femoral vein. This immediately makes superfluous a knowledge of venous anatomy caudad to this point, with one exception. This is that tributaries can, uncommonly, drain directly into the femoral vein and for this reason the anterior and lateral surfaces of the femoral vein should always be

exposed for 2 cm proximal and distal to the saphenofemoral junction. The deep external pudendal vein is the one which most often drains in this manner and it is usually found craniad to the saphenofemoral junction.

Valves

The number of valves in the great saphenous vein is extremely variable – somewhere between five and 25. On average one valve is found every 7 cm and a valve near the termination of the vein is fairly constant. The valves mean that the vein has to be excised and reversed if used as a bypass in arterial surgery. The alternative is to leave the vein in its normal position and break down the valves – a so-called 'in situ' bypass.

Small saphenous vein (Fig. 41.3)

The small saphenous vein forms from veins along the lateral side of the foot and passes behind the lateral malleolus and upwards alongside the tendo Achilles. It passes upwards in about the middle of the calf posteriorly and penetrates the deep fascia at a level between the mid calf and the upper third of the calf, sometimes running within a tunnel in deep fascia before emerging deep to the fascia.

Unlike the termination of the great saphenous vein, which is at a relatively constant level, the saphenopopliteal junction is highly variable with only about 70% of small saphenous veins actually communicating with the popliteal vein.

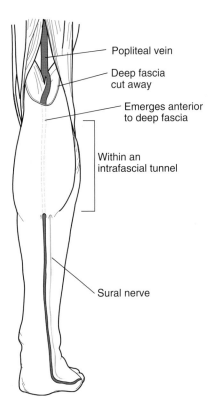

FIGURE 41.3 The small saphenous vein.

The saphenopopliteal junction, when present, may range from the level of the knee crease up to 7 cm above the popliteal skin crease (mean 4 cm).

When it does terminate in the popliteal vein, the termination of the small saphenous vein is not always direct, and it may enter the popliteal vein on its lateral or even its anterior surface.

When there is no communication between the short saphenous vein and the popliteal vein at all, the termination of the small saphenous may be in the great saphenous vein, the femoral vein, the profunda vein or in veins in the gluteal region. (The small saphenous vein represents the postaxial vein of the hind limb bud and in fetal life drains into the internal iliac vein through the sciatic and gluteal veins.)

Frequently the junction has an 'H' type arrangement with a vein ascending from the saphenopopliteal junction into the posterior thigh. This 'Giacomini' vein can often be followed up to communicate with the great saphenous vein or femoral vein.

The sural nerve lies in proximity to the distal half of the vein, although it is quite variable in its relationship.

When tracing the short saphenous vein upwards, it is usually found to pass between the two heads of the gastrocnemius to reach the popliteal vein and it lies close to and usually lateral to the tibial nerve.

As with the great saphenous vein, there are valves in the small saphenous vein. These vary from about four to 12 in number.

The short saphenous vein communicates with the great saphenous vein not only near its termination but also in the leg. The valves in these communications are such that blood flow is towards the great saphenous vein.

As a result of the highly variable nature of the short saphenous vein, preoperative localization of the saphenopopliteal junction by Duplex ultrasound is recommended when an operation on the small saphenous vein is planned.

Perforating veins ('perforators')

Perforating veins are veins passing through the muscular fascia and thus connect the superficial and deep venous systems. Perforators are common in all individuals and may be grouped on the basis of their location in the foot, ankle, leg, knee, thigh and gluteal regions. Perforating veins of the leg (calf perforators) may connect with the main trunk of great saphenous vein, posterior accessory great saphenous vein, short saphenous vein or tributaries.

Some perforating veins are found to be incompetent in patients with varicose veins and it is a matter of some controversy as to whether this is primary or secondary incompetence. The perforating veins may be considered to be of two types depending on the vein in which they terminate. Direct perforating veins end in one of the named or principal deep veins while indirect perforators end in smaller muscular veins. On the medial side of the calf the perforating veins of clinical importance are often found behind the medial border of the tibia at the level of the medial malleolus, about a hand's breadth above the medial malleolus and at the junction of the middle and upper thirds of the leg. These perforators, which terminate in the posterior tibial veins, may communicate directly with the great saphenous vein but more often with a tributary of it.

A more or less constant vein ascends posteriorly about midway between the great and the small saphenous veins. This is the posterior arch vein which was described by Leonardo da Vinci and is now named a posterior accessory great saphenous vein (Caggiati et al 2002). It usually communicates with both the great and small saphenous veins and it is also associated with a large perforator near the upper end of the tibia.

On the lateral side of the leg there are two main perforators that may be of clinical importance. One is in the midline posteriorly, halfway down the calf linking the small saphenous and gastrocnemius veins, and the other joins the peroneal veins with a tributary of the small saphenous vein about a hand's breadth above the lateral malleolus.

In the thigh the number of perforating veins is also variable but the most constant and most clinically significant is one just below the mid thigh level which joins the superficial femoral vein of the deep system with a tributary of the great saphenous vein rather than the great saphenous vein itself.

DEEP VEINS OF THE LOWER LIMB

In the leg the deep veins are usually double and follow their corresponding arteries.

Thus the peroneal veins drain into the posterior tibial veins which join with the anterior tibial veins to form the popliteal vein or veins, as this too is double for much of its course, in about 75% of cases.

A plexus of veins within the soleus muscle usually drains via two tributaries into the peroneal veins so that on venograms the peroneal veins are often the largest veins to be seen.

The veins in the gastrocnemius muscle usually drain directly into the popliteal veins.

The popliteal vein commences its course medial to the popliteal artery and crosses superficial (posterior) to it, to lie laterally, and then as it ascends as the femoral vein, it crosses posteriorly again to lie medially once more in the femoral triangle.

The femoral vein receives numerous muscular branches and the medial and lateral circumflex femoral veins tend to drain directly into it, caudad to the termination of the profunda femoris vein.

There are usually four or five valves in the femoral vein and a similar number in the popliteal vein. The variable nature of the most craniad one or two of these valves is discussed in the section on varicose veins. These valves are damaged when thrombosis occurs in the veins and become incompetent if and when the vein recanalizes. Then when a patient is exercising, the pressure drop that normally occurs is much less than usual. On cessation of exercise there is a more rapid return to the resting pressure, which is approximately equal to that of a column of blood from the heart to the ankle resulting in venous hypertension.

VARICOSE VEINS

Varicose veins generally develop as a result of valvular incompetence (reflux) of the superficial and/or deep venous system. Venous incompetence may be primary (majority) or secondary to an identifiable cause such as DVT. The most common sites of incompetence in primary varicose veins are the saphenofemoral junction and great saphenous vein (approximately 70–80%), the saphenopopliteal junction and short saphenous vein in approximately 20% and deep system in 5–10%. Incompetent perforating veins are frequently present in individuals with varicose veins but are not often present in isolation, i.e. without other incompetent veins.

Individuals with venous skin changes and/or ulcers are found to have deep vein incompetence (± superficial incompetence) in 50–60% of cases and superficial incompetence alone in up to 50% of cases.

Recurrent varicose veins are frequently caused by failure to flush ligate the saphenofemoral junction, recanalization of a saphenofemoral junction, failure to strip or ablate the above knee great saphenous vein, missed saphenopopliteal junction incompetence or unexpected deep venous incompetence.

Most surgeons image the venous system of the leg with duplex ultrasound in both primary and recurrent varicose veins to reduce the incidence of recurrence due to missed sites of incompetence.

REFERENCE

Coggiati A et al 2002 Nomenclature of the veins of the lower limbs: an international interdisciplinary consensus statement. J Vasc Surg 36:416-422.

FURTHER READING

Skandalakis J E et al 1983 Veins of the lower extremity. In: Skandalakis J E, Gray S W, Rowe J S (eds) Anatomical complications in general surgery. McGraw-Hill, New York.

GENERAL SURGICAL
NEUROLOGICAL OPERATIONS

42 | Operations for nerve compression: the anatomy of the carpal tunnel and the lateral femoral cutaneous nerve of the thigh

Glyn Jamieson and Nigel Jones

THE FLEXOR RETINACULUM: CARPAL TUNNEL SYNDROME

The flexor retinaculum is a thick fibrocartilaginous structure which bridges over the concavity of the carpal bones, converting the area into a tunnel known as the carpal tunnel (Fig. 42.1).

The retinaculum is attached medially to the pisiform bone and the hook of the hamate and laterally to the tubercle of the scaphoid and the trapezium.

It divides laterally with the superficial lamina inserting into the scaphoid and trapezium and the posterior lamina inserting into the posterior tip of the groove in the trapezium in which runs the tendon of the flexor carpi radialis muscle. This tendon therefore has its own compartment in this area.

The digital flexor tendons and flexor pollicis longus pass deep to the flexor retinaculum. The median nerve passes immediately deep to the flexor retinaculum lying in front of the tendons.

The median nerve in this position lies behind and slightly to the radial side of the palmaris longus tendon (which is absent in a small number of cases). At the distal margin of the flexor retinaculum, the nerve gives off a branch to the thenar muscles which tends to curve back to enter the muscles (Fig. 42.2).

Several structures cross superficial to the flexor retinaculum (Fig. 42.1). From medial to lateral these are the superficial branch of the ulnar nerve and ulnar artery, the tendon of palmaris longus, the palmar cutaneous branch of the median nerve, and the origin of the thenar muscles.

The tendon of palmaris longus blends with the flexor retinaculum and also contributes fibres to the palmar aponeurosis which is attached distally to the flexor retinaculum.

The diagnosis of carpal tunnel syndrome should always be confirmed by electrodiagnostic tests. Division of the flexor retinaculum can be conducted under local anaesthetic, arm block or general anaesthesia. No tourniquet is necessary. When operating to divide the flexor retinaculum it should be remembered that it is more of a hand structure than a wrist structure and it is situated distal to the flexion creases of the wrist joint.

The skin incision should begin from the flexor crease and run distally along the volar skin crease to a point level with the distal border of the outstretched thumb. The incision is carried deep to divide the palmar aponeurosis and then the firm transverse carpal tunnel ligament which is often partly obscured by the origins of the thenar and hypothenar muscles. Bipolar coagulation should be used for meticulous haemostasis. The median nerve should be carefully identified within its epineurium where it lies immediately beneath the flexor retinaculum. If the division is kept close to the ulnar border of the median nerve this will avoid injury to

FIGURE 42.1 The carpal tunnel and structures at the wrist.

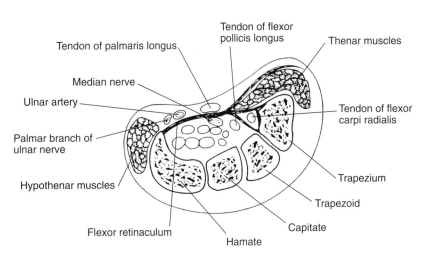

Tendon of palmaris longus
Tendon of flexor pollicis longus
Thenar muscles
Median nerve
Ulnar artery
Tendon of flexor carpi radialis
Palmar branch of ulnar nerve
Trapezium
Hypothenar muscles
Trapezoid
Flexor retinaculum
Capitate
Hamate

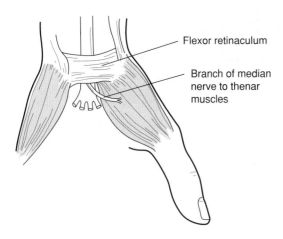

FIGURE 42.2 The branch of the median nerve to the thenar muscles.

the recurrent motor branch to the thenar muscles. The flexor retinaculum should be divided under direct vision distally and then proximally, to the deep fascia of the forearm. It is important to check carefully with a blunt probe that the ligament has been completely divided and that the nerve is quite free. It may be best to make sure the incision is made to one or other side of the palmaris longus tendon attachment (usually lateral) as incision into the attachment has been cited as a cause of recurrent problems. The median nerve itself need not be touched nor its motor branch exposed.

THE LATERAL FEMORAL CUTANEOUS NERVE: MERALGIA PARAESTHETICA

The lateral femoral cutaneous nerve arises from the first three lumbar nerves and exits from the lateral border of psoas major and crosses the iliacus muscle to pass through or below the inguinal ligament about 1 cm medial to the anterior superior iliac spine. It divides into anterior and posterior divisions at a variable point below this emergence.

The tunnel in the inguinal ligament is not unlike that for flexor carpi radialis as it passes under or through the flexor retinaculum in the wrist. The nerve can be irritated as it passes through its compartment in this area, giving rise to a characteristic neuralgic pain on the lateral side of the thigh. This is known as meralgia paraesthetica and perhaps the condition remains well known as much because of its mellifluous name as because of the frequency with which it occurs.

Ninety per cent of cases recover with conservative treatment. In the remainder neurolysis, or even division of the nerve when neurolysis has failed, gives good results.

The nerve passes beneath or through the inguinal ligament, at or near the anterior superior iliac spine, but its course is extremely variable. It then passes through or superficial to the sartorious muscle and pierces the investing fascia about 4 cm below the lateral end of the inguinal ligament. It may enter the thigh, having already divided into up to four branches. Because it is often hard to find, adequate exposure is necessary when operating for the condition of meralgia paraesthetica.

A 4 cm vertical incision beginning just above the lateral end of the inguinal ligament and extending into the thigh is taken through the investing fascia (Fig. 42.3). Some surgeons prefer a skin crease incision about 2 cm below the anterior superior iliac spine – particularly in obese individuals. It must be remembered that the nerve emerges below the inguinal ligament deep to fascia lata and so this structure must be divided in order to find the nerve lying on sartorius muscle. The nerve or its branches are initially sought at the anterior border of sartorius and once found, followed proximally to the entrapment point beneath the inguinal ligament. All constricting bands are divided so that the nerve lies quite free. If neurectomy is to be performed (usually reserved for cases where neurolysis has failed), the nerve should be pulled down and divided close to the inguinal ligament so that the divided end lies above the inguinal ligament and hence above the point of constriction.

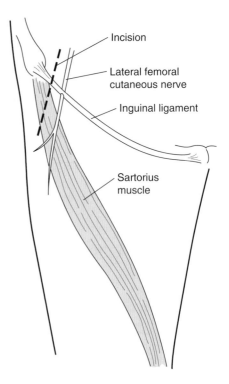

FIGURE 42.3 The lateral femoral cutaneous nerve of the thigh.

43 | Intracranial haemorrhage; extradural and subdural haemorrhage: the anatomy of the vault of the skull, dura and middle meningeal vessels

Glyn Jamieson and Peter Reilly

There is no suggestion that general surgeons still have a role in operations on the skull except in emergencies when no neurosurgeon is available. In this situation an emergency craniotomy can be life-saving so it seems reasonable to include a brief account of the relevant anatomy. When the operation is performed by a non-neurosurgeon, a neurosurgical unit should be contacted so that the procedure can be performed under guidance and plans put in place for a retrieval team which might include a neurosurgeon.

The vault of the skull is of varying thickness and may be only a few millimetres thick in the temporal fossae. It comprises a hard inner and outer table with a cancellous middle layer, the diploe. The outer table is thicker than the inner table which can be fractured in the absence of a fracture of the outer table.

The periosteum of the inner table is fused with an inner dural layer and constitutes the dura mater (Fig. 43.1).

The dura mater is closely applied to the vault bones. However a direct impact can cause the skull to deform inwards and then rapidly spring back. By this process dura can be stripped from the inner table, creating a potential extradural space into which bleeding from torn meningeal arteries or veins can occur.

Extradural haemorrhage occurs most often from trauma to the middle meningeal artery and its branches (Fig. 43.2), although occasionally other meningeal arteries or veins may be torn, giving rise to extradural haemorrhage in other sites. Since extradural haemorrhage is usually caused by a focal

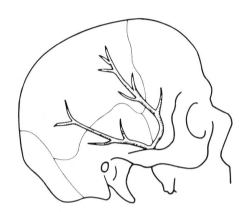

FIGURE 43.2 The surface projection of the middle meningeal artery and its divisions.

impact there may be external evidence of this – such as an abrasion and boggy swelling over the temple – and a skull X-ray may show a fracture line. A fracture may, however, be absent, particularly in children.

In communities where high-velocity impacts are common, acute subdural haemorrhage accounts for 50–60% of all acute traumatic intracerebral haemorrhage. Acute subdural haematomas may be bilateral. They may be remote from the point of impact and there may be no vault fracture.

If a CT scan is not available the side of an intracranial clot may be indicated by the following points

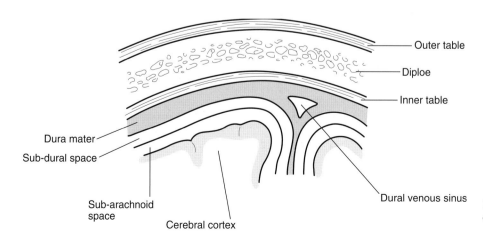

FIGURE 43.1 The layers of the skull and the dura mater.

❶ A boggy temple swelling and a fracture line on lateral skull X-ray.
❷ A contralateral hemiparesis.
❸ The side of the first dilating pupil.

In carrying out cerebral decompression, the best available anaesthetic control is essential. This should aim at normotension and moderate hypocarbia (PA_{CO_2} = 32–35 mmHg). The head should be slightly elevated and the neck free of any constriction. An intravenous line should be established to anticipate a drop in blood pressure when intracranial pressure is suddenly relieved. Blood should be immediately available – preferably in theatre – since blood loss from a middle meningeal artery may be rapid.

The principles of operation are:

❶ Find the clot by drilling a burrhole.
❷ Remove the clot by a wide craniectomy.
❸ Control the bleeding.

Most clots (extradural or subdural) are temporoparietal. Remembering that the floor of the middle fossa is level with the zygomatic arch, the first burrhole should be made in the temple just above the zygoma one finger breath anterior to the tragus. The scalp incision is made down to bone and the edges of the incision are held apart by self-retaining retractors which also help control scalp and muscle bleeding. Bleeding from the superficial temporal artery should be controlled by coagulation and ligation. A fracture should be identified. The burrhole is then made. An extradural haematoma will be immediately obvious. Clot is sucked out through the burrhole to give quick relief of intracranial pressure.

The scalp incision can be continued upwards and forwards as shown in Figure 43.3 and a craniectomy extended to follow the deepest part of the haematoma. It is not necessary to follow the blood clot beyond where it becomes only a few millimetres deep. Meningeal vessels on the dural surface are best coagulated with bipolar diathermy, sealed with Weck clips or carefully oversewn. If the dura is now slack then nothing further need be done. If it is tight then a small opening should be made to see whether there is an accompanying subdural haematoma. If there is a subdural haematoma the dura should be opened over the haematoma, which is carefully sucked out taking care not to damage the brain surface. Small cortical bleeding points may need to be coagulated. The dura is then sutured closed. Extradural haemostasis is very important. Any bleeding dural vessels are diathermied. Bleeding from the bone edge may be controlled by small pieces of haemostatic oxidized cellulose. The dura adjacent to the bone edge may be hitched to the pericranium, taking care to avoid injury to the underlying brain, to tamponade bleeding from beneath the bone edge. A low pressure extradural suction drain is usually wise. Any bleeding in the muscle layers should be diathermied to avoid a recurrent extradural clot.

If no intracranial clot is found beneath the first burrhole then a craniectomy should be extended upwards and forwards to the subfrontal region. If the dura is blue and tense a small opening should be made to determine whether there is a subdural haematoma. The next step is to make other burrholes in the frontal and parietal regions, as shown in Figure 43.3. If no clot is found on that side and the brain is tight the patient must be turned over and the same systematic exploration repeated on the opposite side.

Although most haematomas develop in the lateral frontotemporal region, some occur over the vertex or in the posterior fossa.

Acute subdural haematomas require wider craniotomies than extradural haematomas. Bleeding may come from subdural veins or arteries or from cortical vessels. As for an extradural haematoma, the essential steps are relief of brain pressure and then control of bleeding. If the brain is very tight 1.0–1.5 cm dural slits are made at several sites to remove the clot progressively and provide early relief of pressure. The opening is then turned into a dural flap hinged medially to avoid injury to medial draining veins and the clot removed carefully by suction and irrigation, taking care not to damage the underlying brain. Cortical bleeding vessels are secured by bipolar diathermy. The dura is usually closed, if necessary with an insert of pericranium or temporalis fascia. If the brain is tight the bone may be left out and deep frozen in antibiotic solution for later replacement.

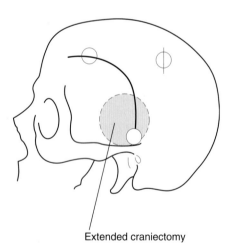

Extended craniectomy

FIGURE 43.3 Site for extension of burr holes to craniectomy. The initial burr hole should be made about 1.5 cm anterior to the external auditory meatus.

SURGERY OF THE SKIN

44 | Skin tumours; paronychia and ingrown toe nails: the anatomy of the skin and some of its appendages

Glyn Jamieson and Dudley Hill

HISTOLOGICAL STRUCTURE OF THE SKIN

The epidermis

The epidermis consists of a keratinized stratified squamous epithelium. The skin is divided into strata which correspond to the progress of skin cells (keratinocytes) from metabolically active cells at the basement membrane to dead cells at the skin surface.

The basal layer (stratum basale) is usually only one or two cell layers thick and provides the metabolically active cells which slowly move towards the skin surface and eventually desquamate.

The successive layers are then the stratum spinosum, the stratum granulosum and the stratum corneum. In some thick skin a stratum lucidum is sometimes added as a layer between the granulosum and the corneum. The metabolic activity of the cells decreases through the skin's layers and the keratin content increases until the stratum corneum is reached. This consists of closely packed layers of dead keratinocytes embedded in lipidic cement. The cytoplasm of keratinocytes of the skin contains vacuoles containing melanin (called melanosomes) the density of which varies depending on the degree of pigmentation in the skin.

The stratum basale and immediately adjacent layers also contain at least three other types of cells. First are melanocytes which usually lie against the basement membrane. They are responsible for production of the melanin which is taken up by the keratinocytes. Freckles represent concentrations of melanocytes and their colour depends to some degree on the proportions of the dark brown pigment, eumelanin, and the more reddish pigment phaeomelanin. Moles (melanocytic naevi) represent benign melanocytic neoplasms.

Second are the Langerhans cells, immunologically active cells, which play a role in antigen recognition of any foreign cells or material which enters the skin. Third are the Merkel cells which are present mainly in hairless skin and are related to certain cutaneous nerve endings.

The dermis

The layer immediately beneath the basement membrane is the papillary dermis which houses a rich network of blood vessels and nerves to the skin. The next layer is the reticular dermis, which is rich in collagen and elastic fibres. Sebaceous glands occur in this layer, usually opening into the apex of a hair follicle, except on the face where they commonly have a separate opening to the skin surface.

The hypodermis/subcutaneous layer

This, also called the subcutis, consists of sparser collagen fibres and contains mainly fat. Skin appendages such as sweat glands and hair follicles may reach into the hypodermis.

Lymphatic drainage of the skin (Fig. 44.1)

Lymphatic capillaries occur in all layers of the skin. A rich network of many blind-ending lymphatic capillaries is found in the reticular dermis.

The nodes to which skin drains are reasonably constant, but at watershed (lymph-shed?) areas drainage can be in several directions, i.e. either to right or left or upwards or downwards. As shown in Figure 44.1, the skin can be divided by two horizontal lines, one corresponding with the clavicles and the other at the level of the umbilicus and then divided vertically by the midline.

Skin above the clavicular lines drains into deep cervical lymph nodes; skin between the clavicular lines and the umbilical line drains into the axillary lymph nodes and skin below the umbilical line drains into the inguinal/external iliac lymph nodes.

Vascular supply to the skin

The blood supply to the skin is derived from the subdermal arterial plexus, which in turn is supplied from a subcutaneous artery through a vertically oriented musculocutaneous perforation vessel.

Skin flaps are considered to be designed in either an axial pattern (in which case they include a larger subcutaneous artery), or in a random pattern (in which case the blood supply is derived entirely from the subdermal plexus). Axial flaps can be longer than random flaps.

There may be an intervening third vascular layer of large, horizontally oriented arteries and veins between the deeper,

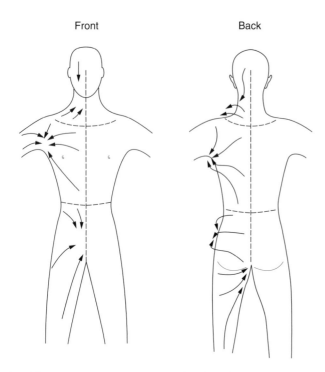

FIGURE 44.1   Directions of flow for the lymphatic drainage from the skin.

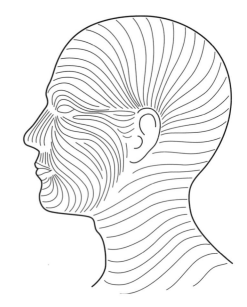

FIGURE 44.2   The relaxed skin tension lines of the head and neck.

larger musculocutaneous vessels and the subdermal vessels. The density of the vessels within this fascial layer varies from approximately every 1 cm on the head and neck to 4–6 cm, in the upper extremities to every 6 cm, on the thorax and abdomen, to every 12 cm on the lower extremities. This accounts for the greater survivability of flaps on the upper part of the body especially the head and neck, and also explains the ability of narrow based random flaps to survive on the face and neck.

The skin lines

Last century it was appreciated that skin was generally held in a state of tension so that a puncture wound with a round object tended to assume an elliptical shape when the object was removed. Langer studied these tension lines extensively in supine cadavers and subsequently published recommended lines along which incisions should be made. However it has since been appreciated that Langer's lines do not always correspond with the lines of greatest tension, with the greatest differences being on the head (Fig. 44.2).

Perhaps the best name for the lines of appropriate incisions in the skin is relaxed skin tension lines. This derives from the fact that relaxing the skin in an area throws the skin into parallel folds which correspond with the tension lines. These are nearly always in the same direction as wrinkle lines, or skin creases over movable areas such as joints; eyelids, etc.

THE NAIL BED

The nail consists of three major parts – its root, its body and its free margin.

There is a fold of skin over the base of the nail and this is prolonged as a thin extension of the stratum corneum forming the cuticle or eponychium (Fig. 44.3).

On both sides the skin also overlaps the body of the nail as the lateral nail folds. The root of the nail blends with a germinative layer called the germinal matrix and this extends under the nail and appears through the nail as the lunule.

The skin beneath the nail – the nail bed – is very vascular and is bound to the nail superficially and the periosteum of the phalanx deeply.

Microscopically nails are part of the stratum corneum which have become densely keratinized.

Infection beneath the lateral nail fold or beneath the cuticle can occur. This is called paronychia in the digits and ingrown toe nail in the foot. The great toe is particularly likely to be affected.

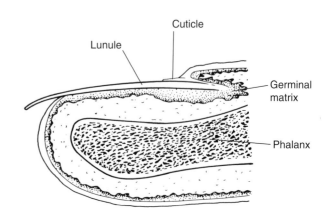

FIGURE 44.3   A nail and its bed.

Index